PRAISE FOR

alchemy
OF HERBS

D1323340

*"In this practical book, **Rosalee de la Forêt** reintroduces us to familiar kitchen herbs and spices, helping us to see them in a new light. Through personal and intimate storytelling, she teaches how to match herbs to people effectively instead of using them as pharmaceutical alternatives. Drawn in by the abundant, delicious recipes, you may come to this book as a home chef, but you will leave as an herbalist, transformed by the power of Rosalee's alchemy."*

— Guido Masé, author of *The Wild Medicine Solution* and *DIY Bitters*

*"Alchemy of Herbs puts the power of some of the most potent herbal medicines on the planet into your hands. These medicines have been tried and tested for millennia. And now, by combining ancient wisdom with modern scientific understanding, **Rosalee de la Forêt** helps you put nature's pharmacy to work. Whether you want more energy, better digestion, deeper sleep, or to get sick less often, Alchemy of Herbs will give you the knowledge you need to restore your health and to contribute to lasting wellness. At once inspirational and deeply practical, this is a book to treasure, and to keep close at hand for the rest of your life."*

— Ocean Robbins, co-host and CEO of The Food Revolution Network

*"It's rare to find a writer who can describe complex ideas with such clarity and skill that anyone can grasp their subject—**Rosalee de la Forêt** is one of those souls. In this book, she's broken down the energetic qualities and medicinal uses of herbs into an accessible and coherent format. If you've ever struggled with matching herbs to people—the true gift of an herbalist—Rosalee gives you the tools to understand how herbs can effectively 'nudge' the body's leanings back into a state of balance. Alchemy of Herbs contains detailed medicinal profiles, zesty recipes, and time-honored plant wisdom. The perfect makings of a top-shelf herbal book that you will treasure for years, and turn to for inspiration time and time again."*

— Juliet Blankespoor, herbalist and founder of the Chestnut School of Herbal Medicine

"This is a wonderfully accessible guide to introducing a medicine chest of healing plants in daily life. The information is presented in a refreshingly approachable way, by an author who loves both herbs and the simple joy they bring into our lives. The abundant recipes show how to access the healing gifts of the herbs as food, created to be both delicious and efficacious. True herbalism!"

— David Hoffmann, herbalist and author of *Medical Herbalism* and *Holistic Herbal*

*"Another green blessing of herbal information from a practicing herbalist. What a delight to look at the herbs that **Rosalee de la Forêt** loves and to encounter her avid desire to include you in the joy of herbal medicine."*

— Susun S. Weed, author of the Wise Woman Herbal series

"I first met **Rosalee de la Forêt** several years ago and was immediately impressed with her knowledge, passion for herbal medicine, and ability to clearly communicate this information. It turns out she is also a very good writer, and it is with great pleasure that I now hold her first book in my hands. Alchemy of Herbs is a wonderful introduction to 29 common herbs and spices, allowing you to understand how to use them safely and effectively for home health care, how to make your own kitchen medicines, and how to make tasty recipes so you can incorporate them into your diet."

—David Winston, RH (AHG), clinical herbalist, ethnobotanist, and
author of *Adaptogens: Herbs for Strength, Stamina, and Stress Relief*

"So many books geared toward those just beginning to explore the world of medicinal plants offer very basic 'take this herb for that problem' information, under the assumption that the foundational underpinnings of herbalism are somehow 'too hard' for beginners to grasp. Here, in plain English, **Rosalee de la Forêt** shows us that the way that herbalists choose herbs for individual people with particular imbalances isn't some magical power or a skill attainable only by those who can devote their lives to intense study. Instead, it is rooted in common sense patterns that anyone can learn to recognize, given a model to do so. That this is done using familiar herbs and spices available to all is an invaluable bonus. A book for everyone."

— jim mcdonald, herbalist and founder of herbcraft.org

"Herbal medicine can offer so much. But where to start? How do you know what herbs are good for you, and how to separate fact from fiction? **Rosalee de la Forêt** presents an excellent approach to learning the rich world of herbs. As an experienced educator and practitioner she weaves together tradition, experience, and science to present a holistic view of each of the plants, while providing specific and practical advice for how you can bring them into your home and life. Alchemy of Herbs is a treasure for any health-seeker's bookshelf."

— Renee Davis, RH (AHG), founder of Goldroot Botanical Medicine

"Many books introduce readers to herbs and their activities, but **Rosalee de la Forêt** skillfully introduces people instead to herbalism—the nuanced art of matching plants to people. Drawing energetic traditions into a modern context and right into our kitchens, she provides a simple and elegant system to look beyond symptoms and generic cures and into the heart of true herbal healing."

— Larken Bunce, clinical herbalist and co-director of
Vermont Center for Integrative Herbalism

"Alchemy of Herbs is a must-read for any herbalist, whether fledgling or experienced! Part reference guide, part recipe book, and part herbal, this is a book that every herbalist will reach for again and again. **Rosalee de la Forêt** has a knack for teaching others how to use herbs in the best way possible by matching people to herbs. This book is the definitive guide for the subject, giving anyone the confidence to use herbs to their fullest potential. Each chapter is engaging, relaying herbal information through a variety of anecdotal stories, scientific studies, and traditional usage, mixed with a variety of unique and inspiring recipes and gorgeous photographs. This is a book you will want to leave sitting out on your desk, coffee table, and kitchen counter, all at the same time."

— Kristine Brown, RH (AHG), herbalist and author/illustrator of *Herbal Roots Zine*

"*Alchemy of Herbs* is a sensory wonder, bringing us our medicines in the most delightful and tantalizing way they can be experienced: as culinary medicines. Step away from the bottle and the capsule and experience herbs in the full richness they can offer both as medicines and as partners in a life rich with plants."

— Bevin Clare, associate professor of Integrative Health at Maryland University
and president of the American Herbalist Guild

"As a French herbalist, I have a particular affinity for herbs that are both culinary and medicinal. We have a long tradition of healing food where I live in the South of France, mainly through the incorporation of aromatic herbs in our daily meals. *Alchemy of Herbs* is what I had been hoping for for years. **Rosalee de la Forêt** sends us a very important message: health does not necessarily mean yucky potions. This book brings together beautiful pictures, tasty recipes, and health recommendations from an expert healer. In a nutshell: this an invitation to cooking for a long and healthy life."

— Christophe Bernard, founder of AltheaProvence.com

"Informative, concise, knowledgeable, and generous . . . **Rosalee de la Forêt**'s sophisticated approach and her personal experience with herbs comes through in her beautiful recipes, which eloquently combine food and herbal medicine. Keep this book on your kitchen shelf—
you'll refer to it for healing and inspiration, always!"

— John Slattery, author of *Southwest Foraging*

"In this inspiring and practical book, **Rosalee de la Forêt** empowers you to awaken your senses in order to choose the best herbs for your needs. And what better way to experience the benefits and pleasures of herbs and spices than in the kitchen? Whether you're brand-new to herbs or have been using them for years, you'll love these enticing recipes for delicious drinks, everyday meals, and simple remedies."

— Emily Han, author of *Wild Drinks & Cocktails: Handcrafted Squashes, Shrubs,
Switchels, Tonics, and Infusions to Mix at Home*

"In *Alchemy of Herbs*, author **Rosalee de la Forêt** joyously shares her deep wisdom of herbs to inspire and empower us to transform our kitchens into nature's apothecary where delicious, healing foods and herbal remedies pour forth. Golden Milk, Hawthorn Cordial, and Nettle Leaf Dukkah are just a sampling of the many tasty, curative recipes offered. She unveils the enchanting, yet readily accessible world of herbalism that makes me fall right back in love with the plant kingdom; and you will too!"

— Dina Falconi, herbalist and author of *Foraging & Feasting: A Field Guide and Wild Food Cookbook*

"In her wonderfully written book, *Alchemy of Herbs*, **Rosalee de la Forêt** encourages the reader to 'break free from the insanity of the One-Solution Syndrome' by choosing personalized herbal formulations based on what our own senses tell us our bodies need. What better scenario is there for using our senses to divine this knowledge than cooking with flavorful and aromatic healing herbs and spices? Self-empowerment begins in the kitchen as Rosalee tempts us with dozens of mouth-watering recipes and encourages us to 'move forward with the mind-set of an explorer.' Those new to plant-based healing as well as experienced herbalists will find that this beautifully illustrated book exemplifies the heart and soul of herbal healing through delicious food as powerful medicine."

— Jeff Carpenter, author of *The Organic Medicinal Herb Farmer:
Ultimate Guide to Producing High-Quality Herbs on a Market Scale*

"*Rosalee de la Forêt* has done a wonderful job of melding both the culinary and medicinal uses of herbs in a way that allows just about anyone to incorporate herbs into their daily lives. The recipes in *Alchemy of Herbs* are not only very appealing, but simple enough for the novice cook or herbalist. For those who are looking to spice up their lives and improve their health, I would say that this is the book for you."

— Natalie Vickery, herbalist and founder of TheFamilyHerbalist.com

"*Rosalee de la Forêt* has broken down some of the more complex parts of herbal medicine into clear and straightforward pieces. It's very practical, but not at the expense of art and beauty. This book will be a classic."

— Traci Picard, herbalist and founder of FellowWorkersFarm.com

"It's exciting to watch more and more people becoming empowered in taking better care of themselves and their families with the use of herbs and spices. *Rosalee de la Forêt* shares concepts like energetics and taste in such a way that makes it easier for people to understand them, and how to find which herbs are best for them as individuals. I'm sure that this book will prove invaluable to those wishing to make that leap into feeling comfortable and confident in making herbs a part of their lives. Everyone will learn something new!"

— Tina Sams, editor of *Essential Herbal Magazine* and author of *Healing Herbs*

"I highly recommend **Rosalee de la Forêt**'s lovely collection of personal stories, recipes, and herbal information. Reading it is like working in the kitchen alongside the delightful Rosalee, whose talent and experience with herbs is expert. Her book is unique in that it explains both the chemistry and the energetics of medicinal herbs and at the same time introduces their use in a friendly and inviting way."

— Holly Bellebuono, author of *The Healing Kitchen* and *The Essential Herbal for Natural Health*

"*Rosalee de la Forêt*'s book is an excellent introduction to the energetics and science behind the use of our most common culinary and medicinal herbs, providing the reader with a solid foundation for further learning and exploration."

— Todd Caldecott, Dip. Cl.H., RH (AHG), CAP (NAMA), Ayurvedic practitioner, medical herbalist, and author of *Food as Medicine*

"I honestly think this might be the best introductory text to herbalism I've seen. It's detailed and relevant, and the recipes look amazing! **Rosalee de la Forêt** is known for her ability to make complicated information simple to understand (the flavor wheel chart she designed is groundbreaking), but this time she's outdone herself. For someone who has no experience with herbs but is interested in exploring plant medicine, this book is going to be a gateway to a wider world! I think it's going to be a smashing success!"

— Thomas Easley, RH (AHG), director of the Eclectic School of Herbal Medicine and co-author of *The Modern Herbal Dispensatory* and *The Modern Herbal Medicine Reference Guide*

alchemy

OF HERBS

ALSO AVAILABLE THROUGH LEARNINGHERBS®

LearningHerbs.com has many free herbal learning experiences, including hundreds of step-by-step, photo-rich remedies and recipes.

For the Beginner

Apothecary: The Alchemy of Herbs Video Companion: Rosalee de la Forêt and John Gallagher bring this book to life by showing you how to create the 15 most essential herbal remedy preparations. Build your own herbal medicine chest!

Herbal Remedy Kit: Find everything you need to start making your own herbal remedies in a single package.

For All Experience Levels

Taste of Herbs: With Rosalee's experience-based online course, you'll learn how to match an herbal remedy to a person.

HerbMentor.com, by LearningHerbs, offers courses designed for busy people, in-depth plant studies, expert-led herb walk videos, and the most supportive community on the web.

For Children

Herb Fairies, by Kimberly Gallagher: A chapter book series for kids, packed with herbal activities.

Wildcraft! An Herbal Adventure Game: A cooperative board game that explores healing herbs.

Please visit:
LearningHerbs: www.learningherbs.com®
Hay House USA: www.hayhouse.com®
Hay House Australia: www.hayhouse.com.au
Hay House UK: www.hayhouse.co.uk
Hay House India: www.hayhouse.co.in

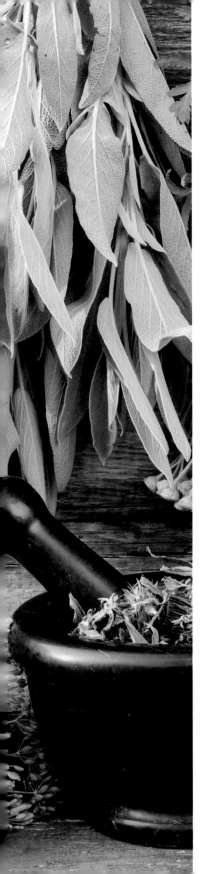
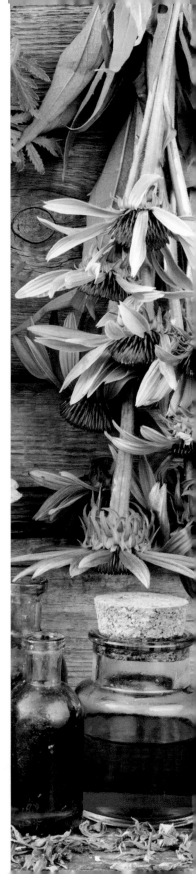

alchemy
OF HERBS

TRANSFORM
EVERYDAY
INGREDIENTS INTO
FOODS & REMEDIES
THAT HEAL

ROSALEE
DE LA FORÊT

HAY HOUSE, INC.
Carlsbad, California • New York City
London • Sydney • New Delhi

Copyright © 2017 by Rosalee de la Forêt

Published in the United States by: Hay House, Inc.: www.hayhouse.com®
Published in Australia by: Hay House Australia Pty. Ltd.: www.hayhouse.com.au
Published in the United Kingdom by: Hay House UK, Ltd.: www.hayhouse.co.uk
Published in India by: Hay House Publishers India: www.hayhouse.co.in

Project Editor: Nicolette Salamanca Young
Cover Design: Jan Bosman; Tricia Breidenthal • *Interior Design:* Bryn Starr Best

All images courtesy of the author, except the following:
Images © Sol Gutierrez: pg. xii, xxi, 355
Image © Matt Burke, www.mattburkephotography.com: pg. 108
Image © Larken Bunce: pg. 306
Images used under license from Shutterstock.com: pg. vii, xxii, 1, 6, 10, 19, 21, 24, 26, 34, 35, 36, 37, 38, 48, 53, 54, 55, 58, 63, 64, 68, 70, 76, 86, 88, 91, 92, 95, 113, 123, 124, 126, 145, 146, 150, 153, 155, 157, 176, 198, 199, 202, 238, 242, 243, 250, 258, 262, 275, 276, 285, 293, 302, 318

All rights reserved. No part of this book may be reproduced by any mechanical, photographic, or electronic process, or in the form of a phonographic recording; nor may it be stored in a retrieval system, transmitted, or otherwise be copied for public or private use—other than for "fair use" as brief quotations embodied in articles and reviews—without prior written permission of the publisher.

The author of this book does not dispense medical advice or prescribe the use of any technique as a form of treatment for physical, emotional, or medical problems without the advice of a physician, either directly or indirectly. The intent of the author is only to offer information of a general nature to help you in your quest for emotional, physical, and spiritual well-being. In the event you use any of the information in this book for yourself, the author and the publisher assume no responsibility for your actions.

Library of Congress Cataloging-in-Publication Data

Names: Foret, Rosalee de la, date, author.
Title: Alchemy of herbs : transform everyday ingredients into foods and
   remedies that heal / Rosalee de la Foret.
Description: Carlsbad, California : Hay House, Inc., [2017] | Includes index.
Identifiers: LCCN 2016037604 | ISBN 9781401950064 (paperback)
Subjects: LCSH: Herbs--Therapeutic use--Popular works. | Self-care,
   Health--Popular works. | Holistic medicine--Popular works. | BISAC: HEALTH
   & FITNESS / Herbal Medications. | MEDICAL / Holistic Medicine. | COOKING /
   Specific Ingredients / Herbs, Spices, Condiments.
Classification: LCC RM666.H33 F664 2017 | DDC 615.3/21--dc23 LC
record available at https://lccn.loc.gov/2016037604

ISBN: 978-1-4019-5006-4

22 21 20 19 18 17 16 15 14 13
1st edition, April 2017

Printed in China

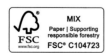

For my husband, Xavier,
my constant source of love and inspiration.

CONTENTS

Foreword by Rosemary Gladstar..xiii

Introduction.. xv

PART I: your introduction to herbs and spices

Chapter 1: The Benefits of Herbs and Spices..........................3
Chapter 2: How Do We Know Herbs Can Do That?..............7
Chapter 3: Matching Herbs to You—Not to an Ailment................11
Chapter 4: How to Get the Most Out of This Book...................27

PART II: the herbs

PUNGENT

Chapter 5: BLACK PEPPER 39
Chapter 6: CAYENNE...49
Chapter 7: CINNAMON..59
Chapter 8: FENNEL..69
Chapter 9: GARLIC...77
Chapter 10: GINGER...87
Chapter 11: HOLY BASIL 97
Chapter 12: LAVENDER...107
Chapter 13: MUSTARD 117
Chapter 14: NUTMEG...125
Chapter 15: PARSLEY..133
Chapter 16: PEPPERMINT 141
Chapter 17: ROSEMARY...149
Chapter 18: SAGE..159
Chapter 19: THYME..169
Chapter 20: TURMERIC..177

SALTY

Chapter 21: NETTLE...189

SOUR

Chapter 22: ELDER..201
Chapter 23: HAWTHORN..211
Chapter 24: LEMON BALM..219
Chapter 25: ROSE...229
Chapter 26: TEA 239

BITTER

Chapter 27: ARTICHOKE 251
Chapter 28: CACAO..259
Chapter 29: CHAMOMILE..267
Chapter 30: COFFEE...277
Chapter 31: DANDELION 287

SWEET

Chapter 32: ASHWAGANDHA..299
Chapter 33: ASTRAGALUS 307

Afterword 315
Metric Conversion Chart 316
Glossary..319
Recommended Resources...325
Endnotes...327
Index 339
Acknowledgments 351
About the Author...355

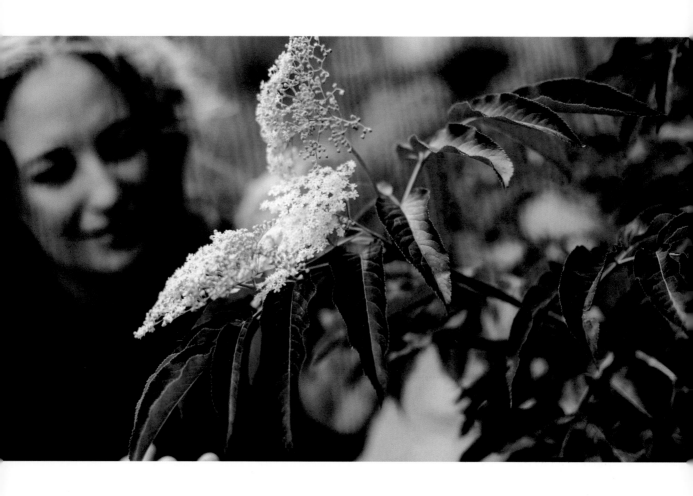

FOREWORD

How wonderful it has been in my more than 40 years as a practicing herbalist to watch herbalism emerge from its place in the "underworld." Interest in herbalism—the art and science of healing with plants—has grown in leaps and bounds, especially in the past few decades. This legitimate healing system had been marginalized and pushed deeply underground by the advent of modern pharmaceutical medicine and the "age of chemicals." But from relative obscurity, it is now flowering and has taken its honorary place among other healing professions.

Herbs offer so much, not only in health and healing but also as a way of life. They provide beauty, balance, and sanity in a world that sometimes seems to have gone awry. Imagine a world without herbs ... It's impossible! Without plants, life as we know it wouldn't exist. We need this chlorophyll-rich, carbon-dioxide breathing, nutrient-dense mass of green matter to breathe, live, and *be*!

Like the tenacious plants that this healing system is based upon, herbalism has rooted deeply in the consciousness of our communities once again—thank goodness! But questions and confusion come along with this rekindled interest in herbalism, as people try to sort through information on herb safety, how to use herbs, which herbs to use, how to prepare them, how much to take. Ultimately, each person is asking, which herb is best for *me*?

Over the thousands of years of herbal usage, people around the world have developed systems that help explain the hows, whens, and whys of using certain herbs. The best of these systems or traditions have been preserved and passed down. In India, Ayurveda medicine, known as the Science of Life, is a composite of over 5,000 years of recorded plant use for health and healing. Likewise, in China a very sophisticated system of healing evolved over several thousand years; the best of that wisdom was encapsulated into a highly effective system termed Tradition Chinese Medicine (TCM). In North, Central, and South America, many different systems of herbal healing were developed by the indigenous cultures that thrived on these plant-rich continents. All around the world in places as diverse as Africa, Western and Eastern Europe, and the Mediterranean, herbal traditions evolved and were passed down through the ages.

No wonder herbalism can seem so overwhelming, confusing, and sometimes even conflicting ... Where does one start to begin to understand this ancient, complex, often contradictory and multifaceted system(s) of health and healing?

Enter Rosalee! In her brilliantly simple yet profound way of teaching, Rosalee captures the essence of some of these great herbal traditions, translates them for us, and makes them accessible for everyone to understand without years of study! At the core of her teachings is the art of matching herbs to individuals through the understanding of constitutional types—in other words, how to match herbs to people rather than to diseases. Often challenging and difficult to grasp, this concept is one that Rosalee presents with ease, calling it an "herbal sweet spot."

Rosalee is a master at teaching the "energetics" of plants, so that we really grasp what these herbs do, how they work in our bodies, and how they affect us as individuals. In *Alchemy of Herbs*, we learn this not through studying chemistry or the complex constituents of plants, but by actually experiencing how the plants work through our senses, especially that of taste. I don't know anyone who is able to teach or write about these concepts quite as simply or clearly as Rosalee does without sacrificing their diverse complexity.

Rosalee also reminds us that there's no "One Solution" to our personal health. This is one of the main problems with modern medicine as well as "modern herbalism": we've been taught that there's a "silver bullet" approach to health where one solution will work for all. But Rosalee's approach is different—and anything but dogmatic. There's no set of rules with "shoulds" and "should nots." Instead, she leads us on a "journey of discovery and awareness" where our personal observations and experiences are of utmost importance in discovering what works best for us as individuals. She reminds us that we truly are our own best asset when it comes to getting the most benefit from herbs. Most importantly, through this journey, we develop a deeply personal relationship with the plants we work with, which really is the heart and soul of herbalism.

In *Alchemy of Herbs*, Rosalee does more than give us facts to ponder; she inspires us to use herbs in our daily lives. She exudes joy and makes learning about herbs fun, practical, and hands-on. She brings herbalism into the kitchen and invites you to play with her as she concocts, mixes, and blends. Her recipes are fabulous; some are already well on their way to becoming classics. She proves that old adage that good health begins in the kitchen and that food is our best medicine.

Great teachers and great herb books, I feel, are those that teach us to think for ourselves and to be self-empowered. Rosalee does just that through all of her teachings and writing. In *Alchemy of Herbs*, Rosalee has hit the "herbal sweet spot" and given us a jewel to treasure.

—Rosemary Gladstar,
herbalist, author, and founder of the Sage Mountain
Herbal Retreat Center and Botanical Sanctuary

INTRODUCTION

More than 2,000 years ago, the Hippocratic school of medicine proclaimed, "Let food be thy medicine." This sage advice still holds powerful wisdom for us today. Thankfully, the concept of making food our medicine is becoming more widely adopted. Eating locally grown, organic, and nutrient-rich foods is gaining in popularity. The number of farmer's markets in the United States has quadrupled since 1994, which means more people are eating locally sourced whole foods.[1] But while we have a growing appreciation for nourishing food, I frequently notice that a critical ingredient is still missing from our dinner table—the herbs and spices!

Herbs and spices can transform a bland meal into a decadent and delicious experience. However, the depth of flavor in a well-spiced meal does more than simply excite our taste buds. As you're about to read in this book, herbs and spices can dramatically revolutionize your health! They can improve your mood, reduce oxidative stress, ensure that you are digesting and absorbing the nutrients from your healthy foods, and prevent many chronic diseases.

I have based this entire book on a very simple premise: You are unique. In our information age, there are "experts" on every corner telling you what foods to eat, what foods to avoid, what miracle drugs can mask your symptoms, and what herbs you and everyone else should be taking. But the truth is that *you* are the best expert when it comes to what works for your own unique body. So rather than tout the next miracle "superfood," I am going to show you how you can personally choose the best herbs for your needs and situation, taking your own special qualities under consideration.

While this book is all about herbs, spices, and food, I promise you that it's not a diet. You don't have to become a vegan or a vegetarian, nor do you have to start eating meat. You won't have to take on a second job in order to afford the ingredients, nor do you need to travel to exotic places to find these healing herbs. This book shows you how to harness the power of herbs and spices in your everyday life by giving you practical and easy recipes: beverages and simple herbal remedies as well as breakfasts, lunches, dinners, and even desserts. After helping you to develop some simple observational skills, this book will start you on a fun journey of personal and herbal discovery that will empower you and transform your health for a lifetime.

OUR CURRENT SITUATION: THE ONE SOLUTION SYNDROME

Our entire modern construct of health is suffering under what I call the One Solution Syndrome. This is the false belief that there is *one solution* for everyone: one medicine for a disease, a single way that you should eat, and just one set of practices that keep you healthy. Another common belief is that Western medicine is the infallible pinnacle of medicine and that traditional or natural therapies are outdated. These two philosophies explain our current state of health care, in which suppressing symptoms with drugs is prioritized over finding the root cause of an illness.

An example of this is Western medicine's approach to eczema. Instead of addressing the factors that may contribute to eczema, such as environment and diet, doctors often prescribe topical steroids to relieve the symptoms. While this can be temporarily effective, long-term use has serious negative consequences while doing nothing to address the underlying cause. Eczema isn't "cured" by the steroids; the symptoms are simply suppressed while the underlying problems continue.

I do believe that Western medicine has its place. For example, I have no doubt that surgeons can fix an astounding number of serious traumas or acute conditions that would otherwise be life threatening. If I break my arm, my first stop would be the hospital, not my local herbalist's shop. However, I am dismayed by our current poor state of health. More than half of our population has some type of chronic disease, and 25 percent of the population has two or more chronic diseases.[2] The United States also spends the most money on health care worldwide, perhaps because many of these chronic conditions are simply managed by a billion-dollar pharmaceutical industry.[3] Something is clearly broken in our society's quest for health.

While modern medicine has advanced health in some powerful ways, it hasn't solved many of our chronic health issues. Some people may be fervently hoping for new advances in technology to save our ailing population, but I know we will never transform our health with a pill. Instead, we need to pay more attention to our past.

THE HISTORY OF OUR CONNECTION
WITH PLANTS AS MEDICINE

For thousands of years, long before the Internet or even books existed, plants were a major source of healing for people all over the world. The use of medicinal plants, referred to as herbalism, has as many traditions and theories as there are cultures on earth. Among the many traditions that exist, in the United States today the three main herbal theories commonly being taught are Western herbal tradition, Ayurveda, and Traditional Chinese Medicine.

Up until the 1900s, herbal medicine was commonly practiced in the United States. Not only was folk medicine popular in the home, but there were also college-trained doctors, called the Eclectic physicians, who primarily used plants as medicine. The Eclectic physicians had colleges across the nation, and they wrote important texts based on their extensive experience that are still referenced today. However, in the early 1900s, the American Medical Association (AMA) single-handedly proclaimed what was "science" and what was "quackery." From this moment on, herbs and other natural healing therapies were routinely dismissed in favor of chemical drugs and invasive interventions. The AMA also decided what could and could not be taught as part of a doctor's curriculum. As a result, the Eclectic colleges began to shut down.

Once antibiotics were created in the 1930s, people began to turn more readily to "better living through science" and used pharmaceutical pills for their illnesses rather than plants. People were so impressed with antibiotics and isolated chemical constituents, such as acetylsalicylic acid in aspirin, that herbalism quickly fell out of favor. In the decades that followed, herbalism continued to exist in isolated pockets throughout the United States, but it was far from mainstream.

With the back-to-the-earth movement in the 1960s, herbs were revitalized. And it's here that we see the beginnings of our current herbal resurgence. Flash forward several decades, and herbs have now become a multibillion-dollar industry within the United States. I hope that one day we will have a fully integrated medical model in which preventing disease through healthy living is prioritized. And when someone does get sick, I hope that diet, lifestyle, and herbs are fully explored as options, leaving pharmaceuticals or surgery as the last resort.

But this book isn't solely about looking back at history, nor is it the One Solution Syndrome dressed up with herbs and supplements. Instead, this book is about making herbs relevant to you in today's world. This book is an invitation for you to break free from the insanity of the One Solution Syndrome and go on your own journey of personal discovery to uncover what works for you as an individual. I hope that this new path will be full of "aha moments" that lead you to immediate and practical benefits, just as it was for me.

FROM MY OWN HERBAL JOURNEY TO YOURS

I've long been interested in natural health, but I didn't always take it seriously. I once thought of it as a fun hobby, perhaps useful for minor ailments. In my mind, Western medicine and doctors were the obvious solution for more serious problems. When I was 23, however, I was diagnosed with a rare autoimmune disease, and my search for answers would forever change the path of my life.

My diagnosis was my first experience with the One Solution Syndrome in the Western medical establishment. Specialists told me there was no cure and that the only available treatment was mass doses of steroids—which, they admitted, would eventually cease to work. I was told to expect a slow decline and a future life expectancy of less than 20 years.

After the initial shock of my diagnosis, I began a more empowered health journey. As I reached out to holistic health practitioners, including herbalists, acupuncturists, and naturopaths, I noticed something very different about their approach to my illness. They seemed less concerned with the diagnosis the doctors gave me and a lot more concerned with getting to know *me*. With their help, along with my own research, I changed my diet, addressed nutritional deficiencies, and used many herbal formulas. After six months I was symptom free, and I have remained that way for more than a decade.

This transformative experience shifted not only my reality but also my path in life. I knew that I wanted to help people who were in positions similar to my own, so I began my own journey into the world of herbalism. My first plant studies were with ethnobotanist Karen Sherwood. We spent lots of time in nature as I learned how to incorporate native and wild plants into our daily lives through food and medicine and even as tools. After that, I began more specific studies in herbalism and immersed myself in an exploration of folk herbalism, which includes using plants as food and to treat minor complaints.

In 2005 I met John and Kimberly Gallagher and began a partnership with them that has dramatically shaped my herbal journey. Early on, I was attracted to John and Kimberly's simple approach to learning about herbs. They emphasized what they had gleaned from their own herbal teachers: explore one herb at a time, and study it closely by using it daily in your life. Shortly after meeting them, I started writing recipe-based newsletters for their company, LearningHerbs.com, and later became part of their community membership site, HerbMentor.com. I am now the Education Director for LearningHerbs, and I continue to be inspired by our mission of keeping herbs simple so everyone can enjoy learning.

As time went on, I knew I wanted to continue my studies, so I headed back to school again, this time focusing on being an herbal clinician. I graduated from the four-year program at the East West School of Planetary Herbology, studying under Michael and Lesley Tierra, then did my professional and mentorship studies with renowned herbalist and former president of the American Herbalists Guild, Karta Purkh Singh Khalsa.

My clinical studies led me into a whole other world of personalized herbal formulas, as I created complex individual health plans and really focused on how to get the best results using herbs and other natural therapies. I love this approach to health, and after a decade of working with people and herbs, I am still amazed at how effective herbs can be for chronic issues. I've seen people ravaged by inflammatory bowel disease regain their lives, and people overcome with pain from rheumatoid arthritis able to move without agony for the first time in years. I've seen weekly migraines disappear, people successfully weaned off diabetes medication (with the supervision of their doctor), and chronic rashes like eczema completely cleared up. In all of these instances there simply wasn't One Solution. (Believe me, if there were one herb or spice that could single-handedly cure any disease, you'd be reading a very different book.) Instead, as I'll keeping reminding you throughout this book, we need to know *who* has the disease, not just *what* the disease is.

Because I have frequently witnessed what herbs and spices can do, it's now strange to think that someone would turn to pharmaceuticals for their health needs rather than using plants first. Luckily, more health care providers, including doctors, naturopaths, and acupuncturists, are beginning to realize the powerful benefits offered by herbs and spices. In a *Hopkins Medicine* article titled "Take Two Carrots and Call Me in the Morning," Dr. Gerard Mullin, one of the nation's top experts on the relationship between food and gut disorders, offered an example of the power of food as medicine: "People who have nausea, or gastric dysmotilities or other GI problems, for them ginger is at the top of my list. It works the same way Zofran does, which is one of our most powerful antinausea drugs. It works on the same receptor in the brain. But a lot of docs aren't aware of it."[4]

Herbs and spices can have a tremendous impact on your health, whether it's improving your digestion or modulating chronic inflammation. As you see benefits to your health, perhaps your doctor may recommend modifying or allowing you to move away from prescription drugs. However, I do *not* suggest that you abandon Western medicine or stop taking any of your prescribed medications without the guidance of your doctor. As you'll see, while it sometimes makes sense to choose herbs instead of or alongside pharmaceuticals, herbs are not going to be as effective if we are stuck in the One Solution Syndrome. In other words, while ginger is great for nausea, it's not great for *everyone* with nausea.

Furthermore, although I am trained in the complexities of herbs, I believe that the most powerful way to use them starts in your kitchen. Sure, you can take a handful of herbal pills or a few squirts of a tincture (an alcohol extract of a plant). But the reality is, herbs and spices will have the most dramatic and positive influence on your health if you maximize their use in your everyday life.

MOVING FORWARD:
THE BENEFITS BEGIN IN THE KITCHEN

One common roadblock on the path to health is that many people assume a "healthy" life is a boring life, devoid of their favorite pleasures. But that is far from the truth, especially when it comes to herbs and spices. A friend recently told me of her experience cooking an herb- and spice-filled meal. As soon as her husband walked through the door, the compliments started coming in. It began with "What's that delicious smell?" and continued with his relishing every bite and asking to have more meals like that in the future.

That is exactly what transforming your health should look like: eating pleasurable food that is filled with nutrients and antioxidants that keep you feeling great! And this book is filled with recipes to help you do just that. While many people in the United States use herbs in their meals, they rarely use a large enough quantity to experience their true power. Using a tiny pinch of herbs in an entire meal doesn't result in flavorful food or in any major health benefits. Whether you're enjoying the calming benefits of Lemon Balm Nourishing Infusion (page 223), savoring every bite of the decadent Cardamom Chocolate Mousse Cake (page 263), or spicing things up with your own Homemade Mustard (page 121), you'll find that there are countless ways to easily get the full benefits of powerful herbs and spices into your diet, whether you are vegan, vegetarian, paleo, locavore, and on and on.

This journey begins with Part I, as you develop your own sense of awareness so that you are empowered to choose the best herbs and spices for you. Part II of the book is divided into five sections, based on the herbal classifications of taste: pungent, salty, sour, bitter, and sweet. Each chapter of Part II focuses on a different herb or spice and includes recipes to help you experience those herbs. At the end of the book you'll find information to help you further, including an Index, Glossary, and Recommended Resources. The Recommended Resources section lists where you can order the herbs found in this book and places you can go to learn more about herbs and spices. (For additional recipes and remedies, book "outtakes," and other fun surprises, be sure to visit www.AlchemyOfHerbs.com/resources.)

The fun with herbs begins right away. Rather than learning through the memorization of complex theories, this is learning through *doing*. As you read, if you find the perfect herb for your situation, you can immediately put it into action with one of the simple recipes. Notice what works, so you can make that a part of your and your family's everyday life.

The focus of this book is transforming your relationship with herbs and spices. I hope it broadens your view and awakens your mind and senses to the powerful effect of medicinal plants, and that it then inspires you to use them abundantly in your daily life. In doing so, you can avoid or even begin to heal some of the chronic problems affecting our population today. This can lead you to a place where you can make empowered decisions about your personalized health care.

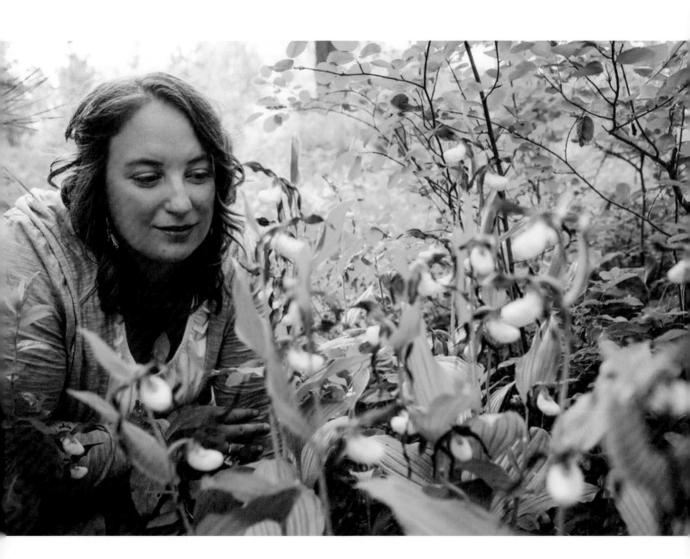

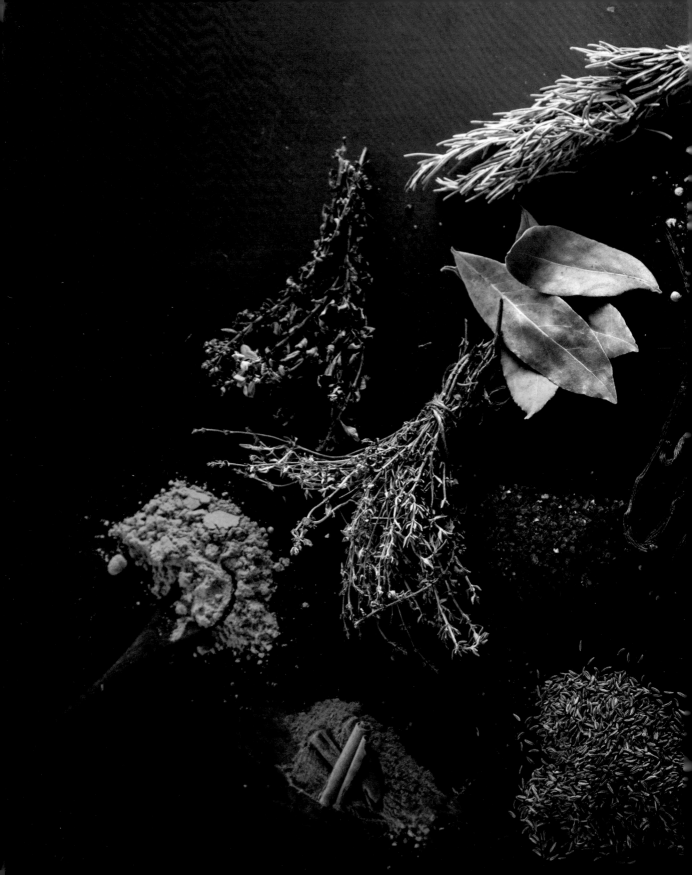

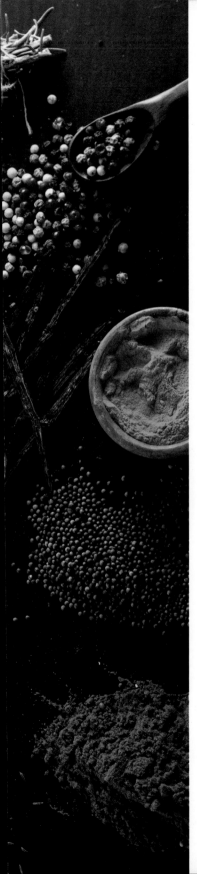

PART I

YOUR
INTRODUCTION
TO

herbs
and
spices

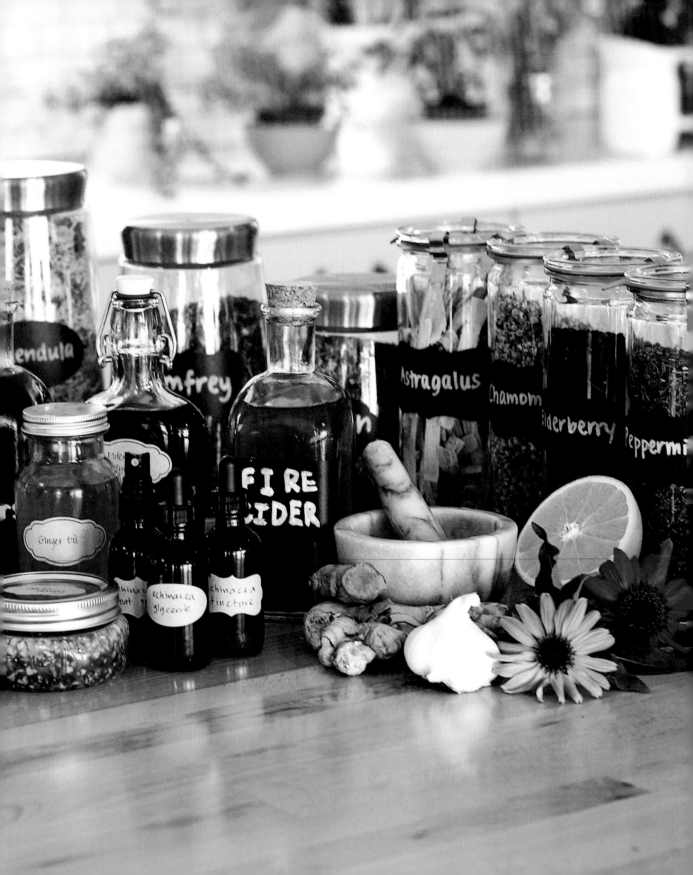

CHAPTER 1

The Benefits of Herbs and Spices

Every meal presents an opportunity to nourish yourself and powerfully support your health. Adding more herbs and spices into your diet comes with many benefits. They provide essential nutrients, support natural energy, promote healthy aging, prevent diseases, aid in the repair of vital processes, and strengthen healthy bodily functions. Furthermore, when used correctly, this form of herbal medicine is safe—and way more fun than popping an herbal capsule or taking an herbal tincture.

You may be wondering how something in your kitchen cabinet can have such a dramatic effect in so many areas of health. Part II of this book will go over the specific gifts of each plant, but before we look at the details, let's examine the general ways in which herbs deliver those qualities.

HERBS STRENGTHEN DIGESTION

A principle in herbalism is that most chronic disease begins with poor digestion. If you can't transform your food into the nutrients your body needs, then how can you have good health? In fact, many culinary herbs have been in use for thousands of years not only because they taste good but also because they help with digestion.

Sadly, all too often, people have had poor digestion for so long that they assume it's a natural part of life. As a clinical herbalist, I've worked with hundreds of people who have come to me for help with various complaints related to chronic illness, and so many will brush off their digestive upsets as "normal." Then, when we work with herbs and spices to strengthen their digestion, they often find that many of their other complaints disappear.

Be aware of the following symptoms, which are clues to poor digestion:

- Bloating
- Gas
- Indigestion
- Heartburn
- Constipation
- Nausea
- Poor appetite
- Recurring diarrhea
- Ulcers

HERBS ARE HIGH IN ANTIOXIDANTS

Herbs and spices are high in antioxidants, which are an important key to limiting the damage done to the body by oxidative stress. Oxidative stress has been linked to heart disease, liver problems, arthritis, premature skin aging, and eye damage. It occurs when the body is overloaded with free radicals, which are any atoms or molecules that has a single unpaired electron. When free radicals come in contact with other cells, they can steal an electron from them, causing the robbed molecule to start the process all over again. This can create a domino effect in the body, leaving a trail of oxidative stress in its wake. Antioxidants have an extra electron that they can give to a free radical and stop this process from happening.

The formation of free radicals is a natural part of living, eating, and breathing. However, it can be dramatically increased by stress, eating processed foods, consuming oils that have been overheated, breathing air pollutants or cigarette smoke, being sleep deprived, or eating charred meats. To minimize oxidative stress, it is important to limit these negative influences and regularly include high-antioxidant foods, such as herbs and spices, in your meals.

HERBS SUPPORT THE NERVOUS SYSTEM

If you take a critical look around you, I think you'll agree that we live in a perpetually stressed culture. How often do you get the response "I'm really busy" when you ask someone how they're doing? Excessive stress is so common that it almost seems normal to run on too little sleep and be rushed, overworked, and overcommitted.

While busyness may have become a normalized part of our culture, our bodies are increasingly showing the effects of constant exposure to chronic stress. Sadly, chronic emotional stress has been linked to the six leading causes of death in the United States: cancer, coronary heart disease, accidental injuries, respiratory disorders, cirrhosis of the liver, and suicide.[1] I hope that as awareness is raised about cultural stress, we can take stronger steps to simplify our modern lifestyle and manage our unrealistic expectations. This will have to include major shifts in our mind-set as well as major policy changes that support hardworking families that are struggling to get by.

Admittedly, herbs aren't going to give you superhuman powers. You won't be able to run on no sleep, zooming from activity to activity on your overly ambitious to-do list. But, as you'll read in this book, herbs and spices can help us modulate the negative effects of stress. They can help shift us from the fight-or-flight response of our sympathetic nervous system to the rest-and-digest state of the parasympathetic nervous system. They can help us get restful sleep at night and reduce levels of anxiety during the day. Along with fresh local food, they offer us high amounts of the vitamins and minerals needed to support our nervous system.

HERBS ARE ANTIMICROBIAL

Some herbs and spices offer a powerful defense against pathogenic bacteria. In an age of pharmaceutical antibiotics, this may not sound all that revolutionary; however, humanity is facing a major problem with antibiotic resistance. As bacteria have evolved, they've adapted to the pharmaceutical antibiotics we use. Now, after decades of rampant overuse of antibiotics, more and more bacteria no longer respond to treatment using antibiotics. In the United States alone, more than 23,000 people die each year from antibiotic-resistant infections.[2] Because plants have been changing and evolving with bacteria for millennia, they have a very complex system that may make it harder for pathogens to adapt to them.

Although it can be necessary to use pharmaceutical antibiotics for certain conditions, doing so can have far-reaching negative effects, particularly on our gut flora, which is the beneficial bacteria in our digestive tract. In recent years, new research has shown the importance of having a healthy and diverse gut flora; however, pharmaceutical antibiotics act by wiping out all bacteria, even the beneficial. The term antibiotic, after all, means "anti-life."

Spices can be strongly antimicrobial without being anti-life. Instead of knocking out everything they come into contact with, plants can be chosen for the specific type of infection. Some herbs more strongly affect one type of bacteria than another. Plants can also be effective against viruses and fungal infections.

Scientists have been studying how plants can make antibiotics more effective. For example, the compound berberine, found in plants such as goldenseal (*Hydrastis canadensis*) and Oregon Grape Root (*Mahonia spp.*), has been shown to make antibiotics more effective for antibiotic-resistant infections.[3]

And that's not all! Herbs can go beyond simply killing a pathogen and also support the ecosystem of the body. They can restore integrity to mucous membranes and support healthy gut flora.

HERBS SUPPORT THE IMMUNE SYSTEM

Another powerful way that herbs can reinforce our health during times of infection is by strengthening or modulating our body's own immune system, which is arguably our best defense against pathogens that lead to illness. Immune system dysfunction can increase our risk of infection and is also implicated in cancer, autoimmune disorders, and seasonal allergies. Herbs can help to strengthen and boost our immune system so that it can do its complex job well.

Herbs and spices aid your health in myriad ways including strengthening your digestion, supporting your immune system, and awakening your senses and bringing joy to your life. To get the most benefits from herbs you'll want to use them every day and in good amounts. This isn't about sprinkling a little bit of herbs and spices into your soup pot. Instead it's looking at every meal as an opportunity to get an abundance of herbs into your life as a powerful way to bolster your health. This is food as medicine at its best!

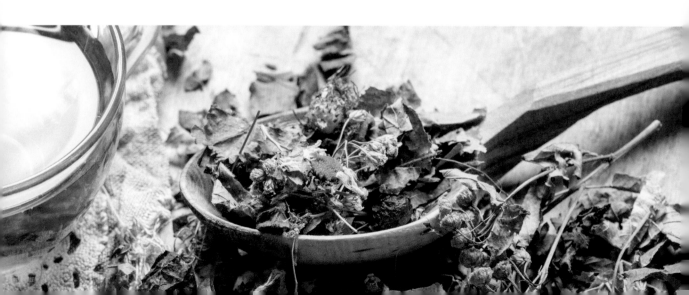

CHAPTER 2

How Do We Know Herbs Can Do That?

As you learn about all the benefits and qualities of herbs, your inquisitive mind may start to wonder, *Do herbs really do that? How do we know it? Is the author just making this up?*

When learning about plants, it is important to realize that there is no one way of knowing. We have historical records of plant use going back thousands of years. Many modern-day herbalists use herbs in their lives and in their practices and share their personal experiences. And, of course, we have a growing number of scientific studies on plants.

FROM HISTORICAL TEXTS TO MODERN-DAY HERBALISTS

The first written record of herbs being used for health dates back more than 5,000 years. Since then, many important texts have been written and preserved that still strongly influence our knowledge. While we certainly want to be skeptical of older texts, we can glean many insights from them that have stood the test of time. Just because some information may be outdated in a text doesn't mean there are no pearls of wisdom to be found.

Modern-day herbalists will often substantiate historical use of herbs through their own personal and clinical experiences. They are rooted in the past while also moving the tradition forward and developing new ways to use herbs. Through apprenticeships, schools, conferences, and organizations like the American Herbalists Guild, herbalists share their experiences along with case studies of their trials and successes. They are a valuable source of information about herbs.

I've been using herbs for myself, my family, and my clients for more than a decade. I have seen how herbs (as well as lifestyle, diet, and counseling) can dramatically shift someone's healing experience. The effect may be as simple as soothing a sore throat or as complex as addressing the root cause of a chronic disease. Woven through this book are stories of my own experiences as well as stories of some people with whom I've had the honor of working over the years. (Names have been changed to protect privacy.)

SCIENCE TODAY

Scientific studies and clinical trials on the use of herbs and spices for health are on the rise. While I've frequently heard people claim that scientific evidence proves that herbs don't work, in reality there are thousands of studies showing their effectiveness. Many of them confirm the traditional use of plants, while others point to new ways of using them.

There are many well-designed studies that use herbs in the way a traditional herbalist would, for example, using the proper dosage and the best extraction (tea, tincture, etc.) and treating the right indications.

However, some studies are poorly designed and these, unfortunately, lead to fantastic headlines that give people the impression that herbs don't work. An unfortunate example was a study published in 2009 in the *Journal of the American Medical Association*. The researchers concluded that gingko does not prevent dementia.[1] Major news outlets across the country ran headlines proclaiming, "Gingko doesn't work."[2] Shortly thereafter, the American Botanical Council issued a press release pointing out the numerous flaws in the study, including the lack of a control group and sloppy statistics that didn't take into account the 40 percent of people who failed to complete the trial. The press release also pointed out that:

> At least 16 controlled clinical trials have evaluated various ginkgo extracts for healthy, non-cognitively impaired adults. A systematic review has shown that in 11 of these trials, the ginkgo increased short-term memory, concentration, and time to process mental tasks.[3]

Unfortunately, critical looks at the flaws in a study aren't sexy enough to make major headlines, so the public is often left with the impression that herbs don't work.

The majority of the studies I've cited in this book are from human clinical trials, also called *in vivo* studies. I've also included a few interesting *in vitro* studies on plants—that is, studies done in a controlled environment outside the living organism, such as the testing of cells in a petri dish. While in vitro experiments can contribute to a better understanding of the effect of a plant, they don't necessarily reflect the effect the plant would have in a human. However, I did not include *any* animal trials for two reasons. First, I question the ethics of many animal studies. Second, the results from animal studies don't often translate to humans.

If we ignore the traditional use of herbs and focus on poorly designed clinical trials, we'll have a dim understanding of the potential of herbs. Conversely, if we rely solely on history and tradition while ignoring scientific studies and the range of experiences of modern-day herbalists, we will be equally misinformed. What's really exciting is when traditional use, modern-day practice, and science converge! The ideal path combines thousands of years of knowledge with the experiences of herbalists today and the many well-designed human clinical trials. In this manner, we begin to get a clearer picture of the many ways that plants can heal.

In keeping with this holistic approach to herbs, I have done my best to present information in this book from the perspective of herbalism while highlighting the ways that science is validating the traditional uses of plants. In the next chapter, we'll learn about the foundation of herbalism: energetics and taste.

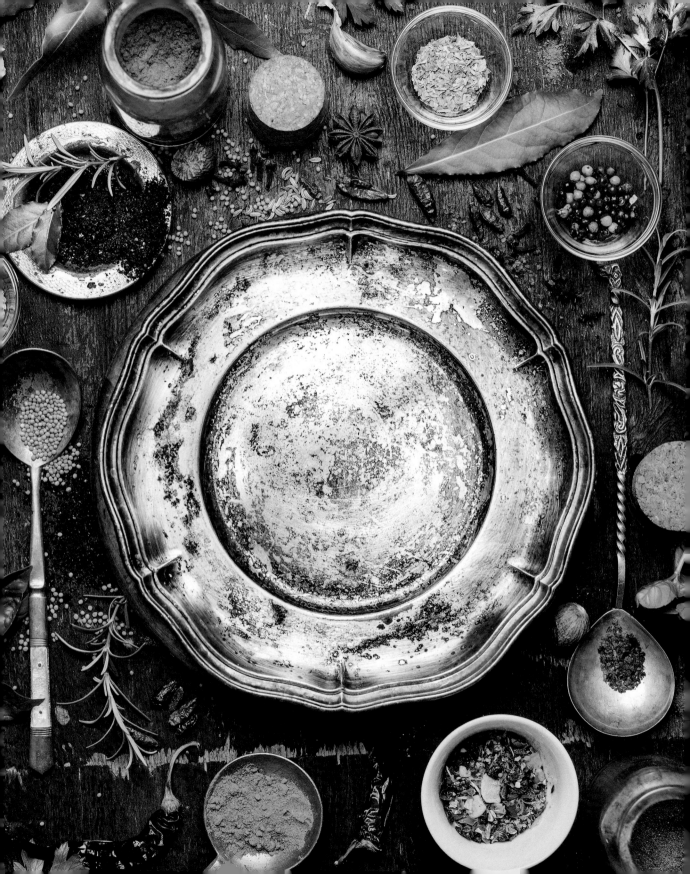

CHAPTER 3

Matching Herbs to *You*— Not to an Ailment

In the United States alone, herbs and supplements are a multibillion-dollar industry. Worldwide it is even bigger—and growing. As popular as herbs are today, however, our mainstream view of them is still missing something. Herbalist and author David Winston likes to say that while *herbs* are becoming increasingly popular, *herbalism* isn't.

In other words, our culture still has the pervasive One Solution Syndrome mentality regarding the use of herbs: "Oh, you have X problem. Then use Y herb." You can readily see this mind-set reflected in the "miracle" cures circulating on social media and in other unethical marketing practices: "Turmeric Cures Cancer!" "Lemon Balm Kills Viruses!" "Echinacea Cures the Common Cold!"

The One Solution Syndrome reflects our culture's approach to health: so many are looking for that *one* thing, either natural or pharmaceutical, that can be the cure for *everyone's* problems. We even see this perspective in diet advice, with every specialized diet out there—whether it's vegan, paleo, South Beach, Atkins, low-carb, DASH, or whatever—all proclaiming to be the *one* way to eat. But if you take this approach with herbs, it's not utilizing key concepts found in traditional herbalism.

Herbal theory has an entirely different approach to health, with principles and diagnostics that go beyond "this for that." Practitioners commonly refer to this as the "art of herbalism." It's important to understand that well-trained herbalists don't treat, diagnose, cure, or prescribe herbs for diseases. Instead, herbalism often takes a more personalized approach, choosing herbs for the *person* rather than simply for a particular ailment.

PERSONALIZING TREATMENT TO THE INDIVIDUAL

At its core, the idea that you and I are different is sort of a "no kidding, Sherlock" obser-vation. There are doubtless many variations between us. Our age, weight, height, eye color, where we live, where we work, fitness level, food preferences, and general life experiences will likely be different. So it makes intuitive sense that even if we had the same diagnosed illness, the solution to our illness could be entirely different.

The idea that we are all individuals, and that herbs, foods, and even lifestyle choices should be selected to match our particular needs, is found in all three of the major herbal systems of today. In Western herbalism we use the four humors: choleric, sanguine, melan-cholic, and phlegmatic. In Ayurveda the tridoshic system is used: Pitta, Vata, and Kapha. Traditional Chinese Medicine uses the five-phases system of Fire, Earth, Metal, Water, and Wood, as well as numerous organ system patterns (Stagnant Liver Qi, Damp Spleen, etc.).

All of these systems are beautiful and complex, and it takes many years of study to reach any sort of comprehension. In this book, I have taken simplified concepts from all of these traditions to create a foundation that anybody can start with—and, conveniently, it doesn't require years of study!

The process of personalized medicine, matching health solutions to the person and not to the disease, can be done in a variety of ways, depending on the herbalist's training. Many herbalists use what is referred to as *energetics* as their underlying diagnostic principle.

THE ENERGETICS OF HERBALISM: HOT/COLD AND DRY/DAMP

So what is energetics? While this term may sound a bit out there or "woo woo," it is based on the physical sensations that you experience every day. At its essence, energetics refers to a classification system based on four complementary qualities: hot/cold and dry/damp.

When it comes to the qualities of hot and cold, I'm not talking about what the ther-mometer is telling us. Instead, it is about the *feeling* of hot or cold. For example, if you've ever eaten a really spicy meal, you've probably noticed that it made you feel warmer, even though your temperature didn't actually change. Similarly, dry and damp sensations are something we can easily observe every day. Does your skin generally feel dry or moist? Have you ever noticed that a cough was dry or moist? Some people notice that the weather can strongly affect them in regards to the humidity. I love the arid desert while others may feel it's uncomfortably dry for them.

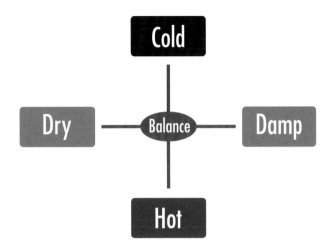

Herbalists assess both people and plants in terms of the four qualities with the goal of supporting health by nurturing energetic balance. If someone is hot, we will use cooling herbs. If someone has excess dryness, we will use moistening herbs. This might sound strange at first, but once you get it, you'll see that you've long perceived energetics in your life without knowing that's what it was. Can you think of people in your life who tend to be hotter by nature? Do you know someone who wears a heavy coat, scarf, and hat when others need only a light jacket? Have you ever met someone who has dry skin and needs to constantly slather on lotion and cream? This is due to their different energetics.

ENERGETICS OF PEOPLE

Every person is born with a unique blend of the four qualities, and the energetics of a person is often referred to as their *constitution*. A person's constitution exists within a moving scale. External influences, such as weather, food, illness, medication, sleep habits, and stress, all have an effect on your evolving inner landscape. Think of your constitution as different shades of gray rather than simply black or white, hot or cold.

Sometimes people's constitutions can be seen in their preferences. If someone tends to be colder, they may enjoy hot weather more than someone who has a warm constitution. Someone with a lot of dryness may be aggravated by the desert but thrive in a more humid environment. The more you pay attention to these things, the more the concepts of energetics will become recognizable within your own life.

Have you ever had someone describe the wondrous benefits she received from the latest and greatest supplement, but when you tried it, you got worse? It's common to have something affect you completely differently from how it affects another person. For example, I have a friend who gets insomnia whenever she has ginger, but ginger has never affected me in that way. Instead, ginger improves my digestion and helps me to keep warm in the winter. Energetics explains why we react to treatments in different ways; each of us is a unique blend of qualities giving us our own unique experiences. When you understand your personal constitution, it opens up a whole new world of awareness of what works best for you.

ENERGETICS OF PLANTS

Just like humans, plants have hot/cold and damp/dry qualities. These qualities can vary depending on where or how the plants grew and how they have been prepared for consumption. For example, fresh ginger is considered to be warm, while dried ginger is considered hot. This isn't an observation measured with a thermometer, which would most likely display the same temperature for each variety of ginger. Instead, it comes from how the herbs act and feel in the body.

While thinking of plants in this way may sound strange at first, I'll bet you already recognize energetics in common foods. Is a cucumber hot or cold? What about a habanero pepper? Is watermelon dry or damp? What about a cracker?

ENERGETICS OF AN ILLNESS

One of the factors that may cause your personal constitution to shift is an illness. As an example, let's say that you generally tend to be cool and dry. But then you come down with an upper respiratory infection, and you develop some dampness in your lungs, such as mucus congestion. You also have a fever, and you're sweating. So while you normally tend to be cool and dry, the effects of this illness leave you feeling more hot and damp. To bring your body into energetic balance, you must understand your personal constitution so you can see how an illness might be affecting it.

An important principle I learned from my teacher Michael Tierra is that you always prioritize acute symptoms. So if you normally tend to be cold and dry but an external influence is giving you more hot and damp symptoms, then you should address the hot and damp symptoms first.

DISCOVER YOUR OWN CONSTITUTION

To help you discover your own constitution, I've created two quizzes that cover the simple basics of hot/cold and damp/dry. Your results will tell you your combination of thermal results and humidity results: hot/dry, hot/damp, cold/dry, or cold/damp.

Remember that these are the very basic principles of personal constitutions. If you went to see a practitioner of herbal energetics, they would likely do a thorough examination to get a more precise understanding of who you are. However, knowing your basic tendencies is all you need to get the most out of this book.

When you fill out these quizzes, keep the following in mind:

- Everyone contains some aspect of all four qualities. But you contain a unique mix of strengths and challenges.

- Look for general tendencies—in other words, how you feel most of the time. For example, if you normally feel warm, but you don't like winter and there was that one time you felt cold in a blizzard, warm wins.

- Although external forces can affect our qualities, we are born with a particular constitution that doesn't change dramatically. If you can't decide on an answer, think back to how you were as a child.

Quiz A:	Determining Hot and Cold

Mark an X next to each statement that feels true to you, then add up the number of true statements in each column. A higher total in the first column indicates more heat qualities. A higher total in the second column indicates more cooling qualities.

❑ I tend to feel warmer than others.	❑ I tend to feel colder than others.
❑ I tend to have a loud voice.	❑ I tend to have a quiet voice.
❑ My entire face can easily get red or flushed.	❑ My face and/or fingernail beds tend to be pale.
❑ My tongue tends to be bright red	❑ My tongue tends to be a pale color.
❑ I have lots of opinions and I'm not afraid to share them.	❑ I often feel like I have a low energy level.
❑ I prefer cold weather.	❑ I prefer warm weather.
❑ I have a large appetite.	❑ I have a small or poor appetite
❑ I am a more active person.	❑ I am a less active person.
Total: _____	Total: _____

Quiz B:	Determining Damp and Dry

Mark an X next to each statement that feels true to you, then add up the number of true statements in each column. A higher total in the first column indicates more damp qualities. A higher total in the second column indicates more dry qualities.

❏ I tend to sweat more easily than others.

❏ My skin and hair are often oily.

❏ My arms and legs can feel heavy.

❏ I often have a stuffy or runny nose.

❏ I tend to have a thick coating on my tongue.

❏ I prefer dry climates and don't like humidity.

Total: _____

❏ My skin tends to be rough and dry.

❏ My hair tends to be dry.

❏ My fingernails are dry and/or brittle.

❏ I often have itchy skin or scalp.

❏ I often have a dry throat, nose, eyes, and/or mouth.

❏ My tongue does not usually have a coating on it.

Total: _____

If you have an equal number of true statements in a quiz, instead of thinking of yourself as predominantly one type or another, you could frame the results as showing how that particular quality manifests in you. For example, perhaps you have signs of dampness in your skin and you don't like humid conditions, but your hair and nails tend to be dry and brittle. In this case, your skin is damp while your hair and nails are dry.

An equal total in your quizzes could also mean that you have a fairly balanced constitution. Someone who is strongly cold/damp will have a lot of signs of coldness and dampness, which makes it easy to determine their constitution. Someone who is only *slightly* cold/damp will have less dramatic symptoms, thus making it more difficult to determine their constitution.

On the other hand, you may be finding it difficult to understand your constitution because of external influences. An illness, medication, the climate, or any number of other factors could be influencing you, thus giving you a mixed result. Letting these concepts soak in a bit, and practicing more awareness, will help you to see your unique patterns.

If you have questions about your constitution, you may want to visit an herbal practitioner to help you see the energetic patterns in your life more clearly. (I also offer a free mini-course on herbal energetics at www.HerbsWithRosalee.com.) However, for the purposes of this book, these very basic quizzes are all you need! You could philosophize about your constitution all day long, but in the end, what really counts is your continuing observation and awareness, particularly of the four qualities.

THE TASTE OF HERBS

Another way to understand the energetics of plants is through their taste. Long before we had the ability to identify isolated constituents, herbalists used their senses to understand and categorize medicinal plants. This concept of taste is most developed within Traditional Chinese Medicine and Ayurveda. The five tastes in Chinese herbal theory are pungent, salty, sour, bitter, and sweet. Ayurveda recognizes the same five tastes, along with *astringent* as a sixth.

This book will lead you on a journey through herbs within each of the five tastes so that you can fully appreciate and experience how particular herbs work for you as an individual.

PUNGENT

The pungent herbs are warming and spicy. They are used to awaken the senses and get things moving. They are ideal for people who tend to feel cold, damp, or sluggish, as they can increase circulation and bring warmth from the core of the body out to the limbs. When it comes to dose, though, easy does it!

You'll see a wide variety of warming qualities among the pungent herbs. Follow a sip of rosemary tea with a sip of cayenne tea and you'll notice a big difference! The heat of cayenne can often force your body to take cooling measures such as sweating.

Did you discover you have a warm constitution? Don't skip this section! While pungent herbs are generally heating, there are a few that are cooling. I've also created the recipes in the pungent section to be broadly balanced and beneficial for most people.

Most of the herbs in this book are pungent herbs. In fact, most of our common culinary herbs are classified as pungent. As I mentioned in Chapter 1, many herbs have become part of culinary tradition because they not only taste good but also support one's health. With a major focus of this book being "food as medicine," I've packed this book with pungent culinary herbs to spice up your life!

SALTY

The salty herbs are high in vitamins and minerals. They are nutrient dense and considered the most nourishing and foodlike of all the herbs.

You might be thinking that these herbs would have the flavor of table salt. However, in herbalism, "salty" refers to herbs that are high in micronutrients; they have a mineral taste rather than an overtly salty taste.

Herbs in this category are known for affecting the fluids in your body. Some are diuretics, helping with the flow of urine; others are lymphatic, helping with the flow of lymph fluid.

Herbs with a salty taste include seaweed, oatstraw, violets, and chickweed. In the salty section, I highlight my favorite salty herb: stinging nettle. Stinging nettle has so many nutrients (even more than kale) that using it regularly in your diet can have dramatic health results.

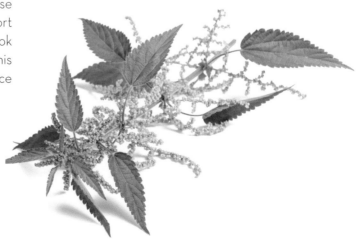

SOUR

The idea of "sour" may make your mouth pucker as you envision biting into a lemon. However, just as with salty, the sour taste in herbalism tends to be more subtle. Most fruits and astringent herbs are classified as sour.

The sour herbs stimulate digestion, build strength, and reduce inflammation. Energetically, they tend to be cooling, but not dramatically so. Because their thermal dynamics are so close to neutral, most people will be able to enjoy these herbs daily.

Many of these herbs are high in antioxidants, the many benefits of which we discussed in Chapter 1. However, while the protective qualities of antioxidants have been making headlines, studies have repeatedly shown that it is not beneficial to ingest antioxidants as supplements. It is ideal to search out your antioxidants in their whole form, and the herbs in the sour section are the perfect way to do that.

Many sour herbs also have an important herbal action: they are astringent, which is the sixth taste in Ayurveda. I think of astringency as a mouthfeel rather than a taste. If you've ever bitten into an unripe banana or drunk a strong cup of black tea, then you've felt the astringent action. While it is often described as a dry sensation in the mouth, astringent herbs are actually tightening the mucosal tissues they come in contact with. Astringency helps with bleeding or swollen gums, swollen throats, healing wounds, and excess discharge such as a runny nose.

SWEET

The sweet herbs nourish and build. They can restore energy levels and modulate the immune system. But before you start dreaming of herbs that taste like sugarcane, I have to tell you that the sweet taste in herbalism is not like visiting a candy store. In fact, your first taste of these plants may not have you thinking about sweetness at all.

Some sweet herbs don't taste overtly sweet but are classified as such because of their building and nourishing herbal properties. Most of our adaptogen herbs, for example, are listed as sweet. Adaptogen herbs are used to broadly support overall health in people with signs of weakness or deficiency. They can also modulate the stress response, which improves a person's negative experience of stress and allows them to feel stronger and less agitated when life throws them a curveball.

Because the negative effects of stress are so far-reaching, these herbs can powerfully support your health in a lot of ways. They can ease inflammation, one of the leading causes of chronic disease. They can help you to sleep deeply every night, which can improve your alertness and energy during the day. They also modulate your immune system, which means fewer illnesses and perhaps even preventive factors against cancer.

Some sweet herbs may be slightly warming or slightly moistening, but most have fairly neutral energetics. People can generally use these herbs no matter their constitution.

BITTER

The bitter herbs stimulate digestion and often have a cooling and draining effect, which can help to modulate inflammation. Many of these herbs are also very important for liver health.

In a popularity contest for the five tastes, my bet is that bitter would not win. In fact, we might call it the taste that most people love to hate. Even our language represents our antagonistic relationship: the bitter truth, bitter tears, a bitter personality. Yet in herbalism, bitter is one of our most important and common tastes.

Herbalists are fond of saying that many digestive problems are due to a "bitter deficiency syndrome." This term was coined by herbalist James Green and refers to the lack of bitter taste in our diets. In doing our best to breed the bitterness out of our vegetables, we've done ourselves a great disservice! The bitter taste is an important part of our digestion.

Your body continues to recognize the taste of bitter long after it hits your tongue. That's because there are bitter taste receptors throughout your body, including in your digestive tract and even in your lungs. The act of tasting even a small something that's bitter activates your entire digestive system. The taste causes you to salivate, which is one of the first steps in the digestive process. It also releases important gastric enzymes that help digest your proteins (among other things) and stimulates bile production, which helps you digest fats. It's amazing, all that bitters can do for your digestion.

I, along with many herbalists, believe that all people can benefit from adding bitters to their life. (As I mentioned, plenty of common digestive problems are due to a deficiency of bitters.) In fact, I recommend experiencing bitter with every single meal you eat.

The energetics of bitter herbs are cooling and drying, making them a great match for those who tend to be warm and damp. However, bitters can be helpful for all types of constitutions, especially if combined with other herbs. In this book, and in many blends you'll find, bitter herbs are often combined with the warming and pungent herbs to improve the flavor and add more warming qualities.

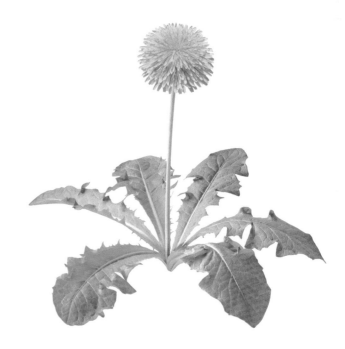

PUTTING THIS ALL TOGETHER

Understanding how to match herbs to people is an integral part of using herbs successfully. While a certain herb may sound like it has a lot of beneficial qualities, if you consistently match the wrong energetics, you may see either unwanted effects or simply a lack of benefits.

Paul Bergner, one of my herbal teachers, relates a story about this in his book *The Healing Power of Garlic*. Many years ago, Paul was interested in the numerous benefits of garlic, so he ate increasingly large dosages of it. However, garlic is very warming and drying, and Paul has a warm constitution. He quickly noticed some benefits, such as a decrease in congestion, but he then began to experience health concerns connected to overly dry tissues and inflammation. That doesn't make garlic a bad herb, or even a dangerous one. Instead, it's a reminder that we need to choose herbs to fit people and not use a one-size-fits-all approach such as the One Solution Syndrome.

Understanding your general constitution, the energetics of your current illness, and the energetics of plants leads us to what I call the herbal sweet spot.

THE HERBAL SWEET SPOT

The search for that perfect sweet spot is instinctive. Do you remember the familiar story of Goldilocks? She finds herself alone in the house of three bears and decides to make herself comfortable. As Goldilocks explores, she is looking for what feels right. She finds three bowls of porridge: one is too hot and one is too cold, so she settles on the one that is "just right" for her. When she is ready for a nap, she tests out the beds. Again, one is too hard and one is too soft, so she snuggles into the one that is just right for her.

The art of herbalism is discovering what is "just right" for the individual. If someone has a lot of heat, we want to cool him down. If someone is too damp, we want to dry her out. This really comes down to common sense, and you've experienced such scenarios before. On a scorching summer day, are you craving a hot bowl of soup or ice-cold lemonade? When you're parched, do you want to eat salty crackers or have a hydrating beverage? If you've been out in a snowstorm, do you raid the freezer for ice cream or have a hot cup of cocoa?

The herbal sweet spot is the culmination of ideas in this book. Rather than jumping to "What herb is good for _____ disease?" you first need to think about who you are as an individual. Within that consideration is your constitution, what your current energetics are, and the herbs that would bring you balance.

To find the herbal sweet spot, you will need to develop a deeper understanding of self to know what works best for *you*. As you read, take note of the energetics of each herb. You'll see which are used for "cold" fevers and which are used for "hot" fevers. You'll see cooling herbs that stimulate digestion as well as warming herbs that do the same. As you experience each herb, ask yourself, *How do I feel?* and then, *How do these herbs make me feel?*

As you start to become more aware of how foods, herbs, and spices affect you, you may have some big realizations. For example, if you tend to feel cold, you may notice that drinking raw fruit juices is increasing your coldness and that you prefer the feeling of warmth after eating a dish with pungent herbs. You may notice that bitter herbs and foods help enhance your digestion. If you have a warm constitution, you may find that bitter herbs decrease heat and bring you comfort. If you have a cooler constitution, you may find that pungent herbs help your circulation. Remember, this book is about experiencing how herbs and spices work for *you*. To get the most out of this book, you have to do some hands-on exploring.

To help you find your herbal sweet spot, this chapter closes with a simple tasting experience to help you observe how herbs and spices make you feel. I highly recommend that you make the effort to experience this yourself, as it will provide a base of reference for the rest of this book.

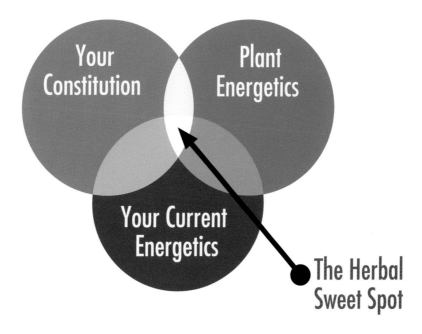

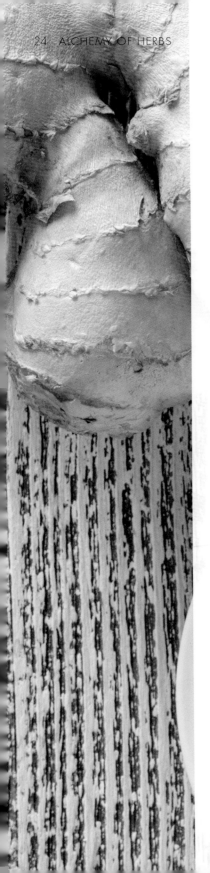
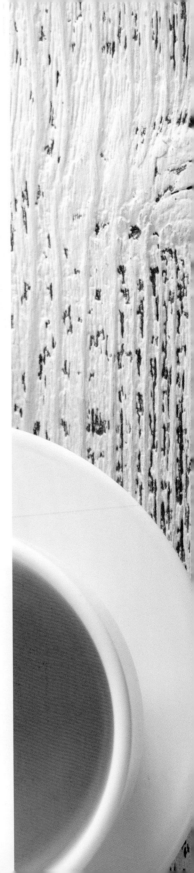

Sometimes noticing how an herb affects us is something that takes place over time. Ginger is a nice herb to start with because it has dramatic energetics that can be immediately felt. If you try this tasting exercise with other herbs, know that the effects may be more subtle. It may take consuming something frequently over a long period of time to get a solid sense of how it makes you feel.

EXERCISE:	How to Know How an Herb or Spice Affects You

This tasting exercise is about noticing how something makes you feel. There are no wrong or right experiences; it's really about your own awareness and observations.

We are going to start by tasting ginger. This is a perfect herb to start with because it's easy to find and its energetics are very pronounced. (Also, most people think it tastes good!)

Start by making a ginger tea. Either fresh or dried ginger will work great; simply use whatever you can most easily find. There is no need to strain either of these preparations, although you may if you wish.

With fresh ginger:

- Put 1 tablespoon of minced fresh ginger into a cup.

- Cover this with 1 cup of just-boiled water.

- Cover the cup and let steep for 10 minutes.

With dried ginger:

- Put 2 teaspoons of dried ginger powder into a cup

- Cover this with 1 cup of just-boiled water.

- Cover the cup and let steep for 10 minutes.

Once your tea is ready, move through these simple steps and observations:

1. Smell your tea.
What do you notice? Does it have a smell? Do you notice any changes in your body when you smell that tea? Is it a pleasurable aroma? Or do you dislike it?

2. Sip your tea.
How does it taste? Sweet? Sour? Salty? Bitter? Spicy?

3. Take another sip.
What do you notice within your body? Do you notice yourself taking deeper breaths? Do you have any sensation in your sinuses? Do you feel the digestive process beginning with salivating and tummy rumbling?

4. Take another sip.
What do you notice about its warming or cooling qualities? Do you feel heat when you sip this tea, on your tongue or in your belly? Or do you feel more cold sensations?

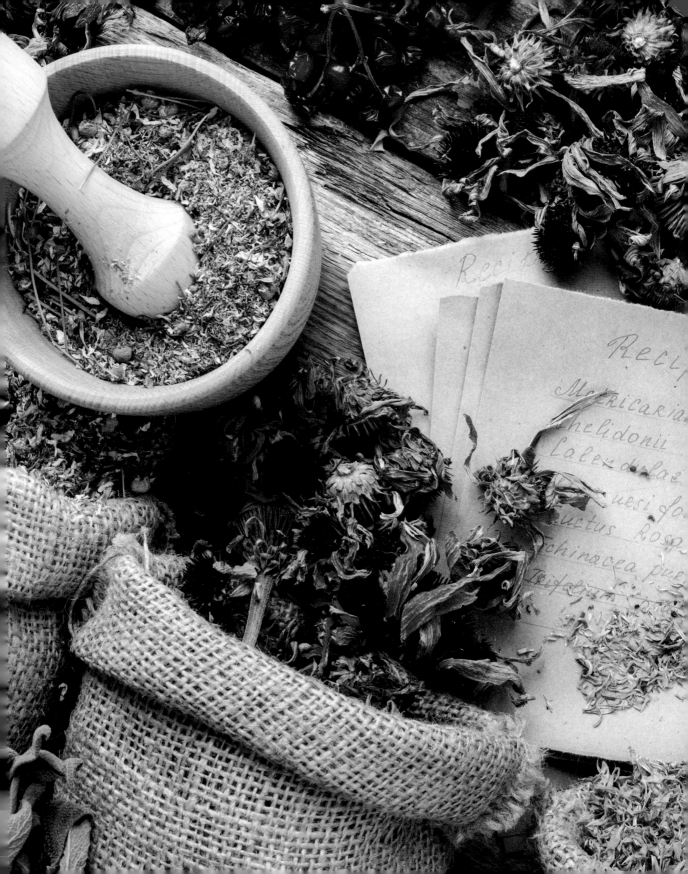

CHAPTER 4

How to Get the Most Out of This Book

To help you get the most benefit out of this book, I encourage you to move forward with the mind-set of an explorer. Still, even an explorer needs the proper setup and tools. In this chapter, I'll discuss how to choose the best ingredients, how to figure out doses and measurements, and what supplies and tools you'll need on your journey.

HOW TO TUNE IN TO YOUR FEELINGS AND EXPERIENCES

As you experience more herbs and spices in your life, remember that herbalism seeks to find balance in the four qualities of hot and cold and dry and damp. Therefore, keeping track of how you are feeling in those areas is a good way to judge if the foods, herbs, and spices you are choosing are working for you. I recommend keeping a journal of your observations because it's easy to forget or miss subtle improvements. It's rare that you take an herb one day and suddenly all your health challenges are gone the next. Instead, it's something that happens over time.

As an example, let's say you feel cold a lot of the time. After reading through the herbs in this book, you decide you are going to incorporate a lot more pungent herbs and spices into your life. After a few months, you think about it and notice you are still feeling cold. It would be easy to then think, *Hmm, this isn't working.*

Let's envision another scenario. Again, say you tend to feel cold. You write in your journal about what exactly that means or how it manifests in your life. For instance, you list very specific ways you feel cold: your feet feel like icicles, you wear a sweater and a hat while others might wear only a T-shirt, and so on. Then you start to incorporate more pungent and spicy herbs in your life. As the weeks and months go by, you continue to write down simple but precise observations about how you feel. You still feel cold, but as you pay close attention, you notice that things are shifting. Perhaps your feet are still cold but you no longer need a heating pad to warm them up in bed. Maybe you still wear a sweater but you no longer need a hat.

Always keep in mind that this experience is about simply noticing how something makes you feel and the changes going on in your body. There are no wrong or right experiences. It's really about your own awareness and observations. Practicing and refining this tasting experience is one of the most important tools you can develop as it can help guide you to making the best choices for you.

HOW TO CHOOSE THE BEST HERBS AND SPICES: TRUST YOUR SENSES

When buying herbs and spices, look for organically grown varieties. You may find high-quality fresh herbs at your farmer's market or dried herbs at a local health-food store. In Recommended Resources I've also listed several companies that sell high-quality dried and fresh herbs online.

There is no set rule as to how long herbs last; some simply store better than others. Exposing herbs to light and heat shortens their potency, and those that are ground into powder have a much shorter shelf life than those left whole. Therefore, as much as possible, buy small amounts of herbs in their whole form and grind them as needed. Store them in a dark space away from heat, and preferably in a glass jar. Storing spices right by the stove, while convenient for cooking, will quickly cause them to lose their potency.

You can be sure that, over time, herbs and spices lose their pizzazz. The best way to judge the quality of your herbs and spices is by using your senses. Dried herbs and spices should retain the same vibrant colors they had when they were fresh, just slightly muted. If a plant was green when fresh, it should remain green (not brown) when dried. If the plant is aromatic, like lavender or holy basil, it should still have a strong scent when dried. Compare its scent to more freshly dried herbs and spices; if it's not vibrant, then the herb is most likely past its prime.

Before getting started on the recipes in this book, I recommend doing a thorough inventory of any herbs and spices you already have on hand. If they are dull and tasteless, compost them! Replace them with fresher, vibrant herbs and spices so you can really get the transformative benefits. Take the time to evaluate the freshness of your herbs and spices at least every six months.

HOW TO USE THE RECOMMENDED AMOUNTS

Each herb chapter in this book has a Recommended Amounts section. These dosages are a combination of my own experience using herbs and considerations from clinical herbal texts. Suggested dosages are admittedly a bit tricky in herbalism, as herbs affect individuals differently. Your age, weight, gender, and current health issues may all play a role in determining the ideal dosage of an herb.

In my own practice I recommend that people start with small amounts of herbs, then slowly increase the amount over time. I like to see people getting the maximum dosage of an herb without experiencing any adverse effects. The listed dosages are safe for most people, yet potent enough for you to notice effects. My intention is that you take these as a starting place to find your own optimal therapeutic dose.

The tinctures will have a ratio listed, which are a set of numbers separated by a colon (e.g., 1:1 or 1:3). These numbers express the amount of herbs used in comparison to the amount of menstruum (i.e., the liquid). A 1:3 ratio, for example, means that a tincture contains 1 part herbs to every 3 parts of liquid. (This is a weight-to-volume ratio, so the herbs are measured out in grams while the liquid is measured in milliliters.) The percentage after the ratio is the tincture's alcohol content.

HOW TO MEASURE DIFFERENT HERBS

Many of us grew up learning the basics of measurement. It's covered in school and anytime you want to make your own batch of chocolate chip cookies. In baking, ingredient measurements are standardized. A teaspoon of baking soda in your house is going to be the same as a teaspoon of baking soda in my house, because it's generally the same size, density, and consistency everywhere.

But measuring in herbalism is a bit different from measuring for baking. The volume of herbs can change dramatically based on how it was harvested and cut. For example, dandelion root can be cut in large, thick chunks or minced up really finely. When the size of an ingredient varies wildly, measuring it by teaspoon and tablespoon won't be consistent. Also, the shape or size of some herbs can make them difficult to measure. Astragalus, for example, is often sold in large, flat slices; it would lead to inconsistent yields if you tried to cram those into a measuring cup. For these reasons, I like to measure certain herbs by weight. I highly recommend that you purchase a small kitchen scale that measures grams, kilograms, ounces, and pounds.

The recipes in this book use a mix of both standard American volume measurements as well as weight measurements. I'll usually choose one or the other—whichever makes the most sense for the ingredient and quantity. For those herbs and spices that would be tricky to get into a measuring cup or spoon, I make sure to use weight measurements but also offer approximate volume measurements, so that you can get started in the kitchen right away—even without any special equipment! For recipes in which it is absolutely crucial to measure an herb by weight rather than volume, I have listed only the weight measurement and included a note in the description.

Those of you more familiar with imperial measurements (ounces, pounds) may be wondering why I chose to measure in the metric system (grams). I find that measuring small amounts of herbs in grams makes more sense than measuring out tiny fractions of ounces (1 gram = 0.04 ounce).

Tinctures are measured in milliliters (mL). This is a handy measurement for small amounts of liquids. Small measuring cups or beakers often have this measurement printed on the side.

You may also want to refer to the Metric Conversion Chart at the back of this book.

HOW TO FIND THE BEST INGREDIENTS

My dad likes to say that the secret to a good-tasting meal is using the best ingredients. That is especially true when you are using your food as medicine. To find the best herbs and spices, please review the Recommended Resources at the back of this book. The following are a few tips on how to source the best ingredients.

Fruits and vegetables: Prioritize local organic fruits and vegetables, whether they are from your own garden or from a farmer's market. They will undoubtedly have more valuable nutrients than those shipped from several states (or countries) away. Many fruits and vegetables start to lose their nutrient content after they are picked. Broccoli, for example, has 50 percent less vitamin C 24 hours after it's been harvested.[1]

Meat from humanely raised animals: It is not necessary to eat meat to use the recipes in this book (nor is it necessary to be a vegan!). However, if you choose to eat meat, you can seek out healthier sources. There are small ranches springing up all over the United States that raise their animals humanely, giving them plenty of room to run around, feeding them healthily, and so on. Seek out meat from cows that are grass-fed and pasture-raised, from free-range chickens, and so on. If you can find it at your local farmer's market, all the better.

Our modern industrial meat industry is nothing short of horrific. Concentrated animal feeding operations (CAFO) result in cheap meat at the grocery store at the cost of the humane treatment of animals and environmental health. Animals raised in these conditions are fed an unhealthy diet and pumped full of antibiotics and hormones. How can we expect to be healthy if we are eating these inhumanely raised animals?

Olive oil: Olive oil is a delicious and healthy oil that is perfect for cooking savory foods. We've recently become aware that a lot of the oil available on the supermarket shelf isn't the quality that it's advertised to be. When sourcing olive oil, look for opportunities to buy direct from a farm (online if necessary).

Honey: Honey is the main sweetener I use in teas and in cooking. I prefer honey, especially local honey, over other sweeteners like cane sugar.* However, I recommend avoiding mass-market honey from the store. Unless the label clearly states otherwise, this honey is most likely not produced in sustainable ways.

On the other hand, when you buy from a local, ethical beekeeper, you're supporting a neighborhood business—and advocating for the bees! Bees are dying at record rates and really need our help right now. Actually, a better way to say it is that we desperately need bees, as they're the pollinators of most of the crops that make up our food. My dear friend Susie Kowalczyk is a beekeeper who is a strong advocate for the bees. She speaks out against the use of pesticides known to kill bees, travels the world to learn about the best beekeeping methods, and keeps her hives strong by using treatment-free methods. That is what I want to support!

A side note on sugar: Sugarcane is often mass-produced using unsustainable agricultural methods. It may need to be shipped long miles to a factory, packaged in environmentally unfriendly materials, and then shipped again to stores hundreds or even thousands of miles away. There is nothing about the sugar industry that I want to support!

We also know that sugar is one of the unhealthiest things we eat. Yet of the 2,000 pounds of food per year that the average American eats, *150 pounds* of that is sugar.[2] The American Heart Association recommends that men get no more than nine teaspoons of sugar a day and women get no more than six, yet we are consuming an average of five times that![3] That's why I call for very little sweetener to be added in most of my recipes.

HOW TO MAKE THINGS A LITTLE EASIER: USEFUL TOOLS AND SUPPLIES

While you could make most of the recipes in this book without any special tools, these inexpensive supplies will make working with herbs easier:

Digital kitchen scale: Using a digital scale is highly recommended for use with some of the oddly shaped herbs and spices. Look for a digital scale that measures grams, kilograms, ounces, and pounds. These can be found in kitchen stores, in hardware stores, and online, with simple ones ranging from $15 to $20.

Spice grinder: A spice grinder allows you to purchase whole spices and grind them as needed, to retain the vibrancy of the spices longer. I use an inexpensive coffee grinder that is reserved exclusively for herbs—but never use it for coffee, as the flavor of the coffee will transfer.

Suribachi: For grinding fresh or small amounts of herbs, I like to use a suribachi. This is a mortar and pestle with a grooved bowl, which makes it easier to grind things than with a smooth version.

Strainers: When making teas or otherwise straining herbs from liquid, strainers and tea balls can be convenient. Look for stainless steel strainers with a very fine mesh. For tea balls and tea infusers, make sure they're large enough to allow the herbs you're infusing to move around. You don't want to have to cram the herbs into a too-small space.

Funnels: Funnels of all sizes are useful for filling jars and bottles with your herbal remedies. Look for funnels made of stainless steel, especially if you are using them for hot liquids.

Cheesecloth: Cheesecloth can catch the fine particles that slip through a regular strainer. I also like that I can really squeeze the cheesecloth to get the most out of the herbs and liquid. Jelly bags can be used for the same purpose and can be used again and again.

Glass jars: Glass jars are indispensable in an herbal kitchen. At all times I have a good supply of pint, quart, and half-gallon jars. These are great for storing herbs, mixing many of the recipes in this book, and then storing what you have made. Note, however, that some glass canning jars on the market have BPA, an endocrine-disrupting chemical, in the lining of their lids. For this reason I use canning jars with a glass lid, such as those by Le Parfait, Weck, or Fido. These are also nice when using a recipe with vinegar, which can corrode a metal lid and ruin the contents.

GOING FORWARD

I recommend that you first read through the entire book to get an overview of how amazing herbs and spices can be for your health. Then choose one herb or spice to immerse yourself in. Spend time with that herb. Taste it, make tea with it, use it in your kitchen. Use it often!

While I hope this book gives you some things to ponder, my wish is that it inspires you to actually use herbs in your daily life. My intent is to give you information that you can put into practice, as well as to motivate and inspire you to try new herbs and spices, and new tastes and recipes. My hope is that your new experiences in the kitchen lead to delicious creations and your own health transformation.

Remember there's no One Solution to your personal health. When it comes to getting the most benefits out of herbs and spices, *you* are your greatest asset. But this can be learned only by your active participation. This isn't a dogmatic philosophy filled with rules and "shoulds" and "should nots." Instead, you are now about to embark on a journey of your own observations and awareness. When you arrive at your destination, you will know the best foods and herbs and spices for you, not because some expert has proclaimed something a superfood that everyone should eat, but because you experienced the benefits within yourself.

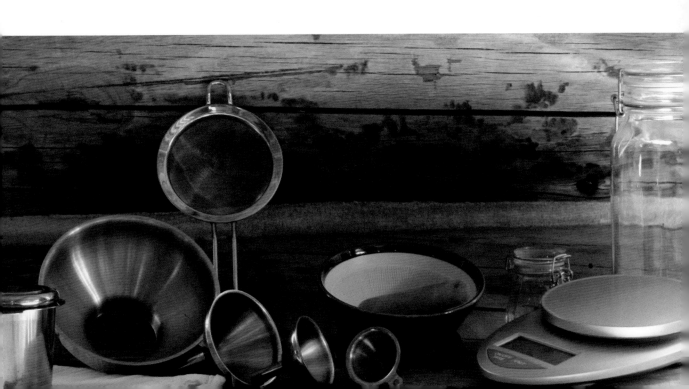

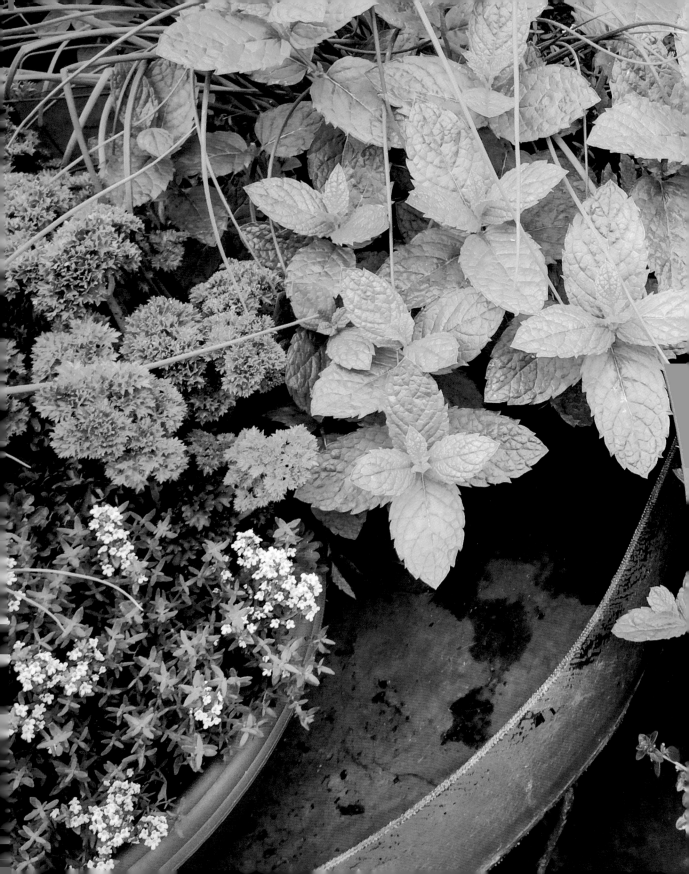

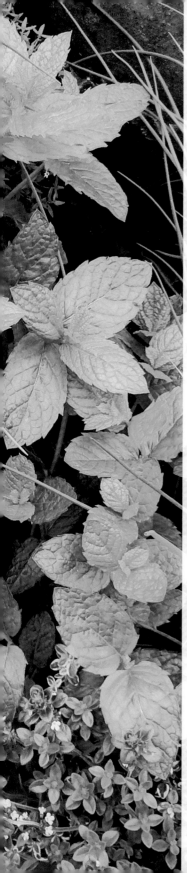
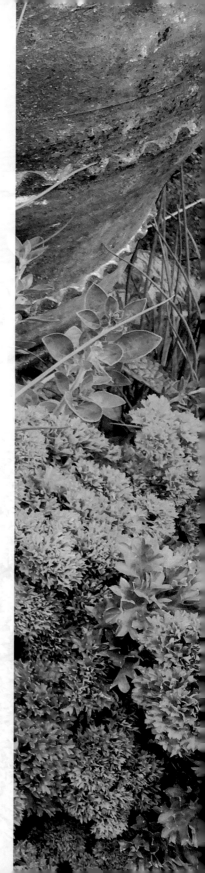

PART II

the
herbs

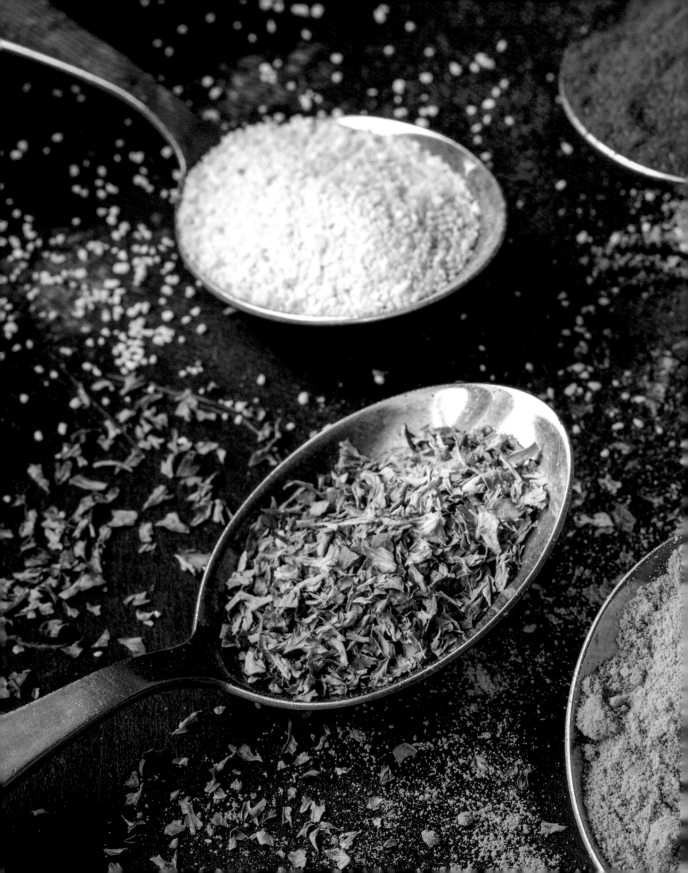

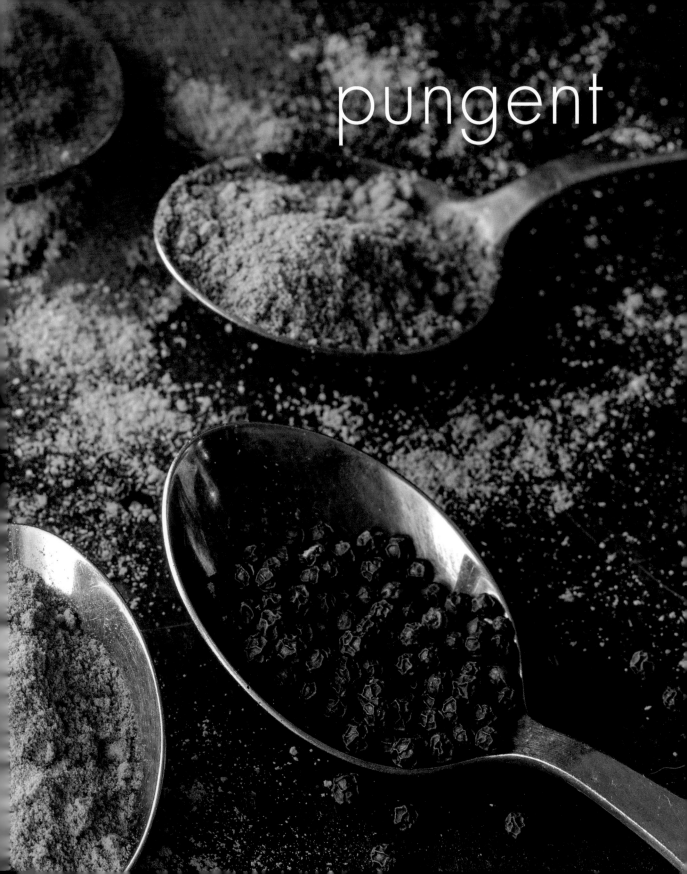

pungent

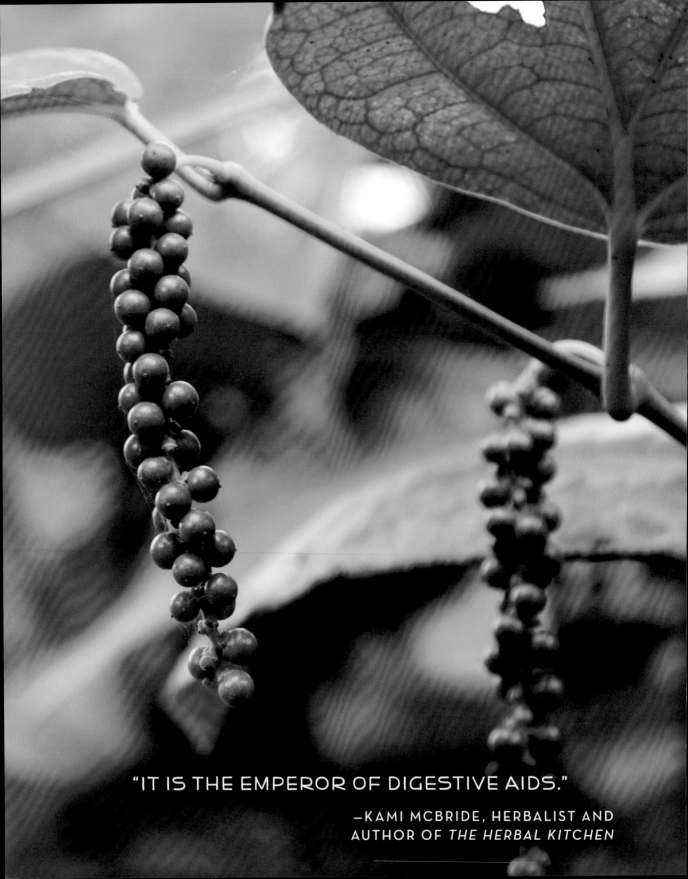

"IT IS THE EMPEROR OF DIGESTIVE AIDS."

—KAMI MCBRIDE, HERBALIST AND
AUTHOR OF *THE HERBAL KITCHEN*

CHAPTER 5

Black Pepper

Black pepper is so common that it's easy to dismiss as a culinary spice used simply for taste, but there's a reason this spice was once called black gold. Besides being flavorful, black pepper strongly supports digestion. As you'll see, it has been used for many different ailments. It is the most popular spice of our modern day and accounts for a fifth of the total spice trade in the world.[1]

What I find most amazing about black pepper is its ability to help you increase your absorption of nutrients from your food. I suggest keeping a pepper grinder full of whole peppercorns near your eating areas so that you can habitually add black pepper as a finishing touch to all your meals.

Botanical name: *Piper nigrum*

Family: Piperaceae

Parts used: berries

Energetics: warming, drying

Taste: pungent

Plant properties: antimicrobial, antioxidant, antispasmodic, carminative, circulatory stimulant, stimulating diaphoretic, stimulating expectorant

Plant uses: fevers, mucus congestion, slow or stagnant circulation, increasing bioavailability of other herbs, hemorrhoids, gentle laxative, arthritis

Plant preparations: food spice, tea, tincture, pastilles

Before we look at the many medicinal benefits of black pepper, let's get some glimpses of its fascinating history. Pepper has been in common use in India for at least 4,000 years, and presumably much longer.

It spread from there to the ancient Egyptians and Romans. Our knowledge of peppercorns in ancient Egypt is limited. After the death in 1213 b.c.e. of the great pharaoh Rameses II, black peppercorns were stuffed in his nostrils as part of the mummification process. Flash forward 1,500 years, and we have a Roman cookbook from the 3rd century c.e. that contains peppercorn in many of its recipes, although it was probably a very expensive spice at the time.

Pepper took a spotlight during the height of the early European spice trade routes. During the Middle Ages, peppercorns were considered an important trade good. They were referred to as "black gold" and were even used like money to pay taxes and dowries.

TYPES OF PEPPERCORNS

When buying whole peppercorns, you will notice red, white, and green varieties in addition to the common black. All of these come from the same plant but are prepared differently to achieve the different looks and slightly different tastes.

Black peppercorns are harvested when unripe, boiled briefly, and then dried in the sun.

White peppercorns are harvested when fully ripe. Their outer flesh is removed so that only the seed remains.

Green peppercorns are harvested when unripe, then treated to preserve the green coloring (usually through freeze-drying, pickling, or other means).

Red peppercorns are harvested when fully ripe, then treated to preserve the red coloring.

MEDICINAL PROPERTIES AND ENERGETICS OF BLACK PEPPER

Black pepper has a broad range of use. Its hot and stimulating characteristics make it useful for a variety of cold and flu symptoms such as fevers with chills (stimulating diaphoretic) and for mucus congestion (stimulating expectorant). Black pepper quickens the circulation by increasing blood vessel size and can be used for signs of stagnant circulation (such as cold hands and feet). It is also used topically for arthritic pain.

FOR INCREASING BIOAVAILABILITY

What I find most amazing about black pepper is its ability to increase the amount of nutrients that you absorb. This is referred to as potentiating bioavailability, and black pepper can do this with herbs, foods, and even pharmaceutical drugs.[2] In practical terms, adding a bit of black pepper to herbal formulas or to your dinner plate means that you have potentiated the qualities and nutrients of the healthy foods you are eating. This is why it's my most frequently used spice. It makes sense to try to get the most nutrients out of our food, and black pepper can help!

A well-known example of black pepper's ability to dramatically increase nutrient absorption is the effect of adding it to curcumin, an extract of turmeric. One study reported that piperine, an extract of black pepper, increased the bioavailability of curcumin by 2,000 percent.[3] Piperine also has been shown to increase the bioavailability of echinacea and berberine-containing plants like goldenseal.[4,5]

Besides increasing the bioavailability of herbs, it has been shown that piperine can dramatically increase absorption of coenzyme Q10, beta-carotene, selenium, and vitamin B6.[6,7,8]

An article in the *International Journal of Recent Advances in Pharmaceutical Research* says it may work for the following reasons:

- It acts as a circulatory stimulant by increasing the size of blood vessels, which helps to transport nutrients around the body.

- It modulates the physical properties of cell membranes, which helps transport nutrients through barriers.

- It produces a thermogenic effect in the gastrointestinal tract, which increases blood supply to the area.[9]

FOR DIGESTIVE ISSUES

Besides adding a pleasant taste to our food, there's another reason that black pepper is found on practically every dinner table in homes and in restaurants. Black pepper supports healthy digestion.

Do you ever feel like food is just sitting in your stomach, or do you have other signs of slow digestion, like bloating or gas? Black pepper's spicy attributes warm digestion to get things moving. On the opposite end of the spectrum, it can also be used to stop diarrhea, even when used externally. One study showed that stir-fried white pepper effectively stopped both chronic and acute diarrhea in infants and children when applied externally over the navel.[10]

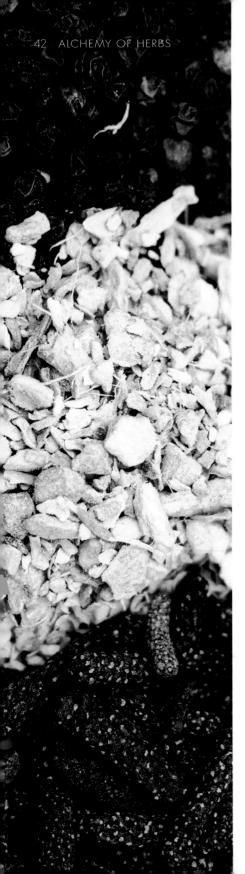

HOW TO USE BLACK PEPPER

Since black pepper dramatically increases the bioavailability of many nutrients, I like to have it freshly ground onto every meal I eat. To get the most out of your pepper, buy whole peppercorns and then grind them as needed. Once they are ground, the aromatics evaporate quickly, so old ground pepper is of little benefit.

RECOMMENDED AMOUNTS

Adding freshly ground pepper to your meals is a great way to enjoy the benefits of this spice. If using black pepper for more therapeutic reasons, such as for arthritis or cold and flu symptoms, the recommended therapeutic amount ranges from 1 to 15 grams per day.

SPECIAL CONSIDERATIONS

Large doses of black pepper may cause nausea and digestive upset. It could potentially act as a synergist with many pharmaceutical drugs, which means it can increase the effects of a drug in unexpected ways. If you are taking pharmaceuticals, consult with your doctor before taking anything more than a normal culinary amount of black pepper.

TRIKATU PASTILLES

Don't be intimidated by the name; *pastille* is basically a fancy French term for pills, while *trikatu* is the name of a famous Ayurvedic herbal formula that is a simple combination of three pungent herbs: black pepper, ginger, and long pepper. (Long pepper, *Piper longum*, is a close relative of the peppercorn.) It is perfect for people with signs of cold or stagnant digestion (such as bloating and gas), or for people with excess mucus. Trikatu can be found in many health food stores, but making your own ensures that it is fresh and potent. Plus, it's really easy!

One of these pastilles can be taken with each meal. If you make them small enough, they can be swallowed whole; if you like things really spicy, you can chew them. You can easily adjust the quantity by remembering that this recipe uses equal parts of each herb (by volume, not weight). The measurements here will give you a small batch of pastilles. To make a large batch, try ¼ cup of each herb and increase the amount of honey too.

Yield: 3 tablespoons

1. Mix together the black pepper, ginger, and long pepper.

2. Very slowly drizzle a small amount of liquid honey, about a teaspoon, over the herbs. (If your honey has crystallized, warm it slightly by placing the jar in a pan of hot water to get it to a completely liquid consistency.) Stir.

3. Continue adding honey 1 teaspoon at a time, stirring in between, until the powdered herbs become a thick, moldable paste. Don't add too much honey or you won't be able to form it into balls. If this happens, add more herbs until you get a pastelike consistency.

4. To make each pastille, take a pea-size amount of paste and roll it gently between your fingertips until it forms a small ball. Roll the pastilles in the licorice or orange peel powder to coat them, if desired. The powder is an optional ingredient, but it does help keep the pastilles from sticking together.

5. Store your pastilles in an airtight container. They should last indefinitely, but for best results use them within six months.

1 tablespoon freshly ground black pepper

1 tablespoon ginger powder

1 tablespoon long pepper powder

1 tablespoon honey

½ tablespoon licorice powder or orange peel powder* for coating the pastilles (optional)

*Orange peel powder is simply orange peel that has been dried and powdered. It is different from store-bought "dried orange peel," which comes in small, uniform chunks. If you make your own, place the dried peels in a spice grinder or food processor and process until it is a fine powder.

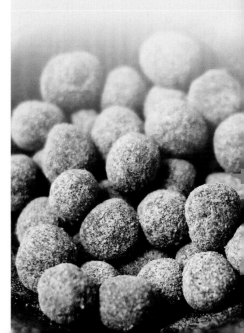

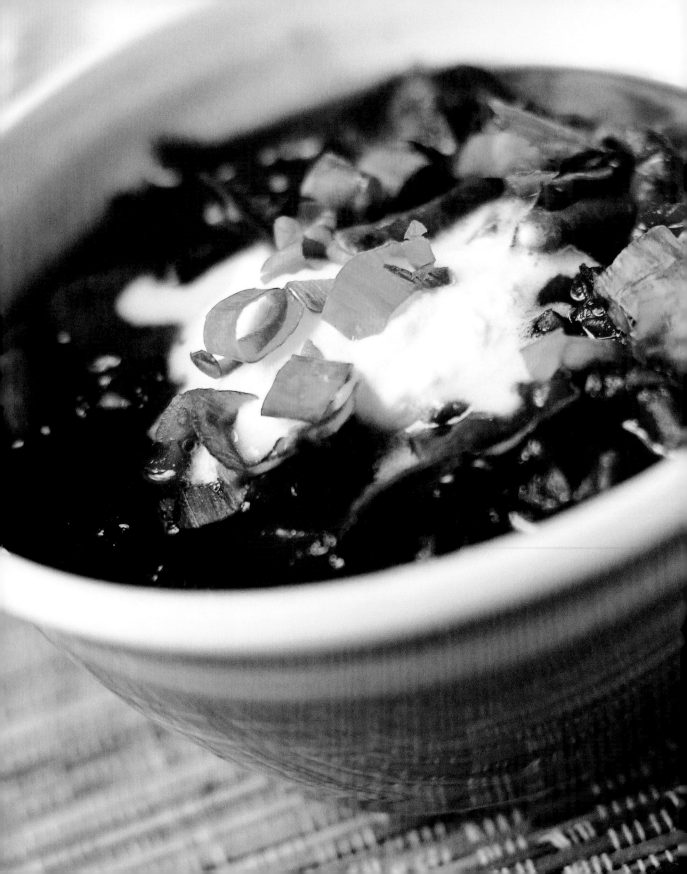

PEPPERY BORSCHT*

Borscht is a traditional beet soup from Eastern Europe. This is a perfect fall and winter soup as it's dense, warming, and filled with winter vegetables. The pepper gives this hearty soup an earthy, spicy taste.

Yield: 10 cups, roughly 5 servings

1. Heat the butter in a large pot over medium heat. Add the onions, and sauté until they are translucent.

2. Add the ground beef to the pan and cook until browned.

3. Add the garlic, caraway seeds, salt, pepper, and bay leaves. Sauté for 1 minute.

4. Add the celery, carrot, cabbage, beets, potatoes, mushrooms, and stock. (You can peel the beets and potatoes if you desire, but I never do.)

5. Bring the mixture to a boil, then lower heat and simmer until all the vegetables are tender, about 30 minutes.

6. Stir in the balsamic vinegar, beet greens, honey, and tomato puree. Cover and continue to simmer for 5 more minutes.

7. Remove the bay leaves before serving. Garnish with green onions and serve with a dollop of sour cream, if desired.

*For a different version of this soup recipe, as well as hundreds of free recipes and remedies, please visit LearningHerbs.com.

2 tablespoons butter

1½ cups chopped onions

1 pound ground beef (preferably grass-fed)

4 garlic cloves, minced

1 teaspoon caraway seeds

2 teaspoons salt, or to taste

2 tablespoons freshly ground black pepper

2 bay leaves

1 celery stalk, chopped

1 large carrot, sliced

3 cups coarsely chopped purple cabbage

2 cups cubed beets

1½ cups cubed potatoes

1 cup chopped fresh shiitake mushrooms

6 cups chicken or vegetable stock

1 tablespoon balsamic vinegar

1 cup chopped beet greens, including stems if desired

1 tablespoon honey

1 cup tomato puree

green onions, for garnish

sour cream (optional)

2 teaspoons peppercorns
(6 grams)

2 teaspoons cinnamon chips*
(6 grams)

2 whole star anise
(2 grams)

1 teaspoon whole cloves
(2 grams)

1 teaspoon fennel seeds
(2 grams)

*You can buy cinnamon chips
or break a whole cinnamon quill
into smaller pieces.

CHINESE FIVE-SPICE BLEND

Chinese five-spice blend is commonly used to flavor many popular Chinese restaurant dishes. This recipe is just one example of many different blends. Over time you may be inspired to create your own. I recommend making this in small batches with whole herbs, ground fresh. (Remember that most powdered herbs lose their flavor and potency within a couple of months.)

Try this on meats, veggies, and even popcorn. It is also used in Lemon Balm and Orange Chicken (page 224).

Yield: approximately 2 tablespoons

1. Toast all ingredients in a dry pan over medium heat until fragrant, about 2 to 3 minutes. Swirl the pan gently and toss the seeds occasionally to prevent burning. Allow to cool.

2. Add the mixture to a spice grinder and grind. (My grinder takes about 30 seconds to get a consistent, soft powder.)

3. Store this blend in an airtight spice jar out of the light.

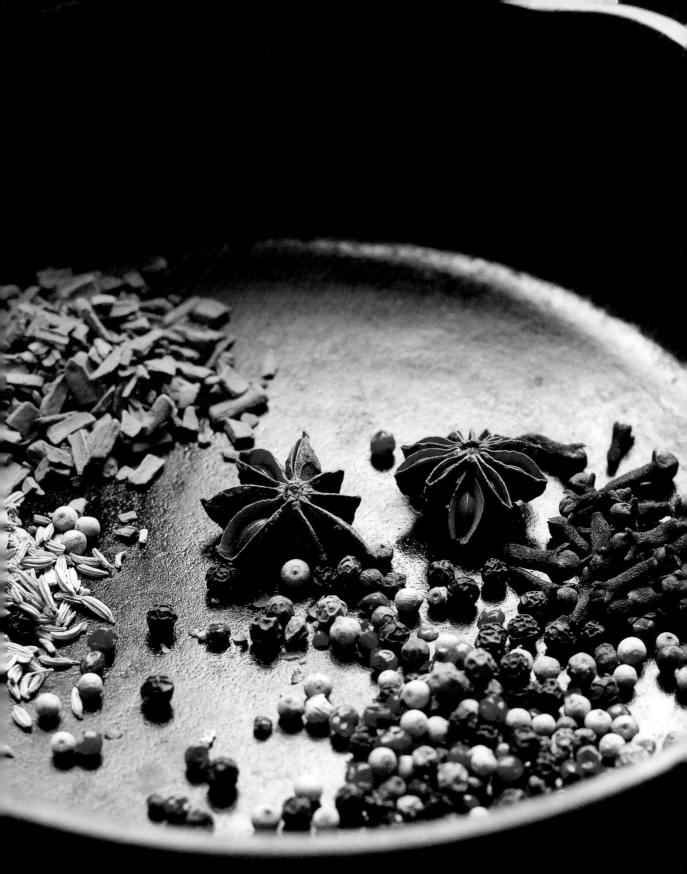

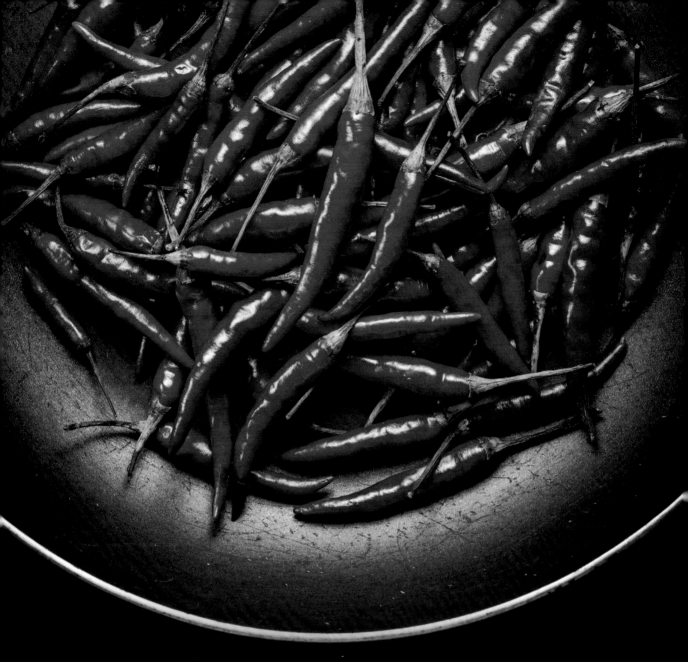

"BECAUSE OF ITS LEGENDARY CURATIVE
PROPERTIES, ITS EXCITING FLAVOR, AND ITS
MAGICAL ABILITY TO SUSTAIN A SENSE OF WELL-
BEING, CAYENNE IS ONE OF MY FAVORITE HERBS
FOR BOTH MEDICINAL AND CULINARY PURPOSES."

–ROSEMARY GLADSTAR, HERBALIST AND AUTHOR OF
ROSEMARY GLADSTAR'S MEDICINAL HERBS: A BEGINNER'S GUIDE

CHAPTER 6

Cayenne

Cayenne is a hot and spicy herb that has countless uses in your kitchen as well as benefits for your health. It can relieve pain, prevent a cold from settling in, dramatically support heart health, and promote healthy weight loss. However, be cautious with the extremely hot energetics of cayenne; success is determined by how well you match the herb to the person.

Other common names: chile, chili pepper

Botanical name: *Capsicum annuum, Capsicum frutescens*

Family: Solanaceae (nightshade)

Parts used: mainly fruits, also seeds

Energetics: warming, drying

Taste: pungent

Plant properties: stimulant, antimicrobial, analgesic, carminative, styptic, antioxidant, stimulating diaphoretic, stimulating expectorant, immunostimulant, rubefacient, antifungal, metabolic stimulant, blood mover

Plant uses: toothache, arthritis, fever, heart disease, poor circulation, parasites, digestive problems, sore throat, depression, low libido, bleeding, inflammation, hypertension, hypotension, headache, neuropathy, shingles, fungal infections, type 2 diabetes, insulin resistance, weight loss, menstrual cramps

Plant preparations: tea, tincture, liniment, oil salve, culinary spice

FOR DIGESTIVE ISSUES

Although we feel the heating effects of cayenne immediately, one study has shown that taking cayenne long term may provide the most benefits. This particular study looked at cayenne's ability to decrease dyspepsia (indigestion) symptoms. Fifteen people were given 2.5 grams of cayenne daily, and 15 people were given a placebo. Starting in the third week, those receiving the cayenne had significantly fewer digestive problems than those receiving the placebo. By the end of the trial, those taking the cayenne had a 60 percent reduction in symptoms while the placebo group experienced a 30 percent reduction in symptoms.[2]

Cayenne and other spicy peppers were once blamed for causing ulcers, but more recent studies show cayenne can have a protective effect on the stomach lining and could possibly prevent peptic ulcers.[3,4]

There are a lot of conflicting studies on cayenne and its ability to resolve or exacerbate common digestive problems like heartburn, gastroesophageal reflux disease (GERD), hemorrhoids, or anal fissures. However, it's important to remember that a person's constitution may play a role in these conflicting results.

FOR INCREASED METABOLISM

Herbalists have long used cayenne to warm people up, whether for chronically cold hands and feet or for acute signs of coldness like chilblains. This increased circulation and metabolic action is referred to as thermogenesis, and it can be beneficial for weight loss or for symptoms associated with colds and upper respiratory tract infections.

In regard to weight loss, one study found that 6 milligrams of cayenne extract aided abdominal fat loss.[5] Another study showed that the most benefits were seen in people who weren't habituated to eating red peppers and in those who tasted the cayenne (as opposed to taking it as a capsule).[6]

FOR HEART HEALTH

The prolific herbalist John R. Christopher, widely known simply as "Dr. Christopher," extolled the virtues of cayenne, claiming that it could powerfully support heart health as well as stop a heart attack. Science has validated the long-term use of cayenne for heart health, although, understandably, no studies have been done on its ability to stop a heart attack!

One four-week study showed a decrease in resting heart rate with regular chili consumption.[7] Another study demonstrated that regular consumption of chili for four weeks supported the body's resistance to oxidation.[8] In vitro studies show that cayenne may reduce platelet aggregation, which potentially reduces the risk of forming a blood clot.[9]

FOR INSULIN RESISTANCE AND TYPE 2 DIABETES

Diet, stress level, and sleep quality are some of the major lifestyle factors related to insulin resistance and type 2 diabetes. However, herbs such as cayenne can play an important role in helping to prevent and reverse the symptoms. Cayenne has been shown to effectively lower blood glucose levels and maintain insulin levels.[10,11] These effects make it a beneficial herb for those wanting to address the insulin sensitivity that can lead to type 2 diabetes.

FOR COLDS AND THE FLU

Karta Purkh Singh Khalsa and Robyn Landis wrote in their book *Herbal Defense*, "You can treat a cold very effectively with nothing but chiles if you can get enough down."[12] Cayenne is an internal heating herbal medicine and one of several long-celebrated ways to stop a cold in its tracks. (Other methods include sweating therapies such as saunas or hot baths.)

If you've ever drunk cayenne tea or added cayenne to your meals, then you've probably felt your sinuses immediately respond. Cayenne promotes mucus secretions from the mucous membranes, causing a runny nose or sinus drainage. Mucus is loaded with antibodies and is a powerful immune system response to an invading pathogen. If a cold or the flu has progressed and there is sinus or lung congestion, cayenne pepper will quickly drain them! Moving congested mucus lessens the possibility of a secondary infection in the sinuses.

FOR PAIN RELIEF

Capsaicin, a major constituent of cayenne peppers, blocks substance P, a neuropeptide that relays pain sensations in the body. Cayenne can be used topically to relieve many types of pain, including low-back pain, diabetic neuropathy (nerve damage), shingles, migraine headache, backache, and arthritis.[13,14,15,16,17]

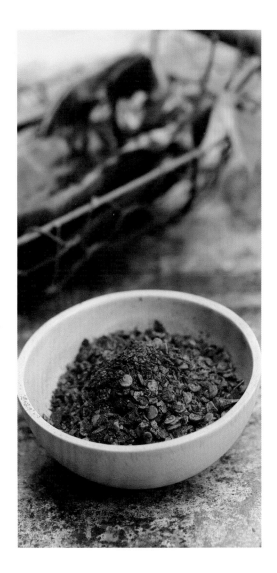

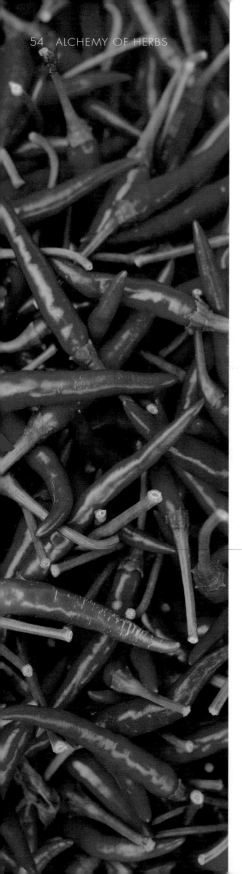

HOW TO USE CAYENNE

Cayenne is a great addition to many culinary dishes. It is most often used dried, either whole or powdered. Because cayenne degrades fairly quickly, make sure you purchase it freshly dried and in small amounts. Ideally, you should restock with freshly powdered cayenne pepper every six months.

The most capsaicin is located in the lining of the seeds and the membrane from which the seeds hang. If using whole cayenne chiles, you can decrease the heat by first removing the seeds.

RECOMMENDED AMOUNTS

To avoid stomach upset, I recommend consuming cayenne with a meal. Depending on your sensitivity and tolerance, you can use just a few sprinkles to spice up your meal or a therapeutic amount of 1 to 10 grams per day.

SPECIAL CONSIDERATIONS

Always start with small amounts of cayenne and then slowly increase as desired.

Cayenne is a hot herb. Taken in large amounts over time could lead someone to feel hot and dry all the time.

Cayenne is very irritating to the eyes and sensitive skin. Avoid touching cayenne or cayenne preparations and then touching the eyes. Consider wearing gloves if preparing large amounts of cayenne.

Cayenne shouldn't be taken in large amounts during pregnancy.

People on warfarin or other blood-thinning pharmaceuticals should talk to their doctor before using large amounts of cayenne.

CAYENNE TEA

Get ready to sweat! Drinking a hot cayenne tea is one of the first things I do when I feel a cold or flu coming on. Not only does this speed the healing process and shorten the duration of a cold or flu, it also feels really good on the throat.

If you have really potent cayenne powder, then start with just ⅛ or ¼ teaspoon. If you can handle that well, then slowly increase the amount. The more cayenne you can use the better, but sip it slowly; you will feel nauseated if you drink something that is too strong.

Yield: 1 cup

¼ teaspoon cayenne powder, or to taste

1 tablespoon fresh lemon juice

1 teaspoon honey, or to taste

1. Bring 1 cup of water to a boil. Place the cayenne powder in a cup, then pour the hot water over it. Add the lemon juice and honey, and stir.

2. Sip slowly once it has cooled a bit. The hotter you drink this, the better.

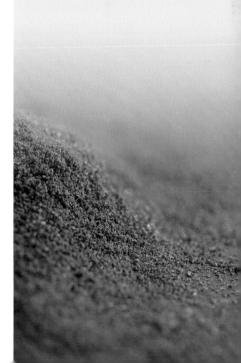

1 cup minced yellow or
brown onions

½ cup grated horseradish

½ cup minced garlic
(approximately 15 cloves)

¼ cup grated fresh ginger

¼-inch piece of fresh
cayenne, or ½ teaspoon
dried, or to taste

2 tablespoons dried thyme

2 teaspoons whole black
peppercorns

½ lemon, thinly sliced into
rounds

¼ cup raw honey,
or more to taste

2⅔ cups raw, unfiltered
apple cider vinegar
(at least 5% acidity)

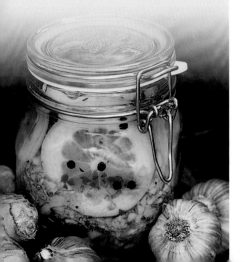

FIRE CIDER

Fire cider is a spicy vinegar that was first created by beloved herbalist Rosemary Gladstar. Since she created this recipe decades ago, thousands of herbalists have made countless versions. If you asked a room of herbalists about fire cider, you'd likely hear that it is a favorite wintertime remedy for most of them.

This vinegar has a bold taste with an interesting combination of spice, sourness, and sweetness. If you are taking it as a preventive remedy, I recommend having it by the tablespoon, one to three times per day. If you are using it to ward something off, I recommend taking a tablespoon every hour. It can be diluted with a little bit of water if desired.

For this recipe, I recommend using pungent yellow or brown onions as opposed to sweet or white onions.

Yield: 2 cups

1. Place the onions, horseradish, garlic, herbs, spices, and lemon into a 1-quart jar. Add the honey.

2. Fill the jar with vinegar, and be sure to cover all the ingredients.

3. Stir well to make sure there aren't any air bubbles.

4. Cover, preferably with a glass or plastic lid. If using a metal lid, place parchment or wax paper between the lid and the jar (vinegar will corrode metal).

5. Let the jar sit for 2 to 3 weeks. For the first few days, shake the jar well once per day.

6. Strain the vinegar into a clean jar. Refrigerate and use within a year.

CAYENNE SALVE

This simple salve can be made very quickly for minor pain relief. It works great for sore muscles and joints, bruises, and even nerve pain. If using for arthritic pain, use it daily, and note that it may take a week or two to see results. This salve can be stored at room temperature for up to a year, but use within six months for best results.

This is a hot mixture! This salve should be used externally only, and not on broken skin, as it may sting open wounds. Even on closed skin, you may feel a bit of burning or heat in the area where it is applied. Sensitive individuals may experience tenderness or blistering. If this happens, discontinue use until the area is healed, then apply less often or in smaller amounts.

Caution: When cayenne comes in contact with your mucosal membranes or eyes, it will burn! Be sure to wash your hands thoroughly after touching cayenne. Consider using gloves to apply the salve to the desired area. If you are using the salve on your hands, consider applying it at night and sleeping with gloves on.

Yield: 4 ounces

½ cup olive oil

2 tablespoons cayenne powder (15 grams)

½ ounce beeswax (14 grams)

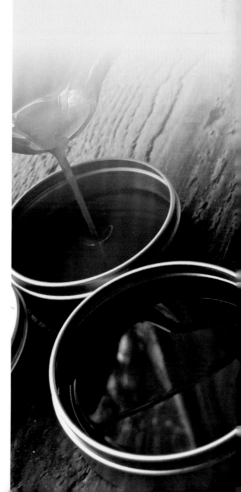

1. The first step is to infuse your oil. You can do this with a double boiler or slow cooker. Take care not to let the oil get too hot or "fry" the herbal material. 100°F is an ideal temperature for the oil.

2. Double-boiler method: Put 1 to 2 inches of water in the bottom of a double boiler. (Alternatively, fill a pot with 1 to 2 inches of water and place a tight-fitting bowl on top.) Place the oil and cayenne powder in the top. Heat over medium-low heat for about 20 minutes, until the oil is fairly warm. Turn off the heat and let stand for 20 minutes to cool a bit. Repeat this warming and cooling process for 2 to 3 hours.

3. Slow-cooker method: Place the mixture in a slow cooker, yogurt incubator, or other low-temperature appliance that can maintain the oil temperature at 100°F for 2 to 3 hours.

4. Pour your infused oil through a strainer lined with two layers of cheesecloth.

5. Gently heat the beeswax over low heat in a small saucepan or double boiler until it is melted. Stir in the infused oil and continue mixing until wax and oil are thoroughly combined.

6. Immediately pour this mixture into jars or tins and let cool, then label the containers.

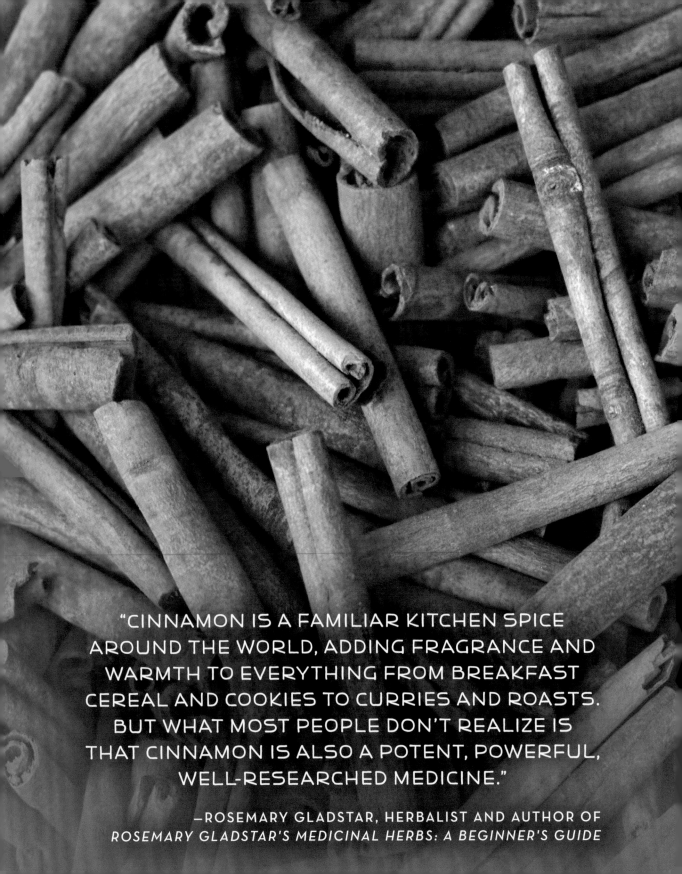

"CINNAMON IS A FAMILIAR KITCHEN SPICE AROUND THE WORLD, ADDING FRAGRANCE AND WARMTH TO EVERYTHING FROM BREAKFAST CEREAL AND COOKIES TO CURRIES AND ROASTS. BUT WHAT MOST PEOPLE DON'T REALIZE IS THAT CINNAMON IS ALSO A POTENT, POWERFUL, WELL-RESEARCHED MEDICINE."

—ROSEMARY GLADSTAR, HERBALIST AND AUTHOR OF *ROSEMARY GLADSTAR'S MEDICINAL HERBS: A BEGINNER'S GUIDE*

CHAPTER 7

Cinnamon

Cinnamon is so often enjoyed in pastries that it might be hard to believe this spice does more than taste good in desserts. Don't be fooled! Cinnamon may be one of the best herbs for improving many common chronic illnesses. It powerfully supports metabolic function, making it an important herb to use alongside diet, exercise, and stress reduction to address the growing epidemic of insulin resistance and type 2 diabetes.

Botanical name: *Cinnamomum cassia* (syn. *Cinnamomum aromaticum*), *Cinnamomum verum* (syn. *Cinnamomum zeylanicum*)

Family: Lauraceae

Parts used: bark (prepared as sticks, chips, powder, or essential oil), twigs, dried flowers

Energetics: warming, drying

Taste: pungent, sweet

Plant properties: aromatic stimulant, warming, demulcent, sweet, astringent, analgesic, hypoglycemic, antioxidant, antimicrobial

Plant uses: toothache, diarrhea, blood movement, infections, arthritis, insulin resistance, colds/flu

Plant preparations: tea, tincture, culinary, tooth powder

The rich history of this aromatic spice reaches at least as far back as 2700 b.c.e., when it was first written about in Chinese texts. In the Bible, Moses is told to make holy anointing oil using two different kinds of cinnamon. The ancient Egyptians used cinnamon not only to flavor food but also in the embalming process.

Nowadays, if given the choice between a bag of cinnamon or a bag of silver, you'd likely take the silver without a second thought. Roughly 2,000 years ago, the opposite would have been true! In the 1st century, Pliny the Elder described cinnamon as having 15 times the value of silver by weight. For centuries, the cinnamon trade was tightly controlled by Arab merchants, who wove fantastical stories regarding its origin and cultivation in order to enhance the magic surrounding this exotic spice and keep prices high. The European entrance into the cinnamon trade began in the 16th century, sparking a violent, centuries-long struggle as countries fought over control of cinnamon plantations.

Cultivation methods for cinnamon trees have been passed down for centuries and remain mostly unchanged to this day. Plantation trees are heavily pruned when they are two years old. This pruning creates a lot of bushy shoots at the base of the tree. These shoots are harvested about twice a year, after heavy monsoon rain makes them easier to process. Then the hard work begins by separating the inner bark of each shoot from the rest of the stalk. Layers of this inner bark are pressed together and then laid out to dry, and during this time the bark curls to form cinnamon "sticks," also called cinnamon quills. After they are properly dried, they are cut to size and shipped around the world. I know it's silly, but every time the flavor hits my tongue, I have to laugh that I am relishing the taste of tree bark.

TYPES OF CINNAMON

There are more than 100 varieties of cinnamon trees, but there are two main species that are commercially available. *Cinnamomum cassia* (cassia cinnamon) is the one you are most likely to encounter on spice shelves in stores across the United States. This cinnamon is native to Indonesia and now grows in tropical climates around the world. *Cinnamomum verum* is commonly called Ceylon cinnamon. Grown in Sri Lanka, some parts of the world consider it "true" cinnamon.

What's the difference between the two? As far as taste is concerned, Ceylon cinnamon has a sweeter and lighter flavor, while cassia is spicier and more pungent. Chefs often prefer cassia for savory dishes such as meats and soups, and Ceylon cinnamon for desserts. In herbal medicine, the two species are used similarly.

MEDICINAL PROPERTIES AND ENERGETICS OF CINNAMON

Herbalist Matthew Wood beautifully describes cinnamon in relationship to its energetics and taste: "Cinnamon is warm and stimulating so it tends to warm up the digestion and the interior, but it is also sweet and astringent so it nourishes and tones."[1]

Cinnamon can ease many digestive complaints, including indigestion, gas, and cramping. It is a common ingredient in chai (tea) blends, which are traditionally drunk after a meal to help with digestion. It's a favorite herb to give to children with diarrhea because it is antimicrobial, tastes good, and gently improves intestinal tone to avoid dehydration.

FOR FEVER

Feeling cold? Feeling hot *and* cold? Cinnamon mildly thins the blood and can be used to increase general circulation, bringing warmth to cold hands and feet. It can also be used in acute situations, such as a cold or flu in which a person is shivering and feels cold. Herbalist Lesley Tierra says that "cinnamon bark also leads the body's metabolic fires back to their source, alleviating symptoms of a hot upper body and cold lower body, such as a flushed face, wheezing, severe sweating, weak and cold lower extremities and diarrhea."[2]

Herbalist jim mcdonald recommends cinnamon for fevers when the body externally feels cold and clammy but there is copious sweating, as well as diarrhea.[3] This makes cinnamon an ideal herb because it warms the outer body, stops excessive sweating, and tones the intestines.

FOR HEALTHY TEETH AND GUMS

Cinnamon has numerous benefits for healthy gums and teeth. When used as a diluted essential oil, cinnamon can alleviate toothaches.

You can also use cinnamon powder as a toothpaste to maintain healthy teeth and gums. Because cinnamon tones tissues and is antimicrobial, it can decrease harmful bacteria levels in the mouth. Herbalist Anne McIntyre elaborates: "The volatile oil in cinnamon is one of the strongest natural antiseptics known. Its antimicrobial properties make it an excellent medicine to prevent and resolve a whole range of infections."[4] (I offer a cinnamon tooth powder in the recipes of this chapter.)

FOR INSULIN RESISTANCE
AND TYPE 2 DIABETES

In 2012 just under 10 percent of the population in the United States had type 2 diabetes, and researchers have found that as many as 30 percent of those in this country have prediabetes or insulin resistance.[5] Millions of people with diabetes and prediabetes are unaware of their condition, and it is affecting people at a younger and younger age. Complications include amputation, heart disease, renal failure, and death.

There are many causes and factors contributing to type 2 diabetes. A deeper discussion of the many holistic approaches are beyond the scope of this book—but the good news is that we can all reduce our risk of developing diabetes by simply using herbs and spices! Cinnamon has been studied extensively, and numerous clinical studies have shown that cinnamon, notably *Cinnamomum cassia*, can dramatically decrease glucose levels and insulin levels.

In a randomized, placebo-controlled, double-blind clinical trial, researchers gave people with poorly controlled type 2 diabetes 2 grams of cinnamon daily for 12 weeks. After 12 weeks, those taking the cinnamon had significantly lower HA1c (a marker that shows average blood glucose levels over time) and lower blood pressure. The researchers concluded, "Cinnamon supplementation could be considered as an additional dietary supplement option to regulate blood glucose and blood pressure levels along with conventional medications to treat type 2 diabetes mellitus."[6]

In another study, cinnamon dramatically improved both glucose and cholesterol levels in adults with type 2 diabetes. The researchers concluded that the results of the study "suggest that the inclusion of cinnamon in the diet of people with type 2 diabetes will reduce risk factors associated with diabetes and cardiovascular diseases."[7]

But you don't have to have insulin resistance or type 2 diabetes to get benefits from cinnamon. Research has shown that taking 3 grams of cinnamon with meals improves metabolic function, thus decreasing your risk of this chronic disease.[8]

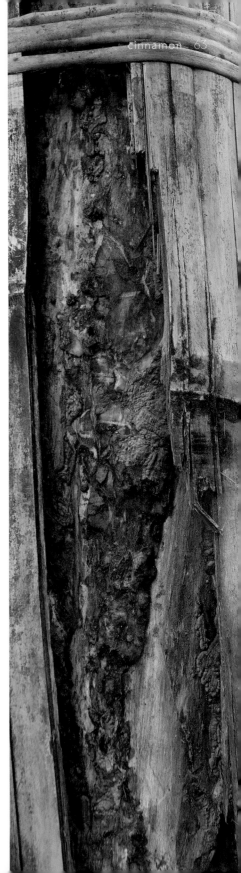

HOW TO USE CINNAMON

The easiest way to take cinnamon is in your food! While most of us are familiar with using cinnamon in sweet recipes, it also goes well in savory dishes such as chili, or on meats. Cinnamon makes a great tea and is commonly added to tea blends. While not native to Mexico, this country has popularized mixing chocolate with cinnamon, which is commonly called Mexican chocolate.

When I make desserts that call for cinnamon, I often triple or quadruple the amount called for in the recipe to get the most benefits from cinnamon while still having a delicious treat.

RECOMMENDED AMOUNTS

Cinnamon can be enjoyed in small amounts in order to flavor food or sweets. The therapeutic amount for cinnamon is 1 to 6 grams per day.

SPECIAL CONSIDERATIONS

Cinnamon shouldn't be taken in large amounts during pregnancy.

Cinnamon can also significantly lower blood glucose levels. While this can be a positive side effect, people with type 2 diabetes should monitor their insulin levels closely if they wish to take this herb regularly.

Cinnamon is an effective blood thinner. It is not advised to take therapeutic doses (i.e., more than common culinary amounts) of cinnamon when taking pharmaceutical blood thinners.

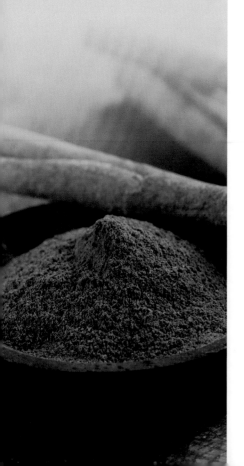

2 tablespoons cinnamon powder

1 teaspoon activated charcoal

1 teaspoon licorice root powder

CINNAMON TOOTH POWDER

Brushing your teeth with powdered herbs may sound strange, but this was common long before we had toothpaste. The powder will not foam, but it will make your teeth feel clean and smooth while supporting the health of your gums. Avoid getting drops of water into your powder, as adding moisture may shorten its shelf life.

Yield: 2½ tablespoons, which should last a couple of months with regular use

1. Blend all the ingredients together and store in a small container with a lid. For best results, discard whatever you don't use within 6 months and make another batch with fresh ingredients.

2. *To use:* Wet your toothbrush. Then, using a small spoon, heap a small mound of powder onto the toothbrush. (I do this over the small container holding the powder so that I can catch any falling powder.) Lightly brush your teeth as you would with a toothpaste.

CINNAMON TEA FOR SOOTHING THROATS

This recipe was inspired by one of my favorite bagged teas, Throat Coat by Traditional Medicinals. There were many years I was never without a box; I thought there was nothing better for soothing a sore throat. Now, I keep these ingredients on hand for a similar-tasting but stronger brew that is also cheaper to make. I use it whenever I have a painful throat, whether from an illness or from a long day of teaching. I recommend making up a large batch and keeping it in a thermos. That way you can sip it hot throughout the day.

This tea contains slippery elm bark, and populations of this tree have been challenged by disease and habitat loss. Buy only sustainably harvested slippery elm bark, and if you can't find an ethical source for slippery elm, then omit it from the recipe and increase the marshmallow root. Because many of the herbs in this recipe are oddly shaped, it's best to measure these by weight rather than volume.

Yield: approximately 1½ cups (1 serving)

---

1. Simmer all the ingredients with 3 cups of water for 20 minutes. Strain off the herbs. Add honey if desired.

2. Sip as needed throughout the day. Drink within 36 hours.

10 grams dried slippery elm bark

10 grams dried marshmallow root

8 grams dried cinnamon chips (or 1½ whole cinnamon quills broken into small pieces)

5 grams dried orange peel*

3 whole cloves

honey, to taste (optional)

*Store-bought dried orange peel comes in small, uniform pieces. If you make your own, be sure to mince the orange peels finely before drying them, as they are difficult to cut once dried.

CHIA SEED PUDDING WITH CINNAMON-MAPLE SYRUP

For the pudding:

⅓ cup chia seeds

1 (13.5-oz.) can coconut milk

⅞ cup plain yogurt

For the syrup:

2 tablespoons butter or coconut oil

1 teaspoon cinnamon powder

¼ teaspoon ground cardamom

¼ cup maple syrup

Chia seeds are nutritious seeds that thicken when soaked in liquid, creating a pudding similar to tapioca. I love this as a simple dessert. It also makes a great breakfast, especially topped with fresh fruit. It may seem strange to put the syrup in the bottom of the glass, but as you pour the chia seeds on top, the syrup naturally folds in throughout the glass.

Yield: 4 cups, or 4 servings

1.   *To make the pudding:* Mix together the chia seeds, coconut milk, yogurt, and ⅞ cup water in a medium-size glass container with a lid. (When measuring out the yogurt and water, you can actually use the empty coconut milk can. Just measure out ½ can of each.)

2.   Let sit, covered, in the fridge for 3 to 5 hours or overnight. When done it should have a thick, puddinglike consistency.

3.   Store in the fridge and eat within 48 hours.

4.   *To make the syrup:* Melt the butter or oil in a small saucepan. Add the cinnamon and cardamom and blend. Add the maple syrup and stir to blend.

5.   Pour equal amounts of syrup into four small jars or cups. Fill the cups with chia seed pudding (the syrup will naturally layer as you add the pudding) and enjoy.

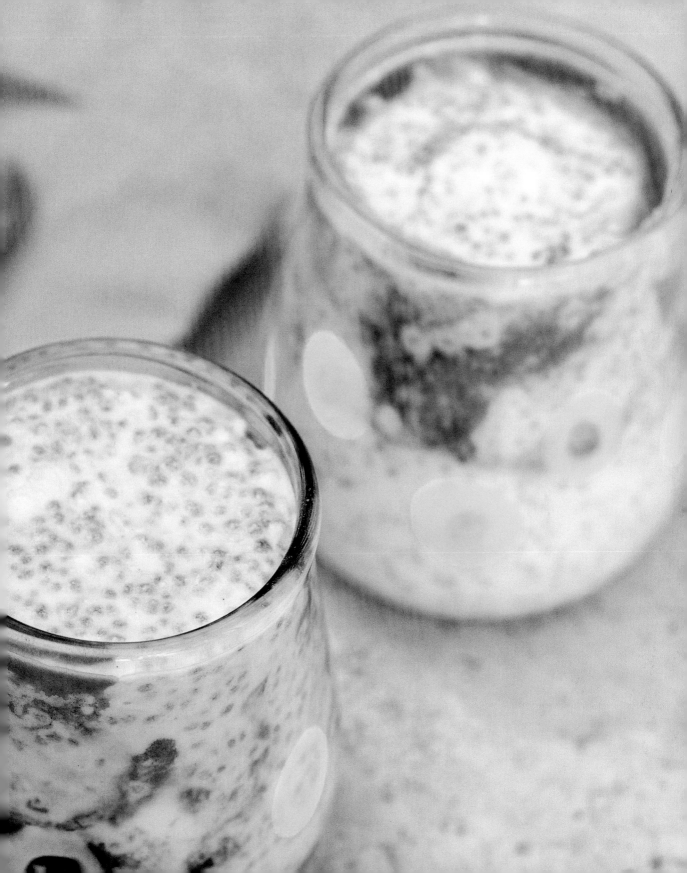

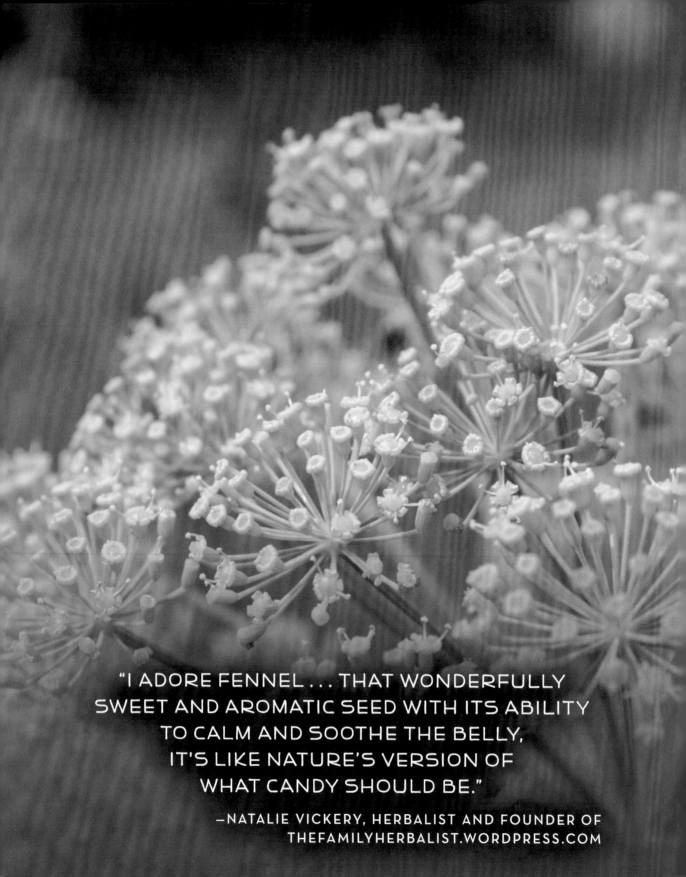

"I ADORE FENNEL . . . THAT WONDERFULLY
SWEET AND AROMATIC SEED WITH ITS ABILITY
TO CALM AND SOOTHE THE BELLY,
IT'S LIKE NATURE'S VERSION OF
WHAT CANDY SHOULD BE."

—NATALIE VICKERY, HERBALIST AND FOUNDER OF
THEFAMILYHERBALIST.WORDPRESS.COM

CHAPTER 8

Fennel

Fennel is an old-world plant that now grows in warm climates across the world. The bulb is a crisp, delicious food, and the seeds have potent aromatic qualities that help to relieve digestive problems, muscle tension, and pain. Both the seeds and the bulb have a mild licorice taste. Fennel is effective and safe for children with colic, for young women with menstrual pain, and for nursing mothers. You can simply chew on the seeds after meals to enjoy better digestion and fresh breath.

Botanical name: *Foeniculum vulgare*

Family: Apiaceae

Parts used: seeds, bulb

Energetics: warming, drying

Taste: pungent

Plant properties: aromatic, carminative, antispasmodic, galactagogue

Plant uses: poor digestion, digestive spasms, menstrual cramps, infantile colic, low lactation

Plant preparations: tea, tincture, syrup, culinary

Fennel originally comes from the Mediterranean, but is now naturalized all around the world, especially in dry soils near a seacoast. Wherever it has grown, it has been widely used as both food and medicine. There is evidence it was used by both the ancient Greeks and the Romans. In her book *Physica*, written in the 12th century, Hildegard von Bingen wrote, "Eating fennel or its seed every day diminishes bad phlegm and decaying matter, keeps bad breath in check, and makes one's eyes see clearly."[1]

MEDICINAL PROPERTIES AND ENERGETICS OF FENNEL

Herbalists attribute many of fennel's abilities to its aromatic qualities, which come from its volatile oil content. Volatile oils are what give plants their strong and aromatic smells. Before we had the ability to recognize individual chemical constituents, people understood herbal qualities through their senses. Aromatic herbs (besides fennel, these include mint, thyme, and basil) have a stimulating quality, which is often used to break up digestive stagnation.

As an antispasmodic herb, fennel is known mainly for soothing muscle tension, digestive spasms, and menstrual cramps; however, it has a variety of other uses as well. It's a mild galactagogue, helping nursing mothers produce more milk. It has been used to support eye health for many centuries, and herbalist David Hoffmann recommends a compress of fennel infusion for conjunctivitis and inflammation of the eyelids.[2] It is also a mild diuretic and can be used in combination with other herbs for edema and urinary tract infections. Fennel is a mild expectorant that can be used in herbal cough formulas.

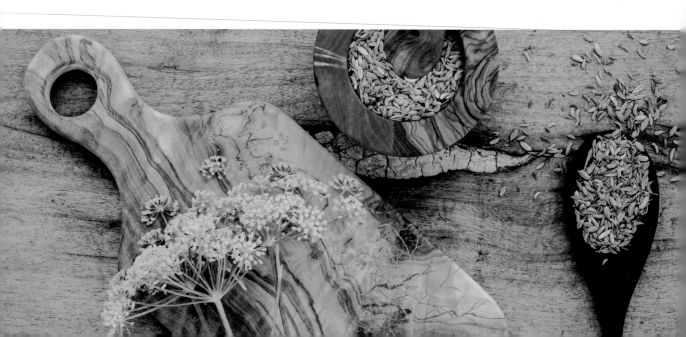

FOR DIGESTIVE ISSUES

Fennel is a favorite herb for a wide range of digestive problems. Feeling queasy after a meal? Try fennel. Having digestive spasms associated with diarrhea? Try fennel. Do you have gas and bloating? Fennel reduces gas and flatulence. It is frequently added to formulas for people with irritable bowel syndrome as it can ease both diarrhea and constipation symptoms. As an antispasmodic, it can relieve gut pain due to intestinal spasms (e.g., cramping associated with diarrhea or gas).

But you don't need to wait until a digestive complaint arises to get benefits from fennel. Chewing fennel seeds after a meal helps to support good digestion and leaves a nice, fresh taste in your mouth.

FOR MENSTRUAL CRAMPING AND FATIGUE

Several clinical trials have shown fennel's effectiveness at reducing cramping and fatigue associated with menstruation. In one study, researchers compared using a fennel extract with using nonsteroidal anti-inflammatory drugs (NSAIDs). Young women were divided into two groups, with one group taking the fennel and the other taking the NSAIDs. After two consecutive menstrual cycles, those taking the fennel had slightly better improvement than those taking the NSAIDs.[3] It's important to note that not only is fennel as effective as the over-the-counter drugs but also it has a far better safety rating than NSAIDs.

FOR COLIC

Colic affects roughly 20 percent of babies and is diagnosed in otherwise healthy babies who cry for more than three hours a day, for more than three days a week, for more than three weeks.[4] Having a baby with colic can be excruciating for parents, who often feel helpless trying to console their distressed little one.

I often wish more families knew about fennel! It is a powerful gift for distressed, colicky babies as well as their parents. This old-time remedy has been used by herbalists, midwives, wise women, and mothers for centuries. Researchers, no doubt impressed with its traditional use, have studied fennel for colicky babies with excellent results.

One study used a fennel seed oil emulsion in babies who were diagnosed with colic. Colic was completely eliminated in 65 percent of the babies receiving the fennel, as compared with 23 percent of the placebo group. There were no side effects in either group, which further validates fennel as being both effective and safe.[5] Another study for babies with colic used an herbal combination of fennel, chamomile, and lemon balm. In this study, 85 percent of the babies receiving the herbal formula cried for an average of 2 hours less per day, while those not receiving the herbal blend saw an average decrease of 28.8 minutes of crying per day.[6]

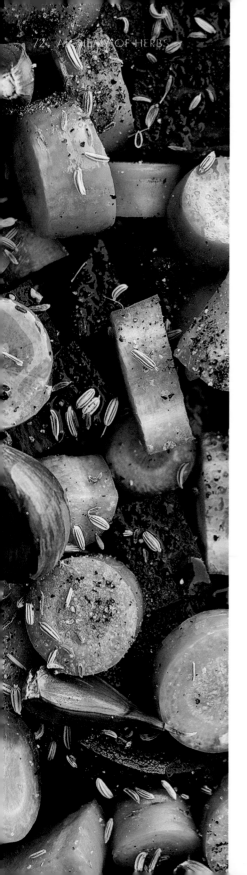

HOW TO USE FENNEL

Fresh fennel bulbs are delicious and a good source of vitamin C.[7] Try adding them raw to salads, or grill them whole.

Fennel seeds have more volatile oils and are considered a more potent herbal remedy than the bulb. Look for light-green seeds that have a slight licorice taste when chewed. Fennel seeds can be eaten whole; powdered for use in cooking; or made into tinctures, teas, syrups, and compresses.

RECOMMENDED AMOUNTS

Fennel seed powder or the whole seeds can be enjoyed as a way to flavor food and generally improve digestion.

The therapeutic amount for different fennel preparations is:

As tea or powder: 1 to 2 grams, 3 times per day

As tincture (dried seeds): 1:3, 60% alcohol, 3 to 6 mL per day

SPECIAL CONSIDERATIONS

Allergic reactions to fennel are rare but have been reported.

ROASTED ROOT VEGETABLES WITH FENNEL

This simple recipe is one of my and my husband's favorites. We do our best to eat locally grown vegetables all year round, so in the fall we buy bulk amounts of keeper root vegetables like beets and carrots and store them in our cellar to enjoy during the snowy winter months. These sweet veggies are enhanced by the aromatics and flavor of fennel.

We love this dish drizzled with high-quality or aged balsamic vinegar. You can peel the carrots and beets if you like, but we never do. The garlic roasts up tender and sweet within its skin; simply remember to remove the skin before eating.

Yield: 6 servings

4 cups cubed beets
  (1-inch cubes)

4 cups cut carrots
  (1-inch half rounds)

1 bulb garlic split into cloves,
  skin on

1 teaspoon fennel seeds
  (2 grams)

¼ teaspoon pepper

½ teaspoon salt

¼ cup olive oil

2 tablespoons balsamic
  vinegar

1. Preheat the oven to 350°F. Combine all the ingredients except the balsamic vinegar in a 13 x 9-inch baking pan and stir well.

2. Place the pan in the oven and bake for 60 minutes, or until the beets and carrots are tender. Stir the vegetables every 20 minutes.

3. Remove the vegetables from the oven and drizzle with balsamic vinegar.

4. Serve warm, and eat leftovers within 3 days.

BITTER FENNEL DIGESTIVE PASTILLES

For the pastilles:

1 teaspoon angelica root powder (*Angelica archangelica*)

1 teaspoon coriander powder

½ teaspoon gentian root powder (*Gentiana lutea*)

½ teaspoon orange peel powder

¼ teaspoon freshly ground black pepper

about 2 teaspoons honey

For the coating:

2 teaspoons fennel seed powder* (6 grams)

¼ teaspoon fine sea salt

*Fennel seeds can be purchased whole or already powdered. If you have whole seeds, simply process them in your spice grinder until you have a fine powder.

Eating something bitter with meals is a tried-and-true way to strengthen and support digestion. While the bitter taste is highlighted in this recipe, the aromatic herbs and spices, along with the honey, temper it so it's more of a treat.

This recipe uses powdered herbs along with honey to form pastilles (a fancy French term for pills). I recommend eating one pastille 15 minutes before each meal.

Yield: approximately 20 pea-size balls

1. *To make the coating:* Combine the fennel seed powder and salt in a small bowl. Mix well and set aside.

2. *To make the pastilles:* In a separate bowl, combine the angelica root, coriander, gentian root, orange peel, and black pepper. Mix well.

3. Gently heat the honey in a small saucepan or double boiler. You don't want to cook the honey; just heat it up enough to give it a thinner, syrupy consistency. This will make it easier to mix with the herbs.

4. Little by little, pour the honey into the powdered herbal mixture while stirring. You'll have enough honey added when the mixture can be molded together without breaking apart.

5. Roll the mixture into pea-size balls. To keep it from sticking to your hands, try putting some of the fennel-and-salt coating on your hands.

6. Roll each pastille in the fennel powder and salt, then store them in an airtight container.

7. These will last for up to three months, but the fresher they are, the more potent the herbs will be.

FENNEL TEA

This tea is perfect for upset tummies, especially those caused by gas. I've also found it to be a great way to stop hiccups! Variations of this tea recipe have long been given to babies with colic, but do not use honey in children under the age of two, due to botulism risk. Adults can drink 2 to 3 servings of this daily. Small children may need only a teaspoon or less, diluted with a little water. Consult with an herbalist for specialized dosing suggestions for young children.

Yield: 1¼ cups (1 adult serving)

1 tablespoon fennel seeds (6 grams)

1 tablespoon dried lemon balm or 2 tablespoons fresh lemon balm

honey, to taste (optional)

1. Bring 1¼ cups of water to a boil. Place the fennel and lemon balm in a mug or large tea infuser. Avoid cramming the herbs into a small infuser; it's better for them to have room to expand and move around.

2. Pour the just-boiled water over the herbs and let the mixture steep, covered, for 5 minutes.

3. Strain, then add honey to taste if desired.

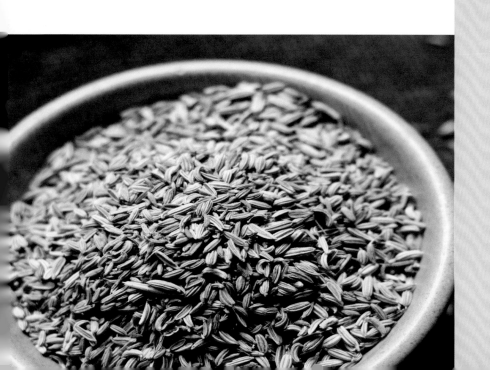

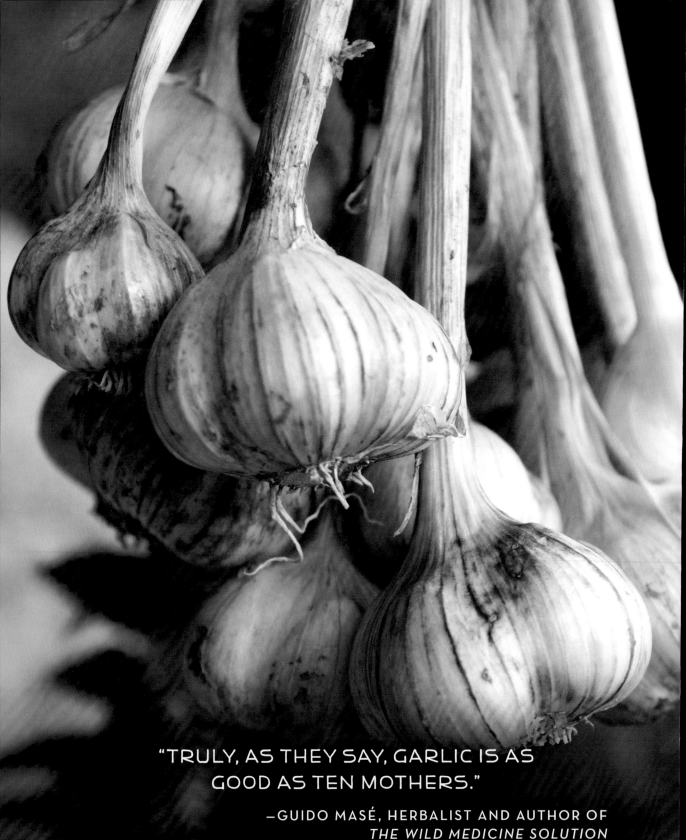

"TRULY, AS THEY SAY, GARLIC IS AS GOOD AS TEN MOTHERS."

—GUIDO MASÉ, HERBALIST AND AUTHOR OF
THE WILD MEDICINE SOLUTION

CHAPTER 9

Garlic

There are few herbs that are as loved or as notorious as garlic. It is renowned worldwide for its healing abilities yet commonly maligned for its strong smell and flavor. Its aromatics are so pungent that it even reputably keeps vampires at bay!

Do you love to eat garlic? If so, you'll know that shortly after enjoying a clove or two your breath and even your skin may reek of garlic. This infamous effect has given garlic the nickname "stinking rose." As you'll see, its permeating effect is an important part of its medicine.

Botanical name: *Allium sativum*

Family: Alliaceae

Parts used: bulb, green scapes (the flower stalks from garlic plants)

Energetics: warming, drying

Taste: pungent

Plant properties: circulatory stimulant, alterative, stimulating diaphoretic, stimulating expectorant, antimicrobial, carminative, immune modulating, vermifuge

Plant uses: hypertension, fungal infections, bacterial infections, optimizing cholesterol levels, colds, flu, bronchial congestion, small intestinal bacteria overgrowth, digestion, asthma, dysentery, plague, cancer, parasites, type 2 diabetes, insulin resistance

Plant preparations: food, oil, vinegar, honey

While Italian cuisine has made garlic famous, it has been cultivated across the globe for thousands of years. The first cultivated garlic is believed to have appeared in central Asia, and was then spread worldwide.

As a medicinal herb, garlic has rarely fallen out of favor. Historically it was used as a panacea for many types of illnesses, including the bubonic plague. Today it is heralded for its ability to support digestion, the immune system, and the heart.

TYPES OF GARLIC

Practically any garlic at the grocery store will work well, but it's important to note that many of the purely white-skinned garlic bulbs sold in the produce section could have been bleached or sprayed with harmful chemicals. You will be most impressed with the heirloom varieties that are emerging all over the United States at health-food stores and farmer's markets. Artisanal garlic farmers are growing a variety of tasty and more powerfully medicinal varieties. Garlic can have as many taste variations as fine wines!

MEDICINAL PROPERTIES AND ENERGETICS OF GARLIC

Garlic bread. Garlic and tomato pasta. Pesto or hummus with lots of garlic. Garlic potatoes. Garlic chicken. Roasted garlic. Aioli. What can't we do with garlic? Not only does it taste delicious in our meals, but it is also a favorite carminative herb. Carminative herbs help with stagnant digestion, which can include bloating, painful stuck gas, a sensation of food sitting heavy in your stomach, and constipation.

Garlic also contains inulin, an important prebiotic. Prebiotics are starchy substances that feed the healthy gut flora of your large intestine. Having a disrupted gut flora has been linked to many health problems, including digestive complaints (especially inflammatory bowel disease), autoimmune conditions, hormone imbalances, and weight gain—and garlic can play a helpful role in relieving these conditions.

Have you ever wondered why the smell of garlic lingers on your breath long after you've eaten it? It turns out that garlic's ability to permeate someone with its scent is an important part of its medicine. Upon being crushed, garlic produces a constituent called allicin. When you eat garlic, your body metabolizes the allicin into several other compounds, and the only way to fully metabolize and eliminate them is through your bloodstream, which releases them through your sweat and through the lungs. It's brilliant, really!

You don't even have to eat garlic to get this effect. This same process can happen when you simply apply garlic-infused oil to your feet. (I offer a recipe for Garlic Oil in this chapter.)

FOR IMMUNE SYSTEM SUPPORT

Garlic has long been heralded as a medicinal herb for infections. It was used during the 1600s against the plague in Europe. Paul Bergner describes its use in the 20th century in his book *The Healing Power of Garlic*: "During World War I, garlic poultices were used for the wounds of soldiers in Europe ... Garlic oil was diluted with water, put on swabs of sterilized moss, and applied directly to the wounds. The lives and limbs of tens of thousands of soldiers were saved in this way."[1] Practically every herbal text in the Western world includes references to garlic's antimicrobial properties, and science has been validating garlic's effects against infections.

Some people refer to garlic as an "herbal antibiotic," but when we look closely, this term doesn't quite fit. When there is an active infection, pharmaceutical antibiotics (literally translated, the word means "anti-life") indiscriminately wipe out bacteria in the body, thus effecting a cure. But that is not how garlic works.

While small to moderate amounts of garlic have been shown to inhibit many types of bacteria, viruses, and even amoebas, you'd have to take ridiculously large amounts of it to negatively affect your healthy gut flora. And garlic isn't something that simply kills other organisms; it also stimulates your immune system. Studies have shown that it increases the natural killer cells of the immune system, reduces inflammatory cytokines (chemical messengers of the immune system), and can decrease specific pathogens such as bacterial cells like streptococcus and fungi such as *Candida albicans*.[2,3,4,5]

Because garlic can support the immune system (and not just kill things), it has been shown to have a positive effect on patients with cancer. One study looked at people diagnosed with inoperable colorectal, liver, or pancreatic cancer. Half of the volunteers were given a placebo and the other half were given aged garlic extract. After six months, those receiving the garlic had increased immune system activity, including an increase in natural killer cells and an increase in natural killer cell activity.[6]

FOR COLDS AND THE FLU

Are you tired of getting every cold that comes around? One study compared a group of children taking long-releasing garlic extracts with another group of children taking a pharmaceutical drug in the hopes of preventing upper respiratory infections. Those taking the garlic had a two- to four-fold reduction in sickness compared with a control group taking a placebo. Incidentally, the pharmaceutical performed no better than the placebo.[7]

Already have a cold or flu? Garlic has been used for colds and the flu for centuries and remains a favorite of herbalists today. Garlic can stimulate the immune system to reduce the severity of the illness, break up lung congestion, and even address ear infections.[8]

It's important to take garlic's energetics into account when using it as an herbal remedy. If you've ever taken a bite of raw garlic, then it will come as no surprise to you that this is a hot herb. After taking that bite of raw garlic and noticing the heating sensation on your tongue, you might also notice your sinuses starting to run. Both garlic's heating and pungent aromatic properties break up mucus in the body. This makes garlic perfect for cold and flu symptoms that include feelings of coldness and for symptoms of congestion in the sinuses and lungs.

FOR HEART HEALTH AND TYPE 2 DIABETES

While garlic has historically been famous for treating infections, these days it often makes the headlines for its numerous positive effects on heart health. Garlic has been shown to lower high blood pressure in people with uncontrolled hypertension.[9,10] You know the common saying that an apple a day keeps the doctor away? I suggest trying a few cloves of garlic a day instead.

One interesting study looked at the effects of garlic on people diagnosed with type 2 diabetes. Both the control and experimental groups were also taking metformin, which is standard antidiabetic therapy. After 24 weeks, those receiving the garlic not only had decreased fasting blood sugar but also showed significant improvement in their levels of cholesterol and triglycerides.[11]

HOW TO USE GARLIC

David Hoffmann, in *Medical Herbalism*, writes: "Used daily, garlic aids and supports the body in ways that no other herb can match."[12]

My husband and I enjoy using a lot of garlic! Every fall we head to the farm of our friends, the Channings, who specialize in growing heritage varieties of garlic. We buy enough braids of garlic to last through the winter, spring, and summer months. We add minced garlic to many of our meals and also use it to make fire cider and garlic honey, two of our favorite remedies for the cold and flu season. (You'll find a recipe for Garlic Honey included in this chapter, and a recipe for Fire Cider on page 56.) Every time I hang our winter supply of garlic braids in the kitchen, I feel grateful and blessed to have such an abundant amount of food and medicine locked up in these cloves. It's so satisfying to know that by simply eating this deliciously pungent herb every day we are dramatically supporting our heart health and our immune system.

When using garlic as an antimicrobial or for cold and flu symptoms, it's best to use fresh, raw garlic. To get the most potency, crush a garlic clove and let it sit for 10 to 15 minutes. Then continue to make it into your desired remedy.

When enjoying garlic to support heart health, you can cook the cloves into meals and still reap the benefits. Cooking also transforms the garlic and decreases some of its heat, making it easier to consume in larger quantities.

Many scientific studies are done using dried and powdered garlic. While these have been shown to have benefits, I recommend using fresh garlic in your kitchen.

RECOMMENDED AMOUNTS

Eating 1 to 2 garlic cloves a day can be a delicious way to get many health benefits from this herb. If using garlic to break up congestion in the lungs or to alleviate the symptoms of a cold or flu, then eating it frequently throughout the day will give the best results. I recommend eating it with other food, especially oils, to avoid nausea.

SPECIAL CONSIDERATIONS

Eating 1 to 2 entire bulbs (not cloves) of garlic for long periods of time has been shown to cause harmful effects such as anemia and bowel flora disruption.

Because garlic is so extreme energetically (it's really hot!), it can readily cause unwanted effects in people who already have signs of heat or dryness. It can lead to nausea, digestive upset, heartburn, or even vomiting when consumed in excess. However, cooking garlic can alleviate these effects.

Eating fresh parsley after consuming garlic may help to decrease the odor of garlic on the breath.

You may commonly see warnings about garlic's effect on thinning blood. These warnings come from in vitro studies (petri dish studies as opposed to human studies). However, several in vivo studies (those done in humans) have shown that dietary garlic does not overly thin the blood and therefore may not be a concern for postoperative patients or for those taking warfarin.[13,14,15] If you are taking any pharmaceuticals or medications that thin the blood (including aspirin, nonsteroidal anti-inflammatories, coagulants, and antiplatelets), please consult your doctor.

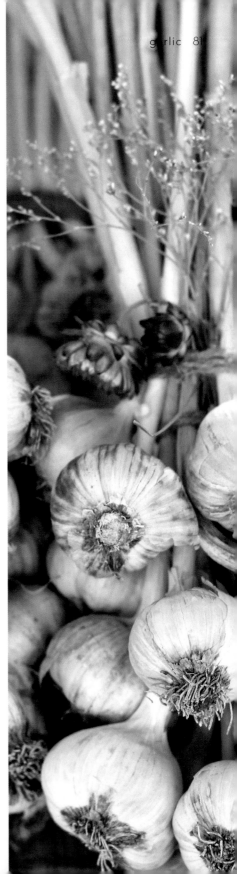

SMOKY GARLIC HUMMUS

1 (15-oz.) can chickpeas

½ cup tahini

¼ cup extra-virgin olive oil, plus extra for drizzling

4 garlic cloves, mashed and minced

2 teaspoons cumin powder

2 teaspoons fresh lemon zest

3 tablespoons fresh lemon juice

1 teaspoon smoked (or regular) paprika powder, plus extra for sprinkling

salt and freshly ground black pepper, to taste

This is my go-to recipe for a quick snack that I can bring to the lake on a hot summer's day or a last-minute appetizer for a potluck. It's easy to whip up and full of flavor. I like to serve it with veggies like carrots, cucumbers, snap peas, and celery sticks. It also goes well with bread or crackers.

Yield: 2½ cups

1. Drain the chickpeas and reserve the liquid. Place all ingredients except the reserved chickpea liquid in a food processor. With the food processor running, slowly add the reserved chickpea liquid until the mixture is smooth.

2. Serve with olive oil drizzled on top and a sprinkling of paprika powder. Store in the fridge and eat within several days.

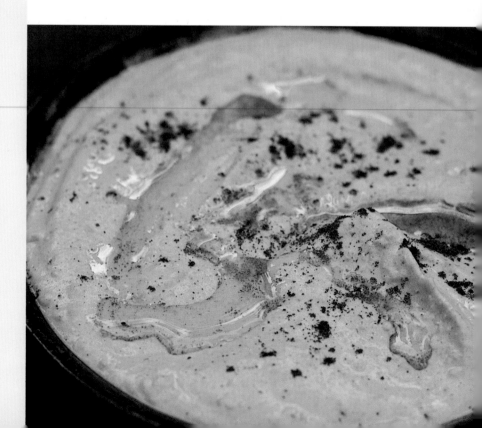

GARLIC OIL

Massaging garlic oil into your feet can be a powerful way to break through congestion in the lungs and sinuses. If putting something on your feet for lung congestion sounds strange, give it a try! You'll notice that within moments, you have garlic breath. As the garlic goes through the bloodstream and then out through the lungs, it will bring its stimulating expectorant and antimicrobial properties right where it is needed most. (You can also place this on your chest, but it will be a lot messier.)

I love this recipe because most folks have garlic in their home. Since this is a topical application, it's great for the younger, pickier crowd, who may not be excited about having to taste herbal remedies!

Caution: Do not eat this garlic oil! There is a risk of botulism when combining fresh garlic and olive oil.

Yield: 1 application

2 to 3 garlic cloves

1 to 2 tablespoons olive oil

1. Peel and finely mince the garlic. Let it stand for 10 minutes.

2. Place the garlic in a small jar. Barely cover the garlic with olive oil.

3. Let this infuse for a minimum of 30 minutes, up to 12 hours. Strain really well.

4. *To use:* Just before bedtime, rub the oil onto the feet. Immediately cover the feet with an old pair of socks, and then another pair of socks. Wear this throughout the night. Repeat as necessary, making a fresh batch of oil for each application.

GARLIC HONEY

½ cup fresh minced garlic
(approximately 15 cloves)

½ cup honey*

* If your honey is thick, you may need to heat it slightly in a double boiler or over very low heat until it is the consistency of a thin syrup, which will be easier to stir into the garlic.

Combining the sweet flavor of honey with the spicy, pungent flavor of garlic may seem like an unlikely combination, but it is surprisingly tasty. The honey also mellows out the raw heat of the garlic, allowing you to enjoy it in larger amounts without getting adverse effects. My favorite way to use it is for a sore throat: take a teaspoon of it every 1 to 2 hours.

This preparation will keep for years. I store my garlic honey on the counter and haven't had any problems with it. I've heard reports from some folks whose mixture fermented with time. If this happens, it's still okay to eat, but if you want to avoid this, store your honey in the fridge.

Over time, the garlic may become rubbery or tough. If this happens you can strain out the garlic and use the remaining honey. For best results I recommend making this in small batches so that you can always have a fresh and potent preparation on hand.

Yield: 1 cup

1. Place the garlic in an 8-ounce glass jar. (Tip: After mincing the garlic, let it stand for 10 to 15 minutes to allow it to react with oxygen and become even stronger medicine.)

2. Put half of the honey in the jar. Stir well, then add the rest of the honey to the jar. The jar should now be filled to the top with the honey and garlic mixture. Add more honey, if necessary, to reach the top. Stir the garlic and honey well, and then put a lid on it.

3. Let the mixture rest in the fridge or on the counter for 24 hours before using. There is no need to strain the garlic from the honey. As time goes on, the flavors of the garlic will infuse the honey even more, but you'll notice that the honey has become thin and taken on the taste of the garlic after only a day.

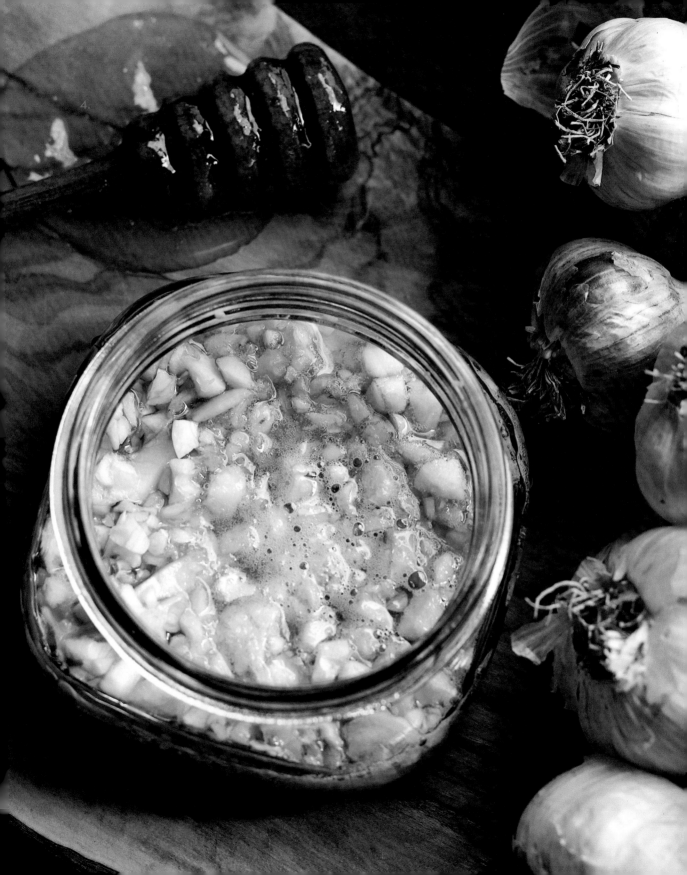

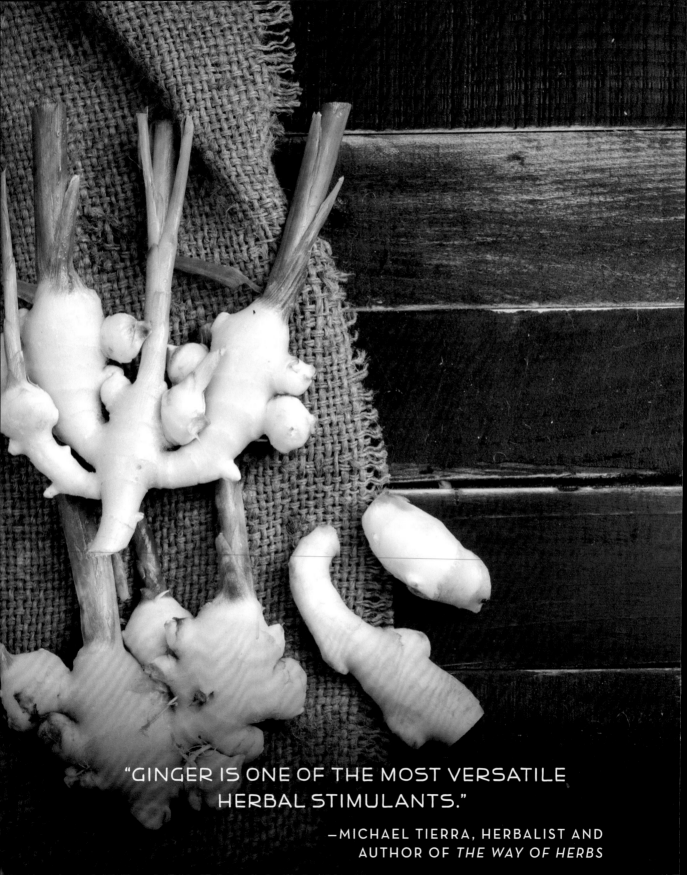

"GINGER IS ONE OF THE MOST VERSATILE
HERBAL STIMULANTS."

—MICHAEL TIERRA, HERBALIST AND
AUTHOR OF *THE WAY OF HERBS*

CHAPTER 10

Ginger

Ayurveda reveres ginger so highly it is referred to as the "universal medicine." It has been used for centuries and is still one of the most popular herbs of our time. It has been widely studied by scientists with positive results for a variety of issues, making it one of the more accepted herbs in Western medicine.

Ginger can be used in an astonishing variety of ways. Because of its heating and drying qualities, it is best used in people with signs of coldness and dampness. Ginger especially affects the respiratory system, digestive system, and circulatory system. It is a powerful anti-inflammatory shown to decrease pain in those with chronic inflammatory pain such as arthritis.

Other common names: gingerroot

Botanical name: *Zingiber officinale*

Family: Zingiberaceae

Parts used: rhizome (commonly called a root)

Energetics: fresh rhizome (warming, drying), dried rhizome (hot, drying)

Taste: pungent

Plant properties: aromatic, anti-inflammatory, diffusive, stimulating diaphoretic, stimulating expectorant, carminative, analgesic, antimicrobial, blood moving, vermifuge, rubefacient

Plant uses: arthritis, migraines, colds and flu, nausea, dysbiosis, menstrual cramps (due to stagnation), ear infections, heart health, inflammation, stomach bugs

Plant preparations: culinary, decoction, powder, tincture, candied, fresh juice

Ginger has been used in Southeast Asia for well over 5,000 years, long before humans were providing written accounts of it. It no longer grows in the wild but is highly cultivated in tropical regions all over the world. As a result, we aren't sure where exactly it originated. The most commonly used part of ginger is the rhizome, or root.

Ginger played an important role in the spice trade between Southeast Asia and Europe. It traveled from India to the Roman Empire more than 2,000 years ago. It's recorded that in the 13th and 14th centuries, a pound of ginger had the same value as an entire sheep.[1] Today, ginger is commonly available as a fresh root, dried and powdered, and candied.

MEDICINAL PROPERTIES AND ENERGETICS OF GINGER

Ginger is used in many ways by herbalists today. But, as I keep reminding you, it really works best when you match ginger to the person. When we move away from thinking of herbs as a simple substitute for pharmaceuticals and toward a clearer understanding of the energetics of herbs, we can better match the herbs to the person, making them more effective.

Hopefully by now you've done the simple tasting experience outlined in Chapter 3 of this book ("Exercise: How to Know How an Herb or Spice Affects You"). You'll know from that experience that ginger is a warm to hot herb with a tendency toward dryness. If you want to get really specific, fresh ginger is considered to be warm while dried ginger is considered to be hot.

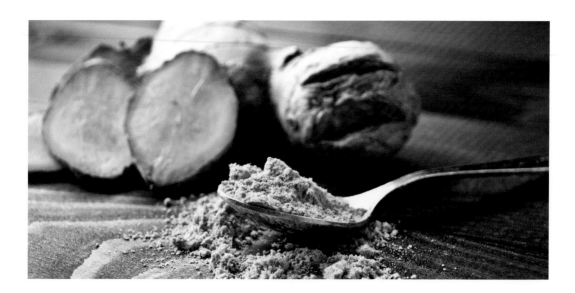

AS A STIMULANT AND SYNERGIST

Ginger is stimulating. When you hear the words *herbal stimulant*, you might immediately think of coffee and its jolt of caffeine. But "stimulant" in this sense means that it moves energy in the body through increasing circulation, promoting digestion, or increasing the flow of fluids in the body; and ginger does all of these.

Ginger is commonly added in small amounts to larger formulas. In fact, it is estimated that more than half of Chinese herbal formulas include ginger in them. This widespread use of ginger is because its stimulating properties make it a synergist, something that increases the potency of other herbs and pharmaceuticals. In his book *Herbal Antibiotics*, Stephen Harrod Buhner reports the way ginger does this: "It dilates blood vessels and increases circulation, helping the blood, and the constituents in the blood from other herbs, to achieve faster and more effective distribution in the body."[2]

MATCHING THE ENERGETICS OF GINGER

Ginger can help to relieve various types of pain, such as the cramping experienced with diarrhea or with menstruation.[3] However, using herbs for pain is not like using over-the-counter medications. Instead, herbs we use for pain have very specific mechanisms of action, and we have to carefully choose which herb to use for a specific type of pain. For example, if there is pain due to muscle tension, we use an antispasmodic herb like fennel or chamomile.

Ginger works especially well for people with signs of coldness. These people may have a pale face or tongue and typically feel colder than others. They may have slow digestion or problems with bloating, and tend toward lethargy or slowness. If someone is in pain and has several of these symptoms, consider ginger.

FOR REDUCING INFLAMMATORY PAIN

One way that ginger relieves pain is through its anti-inflammatory actions. Numerous studies have shown ginger to be effective and safe at relieving pain from osteoarthritis and rheumatoid arthritis both through topical application and internal use. [4,5,6]

FOR MOVING STAGNANT BLOOD

Ginger can be applied topically to relieve blood stagnation. In Traditional Chinese Medicine, pain that is fixed or stabbing is often seen as a symptom of stagnant blood. (A bruise or contusion is an example of stagnant blood that we can easily see.)

Ginger can also be used to treat what herbalists see as stagnant blood in the pelvis, symptoms of which include painful menstruation, delayed menstruation, clots, and fibroids. In this sense, ginger works exceptionally well for menstrual pain with signs of stagnancy and coldness.

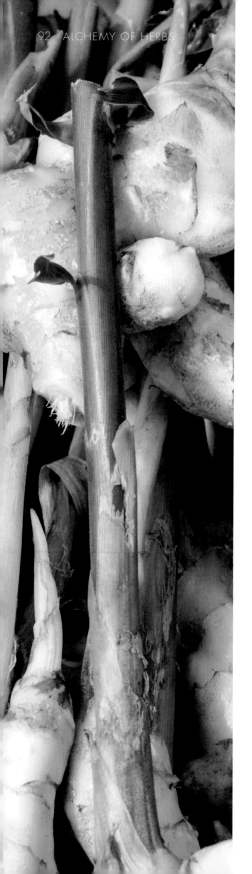

HOW TO USE GINGER

The most common usage of ginger is in cooking, with small amounts being used in both savory and sweet dishes. It is very aromatic with a strong, spicy taste. Fresh ginger, candied ginger, and dried ginger are readily found in grocery stores.

If using dried ginger, be sure to get it from a good source. Dried ginger should be zesty and hot. If it isn't, it may be too old.

When picking out ginger at the store, look for plump pieces with smooth skin. If the ginger looks dried out or has a wrinkly skin, you might look for a fresher choice; however, even when not in ideal condition it's still likely to work. Fresh roots do not need to be peeled, but if you prefer to do so, use a spoon to gently scrape away the thin outer coat.

When treating conditions such as infections or upper respiratory viruses, fresh ginger is preferred to dried ginger.

RECOMMENDED AMOUNTS

Ginger is a delicious culinary spice that can be added in small amounts to both savory and sweet dishes.

The therapeutic amount for ginger is:

Fresh root: 1 to 15 grams per day

Dried root: 3 to 12 grams per day

As tincture (fresh root): 1:2, 60% alcohol, 1 to 2 mL in water, 3 times per day[23]

SPECIAL CONSIDERATIONS

Ginger is very warming and somewhat drying and is therefore not a good match with someone already showing signs of heat and/or dryness.

It should not be used in large amounts during pregnancy.

Patients taking blood-thinning medication should consult with their doctor before taking large amounts of ginger regularly.[24]

GINGER-LEMON TEA

If you could have only one herb on hand for colds and the flu, you couldn't go wrong with ginger. Ginger can relieve a sore throat, decrease aches and pains, clear congestion, warm you up when you feel chilled, shorten the duration of a cold or flu, and ease nausea. It is also a wonderful herb for people with cold digestion or who frequently feel cold. This classic tea can be enjoyed daily.

Yield: 1 cup

1 tablespoon grated or finely minced fresh ginger (6 grams)

squirt of lemon juice

honey, to taste

1. Place the fresh ginger in a mug with the lemon juice and honey.

2. Bring 1 cup of water to a boil, then pour over the ingredients in the mug. Cover and let steep for 15 minutes.

3. Drink while warm. (I like to keep the ginger in the tea and eat it, but you can strain before drinking, if desired.)

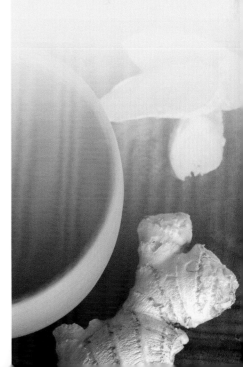

1½ pounds salmon, cut in
  1-inch cubes

1 lemon, thinly sliced into
  rounds

1 tablespoon chopped fresh
  parsley, for garnish

For the marinade:

3 tablespoons tamari
  (or soy sauce)

2 tablespoons minced
  fresh ginger

3 garlic cloves, minced

3 tablespoons olive oil

1 teaspoon chipotle powder

1 teaspoon coriander powder

½ teaspoon fennel powder

1 teaspoon turmeric powder

XAVIER'S GINGERED SALMON

In the Pacific Northwest, we are lucky to have easy access to fresh, wild-caught salmon. This is one of my favorite recipes, which was actually created by my husband (thanks for sharing, honey!). The spiciness of the ginger mixes well with the salty tamari and the other carminative spices.

Yield: 6 servings

1. *To make the marinade:* Combine all ingredients in a bowl.

2. Toss the salmon in the marinade, and let it sit covered in the fridge for 1 hour.

3. Preheat the oven to 350°F. Place the salmon in a 10 x 8-inch baking dish and cover with the lemon slices. Discard excess marinade.

4. Place the salmon in the oven and cook for 25 minutes, or until the fish is flaky. Garnish with parsley just before serving.

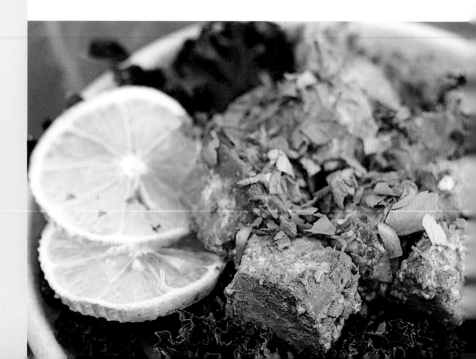

GINGER AND LAVENDER MASSAGE OIL

You can quickly whip up this oil to use on painful joints, an aching lower back, or wherever you want to increase circulation and decrease pain. You can use practically any type of oil. Olive oil is very stable but can have a greasy feel to it. Grape-seed, jojoba, apricot kernel, or almond oil are other possibilities that feel less greasy.

Yield: roughly ½ cup

¼ cup grated or finely minced fresh ginger (30 grams)

½ cup oil

10 to 15 drops lavender essential oil

1. Add the freshly grated ginger to a small jar. Pour the oil over the ginger and stir to combine. Let this sit for 12 to 24 hours.

2. Once the ginger is well infused into the oil, strain off the ginger. Add the lavender essential oil and stir.

3. The water in the fresh ginger will cause this mixture to eventually spoil, so for best results, store in the fridge and use within 1 to 2 weeks.

4. *To use:* Massage a generous amount of the oil into achy joints and sore muscles. Repeat as desired.

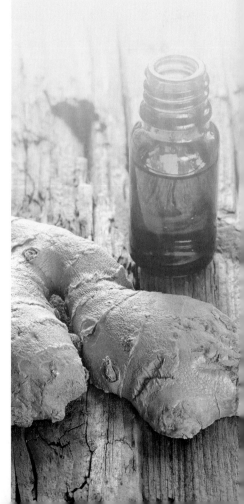

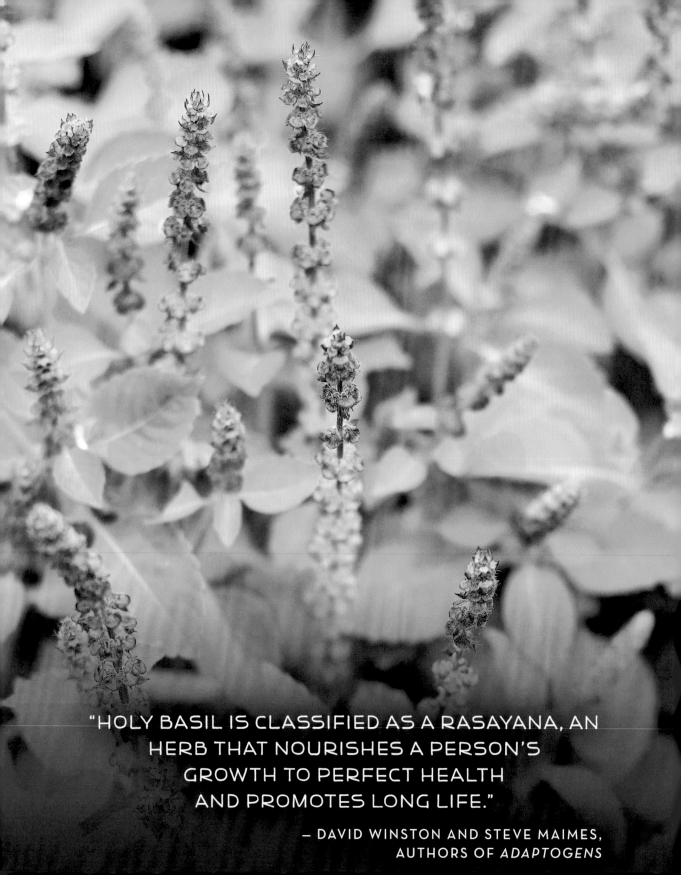

"HOLY BASIL IS CLASSIFIED AS A RASAYANA, AN HERB THAT NOURISHES A PERSON'S GROWTH TO PERFECT HEALTH AND PROMOTES LONG LIFE."

— DAVID WINSTON AND STEVE MAIMES,
AUTHORS OF *ADAPTOGENS*

Holy Basil

I often hear people say that they don't want to be taking herbs for the rest of their life. They equate the herbs with pharmaceutical drugs, thinking of them only as a tool to get healthy, then they can stop using them. However, in other systems of healing like Traditional Chinese Medicine and Ayurveda, specific herbs are taken for a lifetime to ensure vibrant health and longevity.

Holy basil is one of these herbs. It makes a delicious tea (which I include a recipe for in this chapter), and when enjoyed regularly it can have many health benefits including reducing stress and anxiety, regulating blood sugar, and supporting heart health.

Other common names: tulsi

Botanical name: *Ocimum sanctum* (syn. *Ocimum tenuiflorum*), *Ocimum gratissimum*

Family: Lamiaceae (mint family)

Parts used: leaves and flowers

Energetics: warming and drying

Taste: pungent, bitter

Plant properties: adaptogen, antimicrobial, aromatic digestive, relaxing nervine, cardiovascular tonic, expectorant, neuroprotective, antioxidant, immunomodulating, analgesic

Plant uses: stress, anxiety, high blood pressure, viral infections, fungal infections, pain, ulcers, depression, colds and flus, allergic rhinitis, herpes virus, type 2 diabetes, insulin resistance

Plant preparations: tea, decoction, tincture, fresh juice, poultice, powder, infusion in ghee or honey

FOR PAIN RELIEF

Holy basil has been shown to be a COX-2 inhibitor (many modern pain medications, such as Celebrex, are COX-2 inhibitors), making it useful against arthritis and other inflammatory conditions. Tulsi is high in eugenol, a constituent also found in cloves, which is helpful in decreasing pain.[7]

FOR DIGESTIVE ISSUES

Like our common culinary basil, holy basil has many positive effects on the digestive system. As a slightly warming and aromatic herb, it is often paired with dried ginger to relieve symptoms of stagnant digestion, such as bloating, gas, decreased appetite, and nausea. Herbalists also use tulsi for heartburn and to help heal ulcers.

FOR YOUR LUNGS

Herbalists use this herb for serious lung problems including bronchitis and pulmonary weakness. It can also be taken to both prevent and treat upper respiratory viruses, like the cold or flu.

Holy basil's expectorant qualities help move stuck mucus out of the lungs. Add some ginger and honey to holy basil tea to help soothe an irritated sore throat.

FOR IMMUNE SYSTEM SUPPORT

Holy basil helps to strengthen and modulate the immune system. Taken over time it can have a beneficial effect on asthma and can be helpful in alleviating allergic rhinitis symptoms like seasonal hay fever.

In one double-blind, placebo-controlled study, 22 healthy volunteers were given an extract of holy basil daily. After one month their test results showed significant improvements in several immune system parameters as compared to the placebo group.[8]

Two other studies looked at a tea that combined five common herbs from India: holy basil, ashwagandha, licorice, ginger, and cardamom. They gave this tea blend to volunteers aged 55 or older with a history of recurrent coughs or colds. The end results "indicate that regular consumption of the tea fortified with Ayurvedic herbs enhanced NK cell activity, which is an important aspect of the (early) innate immune response to infections."[9]

As an antimicrobial herb, holy basil can be used topically or internally to treat bacterial, viral, and fungal infections. It is frequently used for herpes sore outbreaks (viral infection) and can also be applied externally to fungal infections like ringworm.[10]

In vitro studies of holy basil show it to have anticancer properties.[11] Well-designed human clinical trials would give us more insight into the potential of its used in cancer patients.

Holy Basil

I often hear people say that they don't want to be taking herbs for the rest of their life. They equate the herbs with pharmaceutical drugs, thinking of them only as a tool to get healthy, then they can stop using them. However, in other systems of healing like Traditional Chinese Medicine and Ayurveda, specific herbs are taken for a lifetime to ensure vibrant health and longevity.

Holy basil is one of these herbs. It makes a delicious tea (which I include a recipe for in this chapter), and when enjoyed regularly it can have many health benefits including reducing stress and anxiety, regulating blood sugar, and supporting heart health.

Other common names: tulsi

Botanical name: *Ocimum sanctum* (syn. *Ocimum tenuiflorum*), *Ocimum gratissimum*

Family: Lamiaceae (mint family)

Parts used: leaves and flowers

Energetics: warming and drying

Taste: pungent, bitter

Plant properties: adaptogen, antimicrobial, aromatic digestive, relaxing nervine, cardiovascular tonic, expectorant, neuroprotective, antioxidant, immunomodulating, analgesic

Plant uses: stress, anxiety, high blood pressure, viral infections, fungal infections, pain, ulcers, depression, colds and flus, allergic rhinitis, herpes virus, type 2 diabetes, insulin resistance

Plant preparations: tea, decoction, tincture, fresh juice, poultice, powder, infusion in ghee or honey

For more than 3,000 years holy basil has been honored as one of India's most sacred and powerful plants. When you think about that, it's pretty astounding. One of the oldest and most sophisticated systems of medicine in the world, Ayurveda, reveres this plant. As you might imagine, a plant that enjoys such high esteem must be an amazing plant. This is yet another herb with powerful properties that will leave you asking, "What *can't* it do?"

Holy basil, sometimes referred to as tulsi, grows abundantly in India, western Asia, Malaysia, Central and South America, and even Puerto Rico. The name of one species, *sanctum*, refers to this sacredness. In Sanskrit, tulsi means "beyond compare." It is also referred to as an elixir of life, the queen of herbs, and Mother Nature of medicine.

TYPES OF HOLY BASIL

I'm often asked if the common culinary plant basil is the same as tulsi or holy basil, and the answer is no. While all the basils are aromatic in nature, our common culinary plant, *Ocimum basilicum*, is a different species and is not used in the same way as tulsi. There are more than 60 different species in the *Ocimum* genus.

There are at least three different types of holy basil, and while they can be used somewhat interchangeably, they also have slight differences.

Rama tulsi (*Ocimum sanctum*) has green leaves; it is the most commonly cultivated holy basil and the easiest to find for purchase.

Krishna tulsi (*Ocimum sanctum*) is the same species as Rama tulsi, but has leaves that are more purple in color.

Vana tulsi (*Ocimum gratissimum*) is a perennial basil that is hard to find for purchase. In India it grows in the wild.

MEDICINAL PROPERTIES AND ENERGETICS OF HOLY BASIL

Tulsi's main claim to fame in the Western world is its use as an adaptogen. Adaptogens are transformative herbs that, when taken daily, move a person toward health.[1] These are generally building and nourishing herbs.

FOR REDUCING STRESS AND ANXIETY

Holy basil is especially useful for our stressed population. It has been shown to reduce general anxiety and many symptoms associated with stress such as forgetfulness and sleep problems.

In a two-month study, 35 patients with anxiety were given 500 mg of holy basil twice daily after meals. Before, during, and after the study the patients were assessed clinically using standard questionnaires and different psychological rating scales. The final observations were that holy basil positively affected general anxiety levels as well as the stress and depression that accompany anxiety. The researchers concluded that "*O. sanctum* may be useful in the treatment of GAD [generalized anxiety disorder] in human[s] and may be a promising anxiolytic agent in near future."[2]

FOR YOUR BRAIN

Herbalist David Winston refers to holy basil as a cerebral stimulant and uses it for people with mental fog. He says, "It can be combined with other cerebral stimulants such as rosemary, bacopa, and ginkgo to help people with menopausal cloudy thinking, poor memory, attention deficit disorder (ADD), and attention deficit hyperactivity disorder (ADHD) and to speed up recovery from head trauma."[3]

In the book *The Way of Ayurvedic Herbs*, authors Karta Purkh Singh Khalsa and Michael Tierra elaborate: "Tulsi is considered to expand and sharpen awareness, aid meditation, and promote compassion when taken as a medicine."[4]

FOR INSULIN RESISTANCE AND TYPE 2 DIABETES

Numerous human clinical trials show that holy basil can decrease fasting blood glucose and blood glucose after a meal.[5] A one-month study of 27 patients with non-insulin-dependent type 2 diabetes showed a significant lowering of blood glucose and a significant reduction in total cholesterol, low-density lipoprotein-cholesterol, very low density lipoprotein-cholesterol, and triglycerides.[6]

Holy basil works so well that someone who is taking insulin to control diabetes might need to approach this herb with caution, and adjust insulin levels accordingly with the aid of a health care provider.

FOR CARDIOVASCULAR HEALTH

Holy basil has many beneficial actions on the heart. It is slightly blood thinning and promotes good circulation. Taken daily, it can help optimize cholesterol levels and lower stress-related high blood pressure.

The adaptogenic properties of tulsi can help mediate stress-related damage, which plays a significant role in overall cardiovascular health.

FOR PAIN RELIEF

Holy basil has been shown to be a COX-2 inhibitor (many modern pain medications, such as Celebrex, are COX-2 inhibitors), making it useful against arthritis and other inflammatory conditions. Tulsi is high in eugenol, a constituent also found in cloves, which is helpful in decreasing pain.[7]

FOR DIGESTIVE ISSUES

Like our common culinary basil, holy basil has many positive effects on the digestive system. As a slightly warming and aromatic herb, it is often paired with dried ginger to relieve symptoms of stagnant digestion, such as bloating, gas, decreased appetite, and nausea. Herbalists also use tulsi for heartburn and to help heal ulcers.

FOR YOUR LUNGS

Herbalists use this herb for serious lung problems including bronchitis and pulmonary weakness. It can also be taken to both prevent and treat upper respiratory viruses, like the cold or flu.

Holy basil's expectorant qualities help move stuck mucus out of the lungs. Add some ginger and honey to holy basil tea to help soothe an irritated sore throat.

FOR IMMUNE SYSTEM SUPPORT

Holy basil helps to strengthen and modulate the immune system. Taken over time it can have a beneficial effect on asthma and can be helpful in alleviating allergic rhinitis symptoms like seasonal hay fever.

In one double-blind, placebo-controlled study, 22 healthy volunteers were given an extract of holy basil daily. After one month their test results showed significant improvements in several immune system parameters as compared to the placebo group.[8]

Two other studies looked at a tea that combined five common herbs from India: holy basil, ashwagandha, licorice, ginger, and cardamom. They gave this tea blend to volunteers aged 55 or older with a history of recurrent coughs or colds. The end results "indicate that regular consumption of the tea fortified with Ayurvedic herbs enhanced NK cell activity, which is an important aspect of the (early) innate immune response to infections."[9]

As an antimicrobial herb, holy basil can be used topically or internally to treat bacterial, viral, and fungal infections. It is frequently used for herpes sore outbreaks (viral infection) and can also be applied externally to fungal infections like ringworm.[10]

In vitro studies of holy basil show it to have anticancer properties.[11] Well-designed human clinical trials would give us more insight into the potential of its used in cancer patients.

HOW TO USE HOLY BASIL

Herbalists often prefer to use fresh holy basil. However, the dried leaves can also make a lovely tea.

The most common way to prepare holy basil is as a tea. Because of its high volatile oil content, do not steep it for longer than 5 to 10 minutes, covered.

RECOMMENDED AMOUNTS

You can start with 1 teaspoon of the leaf and increase as desired. It will be difficult to take too much of this herb; I've seen daily recommendations of up to 4 ounces (approximately 2 cups)! (Larger quantities are more accurately measured by weight; however, a teaspoon of herbs is too light to measure accurately on the average kitchen scale.)

The therapeutic amount for holy basil is:

As tincture (fresh herb): 1:2, 75% alcohol, 3 to 5 mL, 3 times per day

As tea: 1 teaspoon to 2 cups (by volume) or 2 grams to 113 grams (by weight)

SPECIAL CONSIDERATIONS

Holy basil may have an antifertility effect on both men and women and therefore should not be used regularly by pregnant women or couples wishing to conceive.

It is slightly blood thinning and should not be taken by those who are currently taking warfarin.

Those who are taking insulin to control their diabetes may need to consult with their doctor about adjusting insulin levels while taking holy basil.

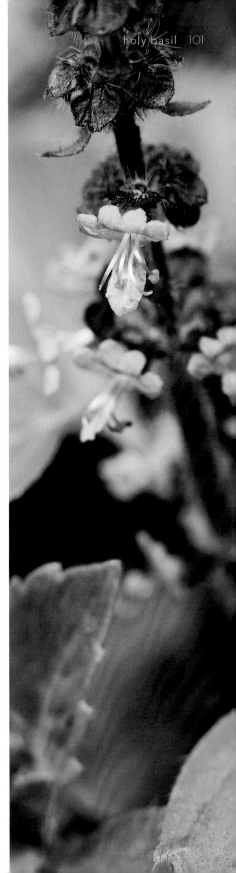

HOLY BASIL–GINGER JULEP

1 sprig fresh mint

1 sprig fresh holy basil

1½ tablespoons Holy Basil–
Ginger Syrup
(see page 104)

1½ tablespoons fresh
lemon juice

¼ cup bourbon

sprig of fresh holy basil or
mint, for garnish

I am very happy to be able to include this recipe created by my friend Emily Han, who is the author of *Wild Drinks & Cocktails: Handcrafted Squashes, Shrubs, Switchels, Tonics, and Infusions to Mix at Home*. Her unique drinks are fun and tasty, and this one is no exception. You can see more great recipes from Emily at www.EmilyHan.com.

Here's what Emily says about this recipe: "Holy basil, or tulsi, has a peppery, spicy taste that brings complexity to a cocktail. Here I've emphasized the herb's warming qualities by pairing it with ginger to make a honeyed syrup that's fantastic in a julep. For an even more peppery drink, substitute rye whiskey for the bourbon. Leftover Holy Basil–Ginger Syrup (page 104) may be used to punch up a glass of lemonade, too."

If you have only dried rather than fresh holy basil, you can still make this recipe. Simply substitute the sprigs of fresh holy basil for fresh mint, and proceed to make the Holy Basil–Ginger Syrup with your dried holy basil.

Yield: 1 serving

1. Muddle the mint sprig, holy basil sprig, Holy Basil–Ginger Syrup, and lemon juice in a julep cup, collins glass, or other tall glass.

2. Fill the glass with crushed ice, and pour the bourbon over the ice.

3. Garnish with the remaining holy basil sprig.

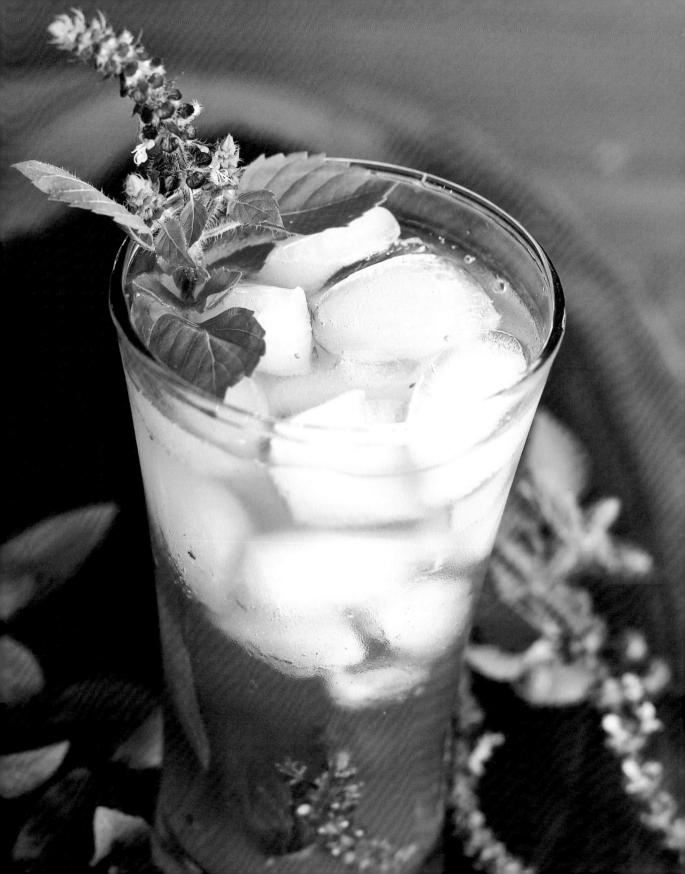

HOLY BASIL–GINGER SYRUP

2 tablespoons finely chopped fresh holy basil leaves, or 1 tablespoon dried holy basil

1½ teaspoons grated fresh ginger

½ cup honey

Yield: about ¾ cup

1. Bring ½ cup water to a boil. Combine the holy basil and ginger in a heatproof ceramic or glass container.

2. Pour boiling water over container and cover. Steep for 15 minutes.

3. Strain through a fine-mesh strainer, squeezing to extract all the liquid; discard the solids.

4. Stir the honey into the warm liquid until dissolved.

5. Store in the refrigerator for up to 2 weeks, but use within 1 week for best flavor.

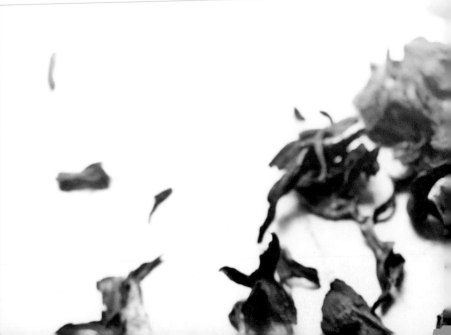

HOLY BASIL TEA

This loose-leaf, aromatic tea is a nice afternoon pick-me-up or a great way to start the morning. I especially love this with fresh holy basil, but dried works as well.

Rooibos is an herbal tea that originally hails from Africa. Its vanilla notes blend well with the more aromatic qualities of holy basil and the tang of the hibiscus.

Yield: 1¼ cups, 1 serving

1. Bring 1¼ cups water to a boil. Place the herbs in a tea mug or large infuser. Avoid cramming the herbs into a small tea infuser; it's better for them to have room to expand and move around.

2. Pour the just-boiled water over the herbs. Let steep, covered, for 5 minutes. Strain. Add stevia or honey if desired, for sweetness.

1 tablespoon chopped fresh holy basil, or 2 teaspoons dried holy basil

2 teaspoons rooibos tea leaves

1 teaspoon dried hibiscus

stevia or honey, to taste (optional)

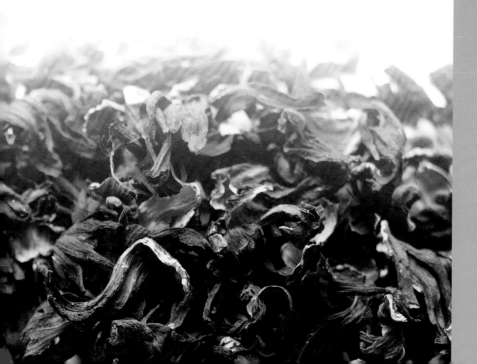

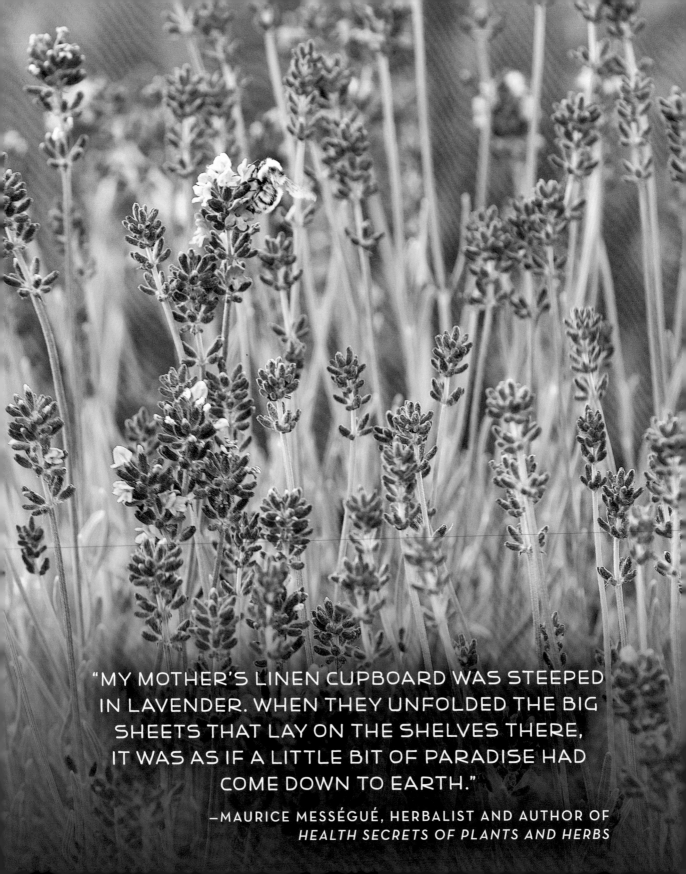

"MY MOTHER'S LINEN CUPBOARD WAS STEEPED IN LAVENDER. WHEN THEY UNFOLDED THE BIG SHEETS THAT LAY ON THE SHELVES THERE, IT WAS AS IF A LITTLE BIT OF PARADISE HAD COME DOWN TO EARTH."

—MAURICE MESSÉGUÉ, HERBALIST AND AUTHOR OF
HEALTH SECRETS OF PLANTS AND HERBS

CHAPTER 12

Lavender

When was the last time you smelled lavender? Not lavender-scented candles, body care products, or potpourri, but real lavender? If you have savored the aroma of lavender, then you'll know it has as many different scents as there are plants! A wild shrub growing on a sunny hillside in the rocky soil of southern France will smell different from the flowers in your garden. The conditions in which lavender grows and the type of plant all contribute to a unique fragrance.

Whenever I see lavender growing, I like to stop and sniff its delicate and unique perfume. Although some might dismiss lavender as simply a pretty-smelling plant, I love that it teaches us how important smell can be. While we know that eating or drinking things can have an effect on our health and how we feel, lavender shows us how the simple act of smelling something can dramatically alter our mood by reducing anxiety and pain and promoting sleep.

Other common names: true lavender, English lavender

Botanical name: *Lavandula angustifolia*

Family: Lamiaceae (mint)

Parts used: flower buds, aerial portions

Energetics: warming

Taste: pungent, bitter

Plant properties: aromatic, antimicrobial, analgesic, relaxing nervine, carminative

Plant uses: bacterial and fungal infections, tension, poor sleep, anxiety, pain, wounds, burns, depression, headaches, dyspepsia, bug bites

Plant preparations: tea, tincture, essential oil, culinary

Lavender has long been loved for its pleasing and relaxing scent. We know that it was used by people in the Mediterranean for at least 2,500 years, and it was commonly used in bathing and laundry. Its popularity spread through northern Europe. The beloved French king Charles VI lay on satin pillows filled with lavender, and Queen Elizabeth I of England reputedly required lavender preserves to be available daily. Judging by our continued frequent use of lavender in candles, bath products, and even detergents, lavender isn't going out of style.

TYPES OF LAVENDER

There are several species of lavender, but the best one for healing is *Lavandula angustifolia*, which is also commonly referred to as English lavender or true lavender.

The common hybrid *Lavandula x intermedia* is widely cultivated for commercial use but has different properties from true lavender. (The *x* in the name denotes that a plant is a hybrid.) It is often referred to as *lavandin*. Essential oil of lavandin is fine for adding scent to your laundry detergent, for example, but not ideal when using it as an herbal remedy.

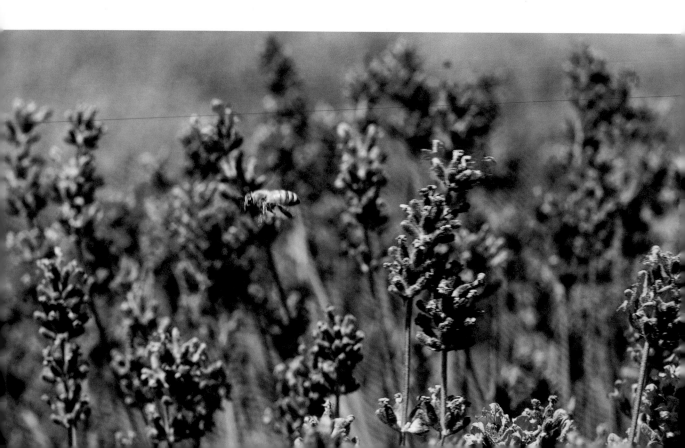

MEDICINAL PROPERTIES AND ENERGETICS OF LAVENDER

If we didn't know better, we could dismiss lavender as a good-smelling plant and leave it at that. But lavender has two stories to tell. The first is that the smell is a surprisingly important part of its medicine. The second is that this complex plant has many benefits beyond its scent.

FOR RELAXATION AND SLEEP

Lavender has long been used to decrease anxiety, induce relaxation, and promote sleep. Herbalist Kiva Rose Hardin explains, "Lavender is appropriate as a [relaxing] nervine when a person is anxious, confused, and has a wrinkled forehead that can't relax. The forehead will give it away every time."[1] (In herbalism, a nervine is broadly used to describe an herb that affects the nervous system. Herbalists break them down into two categories: relaxing and stimulating.)

Studies have shown that simply smelling lavender can bring relief even in one of the most anxiety-inducing situations: the dentist's office! In one study, 200 people were divided into four groups and assessed for anxiety, mood, alertness, and calmness while waiting for their dentist appointment. One group smelled lavender essential oil, one group smelled orange essential oil, one group listened to music, and the control group was exposed to no scents or music. Both the lavender and orange scents were found to reduce anxiety and improve the mood of the waiting patients.[2]

Lavender is also well known for promoting sleep. During a study in an intermediate-care hospital unit, researchers found that the patients who had the scent of lavender in their rooms all night showed modest sleep improvement and lowered blood pressure as compared to the control group.[3] Personally, I love sinking into the scent of the lavender-filled pillow I keep on my bed—and, for the record, I sleep really well.

One study demonstrated that capsules of lavender essential oil were as effective for addressing generalized anxiety disorder (GAD) as lorazepam, a common pharmaceutical drug. Not only that, but it also has a better safety record! Unlike lorazepam and other benzodiazepines used for GAD, lavender does not cause extreme drowsiness, nor is their a risk of abuse or addiction.[4]

Are you wondering how simply smelling lavender can so dramatically change our emotions and quality of sleep? Researchers decided to investigate the effects of lavender essential oil on the autonomic and central nervous systems. As compared to the control group, participants who smelled lavender had a significant decrease in blood pressure, heart rate, and skin temperature, which means they had a decrease of autonomic nervous system arousal. They also had stronger theta and alpha brain activity, which are the calmer, more relaxed brain waves seen during sleep and meditation.[5,6] Another study showed that smelling lavender essential oil protected the body from oxidative stress and decreased levels of the stress hormone cortisol.[7]

FOR DEPRESSION

Lavender can relieve certain types of depression. Herbalist David Winston uses lavender for people who feel they are in a fog and for those experiencing stagnant depression, which he defines as a fixation on a specific traumatic event. For these purposes, he recommends using it internally as a tea or a tincture and likes to combine it with lemon balm.[8] (For more information about lemon balm, see Chapter 24.)

One study looked at the effects of lavender and rose aromatherapy in women who were at high risk for postpartum depression. After two and then four weeks, the women receiving aromatherapy treatments showed significant improvements over those in the control group.[9]

FOR DIGESTIVE ISSUES

Lavender is slightly warming and aromatic, so herbalists often use it for cold and stagnant digestion or for calming digestive spasms. It works well for nervous stomachs since it both helps digestion and helps to calm the nerves. Because it's not as hot as garlic, ginger, or cayenne, it can be tolerated better by a broader range of people. I like to combine it with chamomile as an after-dinner tea.

FOR HEALING

In 1710 the physician William Salmon recommended that lavender be used "against the bitings of serpents, mad-dogs and other venomous creature, being given inwardly and applied poultice-wise to the parts wounded."[10] Herbalist Maud Grieve wrote that lavender was frequently used to treat wounds in World War I.[11] Since then, many researchers have validated its pain-relieving and antiseptic qualities.

Two different studies of women recovering from an episiotomy found that lavender essential oil applied topically was as effective as a standard antiseptic in reducing pain and preventing complications, and even better at reducing redness.[12,13] Lavender oil was shown to have strong antimicrobial effects and was effective in reducing ulcers, promoting healing, and calming inflammation when used topically on canker sores.[14]

The miraculous story of French chemist René-Maurice Gattefossé is often repeated in aromatherapy texts. He made lavender essential oil famous for healing when he used it for his own serious burns from a laboratory explosion in 1910. He reported that one rinse of the essential oil stopped the gas gangrene that was quickly covering his hands.[15] I've used lavender essential oil for my own minor burns and am always amazed at how quickly it reduces the pain.

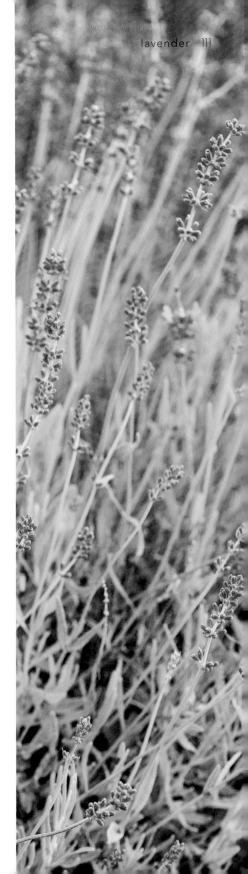

FOR REDUCING PAIN

Lavender has been used for relieving pain, especially headaches, for centuries. Herbalist Nicholas Culpeper recommended using lavender on the temples as far back as 1652.[16] Modern research has shown that inhaling lavender essential oil is an effective way to address migraine headaches. In a study of people diagnosed with migraine headaches, out of 129 headache episodes, 92 responded entirely or partially when the subject smelled lavender essential oil.[17]

The scent of lavender has been shown to be a safe and effective way to reduce even the pain after a cesarean.[18] Another study of 48 post-tonsillectomy patients aged 6 to 12 years old found that those given lavender essential oil to smell used significantly less acetaminophen than those in the control group.[19]

Applied topically, the essential oil can decrease the pain and itch associated with bug bites and bee stings. A beekeeper friend of mine keeps a bottle of lavender essential oil with her at all times so she can apply it immediately after being stung. She says it quickly reduces the pain and prevents excessive swelling. Massages with lavender essential oil were found to be effective in reducing the pain of women with painful periods.[20]

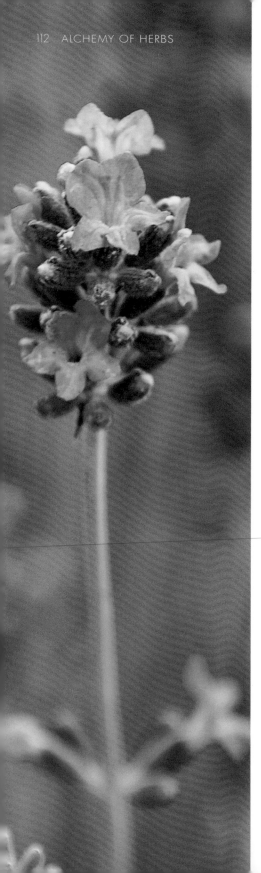

HOW TO USE LAVENDER

My best tip for using lavender is to make sure you have real lavender; it should be labeled with the scientific name *Lavandula angustifolia*. (Lavandin can be used just for its pleasant scent, if desired.)

RECOMMENDED AMOUNTS

When using lavender in food or tea, it is best used in smaller amounts. Too much lavender gives an unpleasant, bitter taste.

The therapeutic amount for lavender is:

As tea: 1 to 3 grams per day

As tincture (dried flowers): 1:5, 70% alcohol, 1.5 to 2 mL, 3 to 4 times per day[21]

As essential oil: inhaled or diluted in a carrier oil for external use

SPECIAL CONSIDERATIONS

Lavender essential oil is very powerful, and one should be cautious when using it externally and internally. While many people consider the oil safe to use undiluted on the skin, I've personally seen this method cause chemical burns. A 1 percent dilution in a carrier oil is safest for sensitive skin.

Lavender essential oil should be consumed only under the guidance of a trained clinician. It should not be used internally during pregnancy.

Do not eat lavender from florists or garden shops. These flowers have likely been sprayed with chemicals that haven't been approved for food use.

There have been some unsubstantiated reports that lavender-scented products have adversely affected young boys due to estrogenic effects. These isolated cases have been questioned. Currently, the *Botanical Safety Handbook* gives lavender its highest safety rating.[22]

LAVENDER BATH SALTS

One of my favorite ways to relax and relieve stress is to take a lavender bath. This blend is especially suited to muscle aches and pains. I add a lot of salts to the bath to make it therapeutic, as I've found the small amount of salts that some recipes call for to be ineffective.

To cut down on cost, look for sea salt and Epsom salts being sold in bulk. You can find Epsom salts at many drugstores, or order them online.

Yield: 3 cups salts for 1 bath

1 cup sea salt

2 cups Epsom salts

20 to 30 drops lavender essential oil

1. Mix all the ingredients together in a large bowl. Use immediately, or store the salts in an airtight container for later use.

2. *To use:* Add the entire batch to a bath of warm water, and soak as long as desired. I suggest taking a quick shower afterward to rinse off the salts.

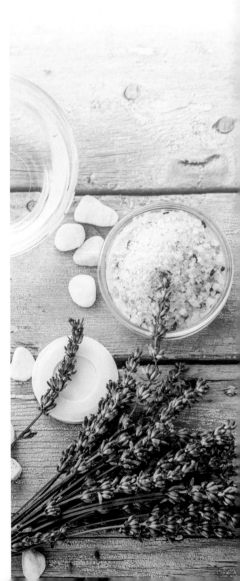

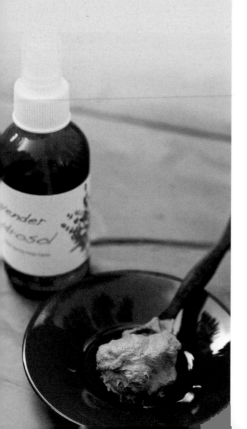

1 tablespoon lavender flowers

2 tablespoons cosmetic clay

lavender hydrosol

LAVENDER AND CLAY FACIAL

These three simple ingredients combine to create a luxurious facial spa experience without any strange additives. Practically any cosmetic clay will work. I like French green clay, but kaolin and bentonite clay are also good options.

Hydrosols are a by-product of essential oil creation. When plants are steam-distilled, the oils are extracted and the water from the steam becomes the hydrosol, which has picked up unique properties from the plant. You can find them at online retailers listed in the Recommended Resources. Plain water can also be used in place of the lavender hydrosol.

Yield: 1 generous application (enough to thickly coat your face and neck), or 2 applications spread more thinly

1. Powder the lavender flowers and mix together with the clay. Add small amounts of lavender hydrosol slowly, stirring and checking the consistency after every addition. You want the end product to be a thick paste that spreads easily.

2. Spread the mixture on clean skin. Cover your face as well as your neck, if desired. Let sit until the mixture dries, about 15 minutes depending on thickness.

3. Rinse the mask off with warm water. Pat dry, and follow up with Elderflower Facial Serum (page 208) or Green Tea and Rose Facial Cream (page 246), if desired.

LAVENDER AND ORANGE CUSTARD

This is a simple yet delicious custard that pairs the relaxing flavor of lavender with the bright citrus flavor of orange. This is a great dessert to make a day ahead for a stress-free dinner party. If you don't have access to vanilla bean powder, substitute 1 teaspoon of vanilla extract.

Yield: 5 servings

1. Add the milk and lavender to a saucepan, and heat on medium-low until the milk starts to bubble, about 10 minutes. Turn off the heat and let the lavender infuse for another 10 minutes. Strain out the lavender, and let the milk cool for about 20 minutes.

2. While the milk is cooling, preheat the oven to 350°F. In a separate bowl, mix together the eggs, honey, salt, vanilla bean powder, and orange extract until well combined. (Do not beat the eggs; you don't want them to be fluffy.)

3. Once the milk has cooled, slowly add it to the egg mixture, stirring constantly.

4. Fill five 6-ounce ramekins with the custard, and place them in a deep baking dish. Pour hot water into the baking dish until the water reaches halfway up the sides of the ramekins.

5. Place the baking dish in the oven and bake for 30 minutes. The custard is done when it has just a very slight jiggle and the top shows some hints of darkness.

6. Remove from the oven, let cool completely, and then store in the fridge overnight. Serve cold.

2 cups whole milk

1 tablespoon dried lavender flowers

4 eggs

⅓ cup honey

½ teaspoon salt

1 teaspoon vanilla bean powder

1 teaspoon organic orange extract

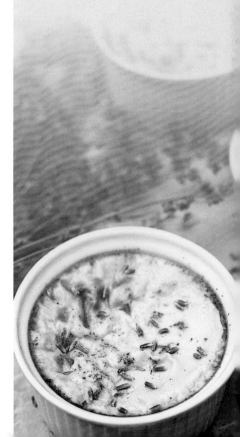

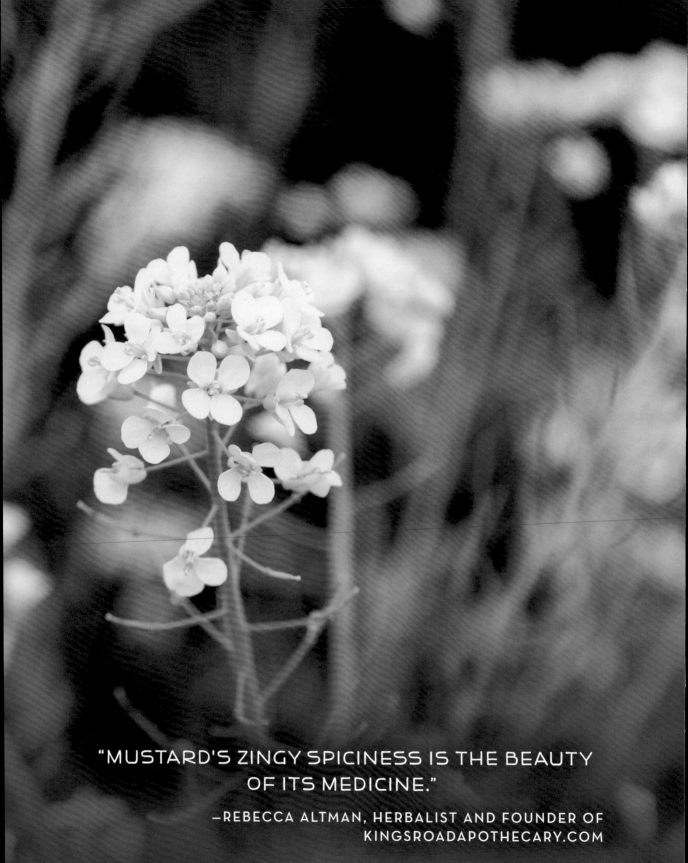

"MUSTARD'S ZINGY SPICINESS IS THE BEAUTY
OF ITS MEDICINE."

—REBECCA ALTMAN, HERBALIST AND FOUNDER OF
KINGSROADAPOTHECARY.COM

CHAPTER 13

Mustard

A couple of years ago my husband and I were traveling through France to visit our family. The trip had gone perfectly until I caught a cold our last week there. I quickly used all the herbs I had brought with me, but I was still a stuffy, foggy-headed, miserable mess. I really wanted to get the most out of every second of my trip, so I was desperate for something to help me.

While standing in the kitchen, bemoaning my stuffy sinuses, I suddenly realized I'd overlooked the very potent herb found in practically every French kitchen: mustard! Sure enough, I found several different kinds in the fridge and took a spoonful out of one of the jars. My sinuses immediately started to drain, and I started to sweat. Mustard—especially well-prepared, authentic mustard—is pungent, spicy, and downright hot! Regular spoonfuls of mustard had me feeling a lot better in no time.

Mustard seeds go beyond helping us with cold and flu symptoms. The small and humble mustard seed protects us against DNA damage and oxidative stress, thus offering us a powerful ally for preventing cancer and improving heart health.

Botanical name: *Brassica alba, Brassica juncea*

Family: Brassicaceae

Parts used: seeds

Energetics: warming, drying

Taste: pungent

Plant properties: stimulating expectorant, rubefacient, analgesic

Plant uses: congestion in sinuses and lungs, arthritic pain, fever, cancer prevention, muscle aches and pains

Plant preparations: mustard condiment, plaster, bath, culinary

Many different mustard species have been cultivated and harvested for thousands of years. There's archaeological evidence that one related species was used as a spice more than 6,000 years ago in northern Europe.[1] Another species was most likely cultivated in China as far back as 5,000 b.c.e.[2] Ancient Romans are credited with creating the first recipes that resembled the prepared mustard condiments we are most familiar with today, as well as with spreading the seeds throughout their empire. At some point, mustard traveled to Gaul (present-day France), where making it was developed into an art. Dijon, a city in the Burgundy region, is famous for its preparation of mustard, created by Jean Naigeon in 1856.

Mustard grows practically everywhere, like a weed. That's why, historically, it's been both popular and readily available—unlike many spices that were reserved only for those with deep pockets, such as black pepper, nutmeg, and ginger.

TYPES OF MUSTARD SEEDS

The two types of mustard seeds that are readily available commercially are *Brassica alba* and *Brassica juncea*.

Brassica alba produces seeds that are referred to as either white or yellow. They have a milder flavor, and most mustards in the United States are made from them.

Brassica juncea produces seeds that are referred to as brown, and these have a sharper, more pronounced heat that especially affects the sinuses.

MEDICINAL PROPERTIES AND ENERGETICS OF MUSTARD

While mustard is often brushed aside as a simple condiment to have with your hot dog or pastrami—certainly not a headline health food—it packs a secret punch.

Due to certain nonsustainable agriculture methods, our food supply today contains a fraction of the nutrients it once did. Many of our favorite fruits and vegetables, such as tomatoes, apples, and lettuce, have been selectively cultivated for certain traits that are better for business than our health. But not the brassicas!

Brassicas, also known as cruciferous vegetables, are a genus within the Brassicaceae plant family. It includes broccoli, cabbage, and kale. In her book *Eating on the Wild Side*, author Jo Robinson explains that brassicas are some of our healthiest foods because they most resemble their ancient ancestors.[3] The brassicas have not changed significantly from their predecessors and still contain an impressive amount of phytonutrients, which have been shown to have strong cancer-fighting potential: mustard included!

FOR CANCER

Mustard has been studied extensively for its various anticancer properties. Compounds found in mustard seeds, allyl isothiocyanates (AITCs), have shown promise for use in cancer prevention and treatment.

One clinical trial gave volunteers 20 grams of a mustard preparation. After only three days they showed a significant reduction in DNA damage and even had a decrease in total cholesterol. The researchers concluded that "even short-term intake of ITC-containing vegetables [like mustard] might indeed be associated with reduced cancer risk."[4]

FOR HEART HEALTH

Mustard seeds and mustard seed oil support heart health, possibly because their high levels of omega-3 fatty acids reduce oxidative stress.

A trial that included 360 patients tracked their progress for one year after a heart attack. The groups that received fish oil or mustard oil showed significant improvements in their cardiovascular health as compared with the placebo group, including fewer cardiac events and a reduction in arrhythmias. The researchers concluded that both oils may provide rapid protective effects in patients at risk for heart attacks.[5]

FOR YOUR LUNGS

Using a mustard seed poultice directly over the lungs has been a long-lived tradition to help people with congested lungs and bronchitis. The spicy, stimulating properties of the mustard seeds increase and thin mucus secretions, making it easier for the body to expel them from the lungs. This action causes herbalists to call mustard a stimulating expectorant. It makes mustard a wonderful aid in breaking up congestion in the body.

Chinese researchers put this old folk remedy to the test. They performed a study on people with chronic bronchitis using a plaster made from various herbs including mustard seeds. Those receiving the treatment had significant improvement in their symptoms as compared with the control group.[6]

FOR PAIN

Historically mustard was used frequently to treat arthritis, especially arthritis that gets worse in cold weather. It is often used in the form of a plaster to reduce pain and speed the healing of injuries like an ankle sprain or muscle strain.

Mustard relieves pain by being a topical counterirritant or rubefacient; in other words, it works by irritating tissues, thus bringing circulation and heat to the affected area.

One way to use mustard topically is to take a mustard bath. (I include a recipe for one in this chapter.) It warms tired and sore muscles and relieves all-over body pain. This is a traditional remedy to support the fever process when someone is feeling chilled (though *not* when someone is feeling hot or restless).

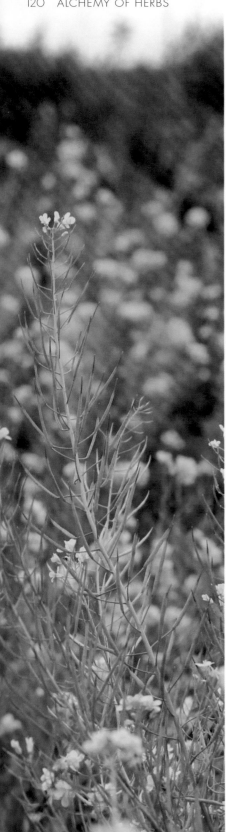

HOW TO USE MUSTARD

The yellow or white seeds tend to have a subtler and milder flavor. I like to use the brown seeds for more of a hot and stimulating effect.

Mustard oil can be found in specialty shops. This makes a nice cooking oil and a great way to get mustard into your diet.

RECOMMENDED AMOUNTS

Enjoy mustard seeds as a regular part of your diet to get the most benefits. There are no firm therapeutic amounts for mustard seeds.

SPECIAL CONSIDERATIONS

Eating excessive amounts of mustard might cause stomach upset.

HOMEMADE MUSTARD

Making your own mustard is really easy! As you get the hang of the basic steps, you can improvise with many different herbs for a variety of tastes. For this recipe I chose to go with the smoky and spicy flavor of chipotle. While the steps are super simple, note that the mustard seeds need to be soaked for 2 days prior to release the flavor of the seeds.

The following recipe uses both yellow and brown mustard seeds, but if you prefer a milder taste, omit the brown and double the amount of the yellow.

Yield: 1¼ cups

1. Place $^1/_2$ cup water, the mustard seeds, and the apple cider vinegar in a glass bowl. Cover and let sit for 2 days.

2. Place the seeds, including the liquid, into a food processor or blender. Add the rest of the ingredients and blend until the mustard is ground into a paste.

3. This mustard will keep in the fridge for about six months.

¼ cup brown mustard seeds

¼ cup yellow mustard seeds

½ cup apple cider vinegar

1 teaspoon honey

1 teaspoon turmeric powder

2 teaspoons paprika powder

1 teaspoon chipotle powder

1 teaspoon salt

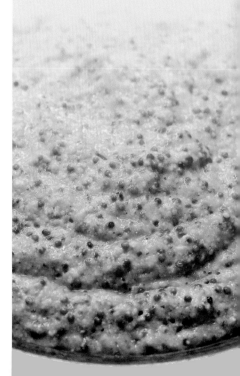

SQUASH SOUP WITH MUSTARD SEEDS

2 pounds winter squash

2 tablespoons olive oil

½ teaspoon whole
  cumin seeds

1 teaspoon brown
  mustard seeds

1 medium onion, minced

1½ teaspoons salt

1 tablespoon minced
  fresh ginger

2 garlic cloves, minced

2 (13.5-oz.) cans coconut milk

2 tablespoons lemon juice

The credit for this delicious fall soup goes entirely to my husband. One year we were gifted loads of winter squash, and he took on the important role of finding interesting ways to enjoy this hearty vegetable. Out of his many delicious dishes, this soup was one of my favorites. Practically any winter squash will work, although acorn squash may be hard to peel.

Yield: 8 cups, 4 servings

1.   Remove the peel, stem, and seeds of the winter squash, then roughly chop it into medium-size pieces.

2.   Pour the oil into a large saucepan on medium heat, then add the cumin and mustard seeds. When the seeds begin to sizzle, add the onion and salt and fry for 3 to 5 minutes, stirring occasionally. Add the ginger and garlic and fry for another couple of minutes, until aromatic.

3.   Add the squash and coconut milk and turn up the heat a bit until the mixture reaches a slight boil. Then reduce the heat to low and simmer for about 30 minutes, until the squash is soft.

4.   When done, pour the soup into a food processor. You may need to do it in two batches so the food processor doesn't overflow with the hot liquid. Process on low for about 2 minutes, until the soup is smooth. Stir in the lemon juice.

5.   Serve warm.

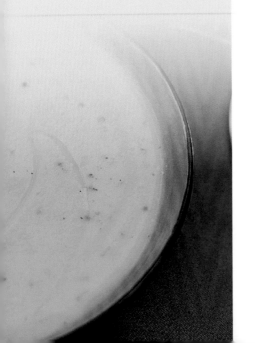

MUSTARD AND GINGER BATH SALTS

Rebecca Altman, from Kings Road Apothecary, is a brilliant herbalist who creates synergistic herbal formulations like teas, tinctures, ointments, and many others. She graciously agreed to create this stimulating bath recipe featuring the spicy and invigorating qualities of mustard exclusively for this book. You can see more great products from Rebecca at www.Kings RoadApothecary.com.

Here's what Rebecca says about this recipe: "Mustard powder stimulates circulation and warms the muscles. It's a lovely addition to a bath in the winter, when the cold is seeping into your muscles, making you feel stiff and sore. I also love to use it after a difficult workout or when I've been injured in some fashion. I've also added ginger—another spicy, warming herb—and some essential oils that help stimulate circulation."

Yield: 3 cups salts

1 cup Dead Sea salt

¾ cup Epsom salts

¼ cup baking soda

¾ cup mustard powder

¼ cup ginger powder

10 drops eucalyptus essential oil

10 drops peppermint essential oil

10 drops cedar essential oil

10 drops lavender essential oil

10 drops rosemary essential oil

1. Mix the salts and baking soda together in a big bowl.

2. Run the mustard and ginger powders through a sieve to separate out any lumps, then add them to the salts. Mix thoroughly.

3. Add the essential oils to the salt blend and stir in well. Store in an airtight container.

4. *To use:* Add one to three cups to a hot bath.

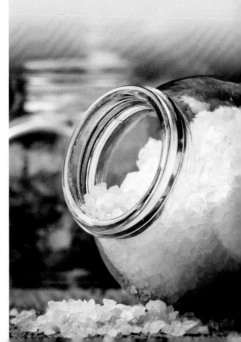

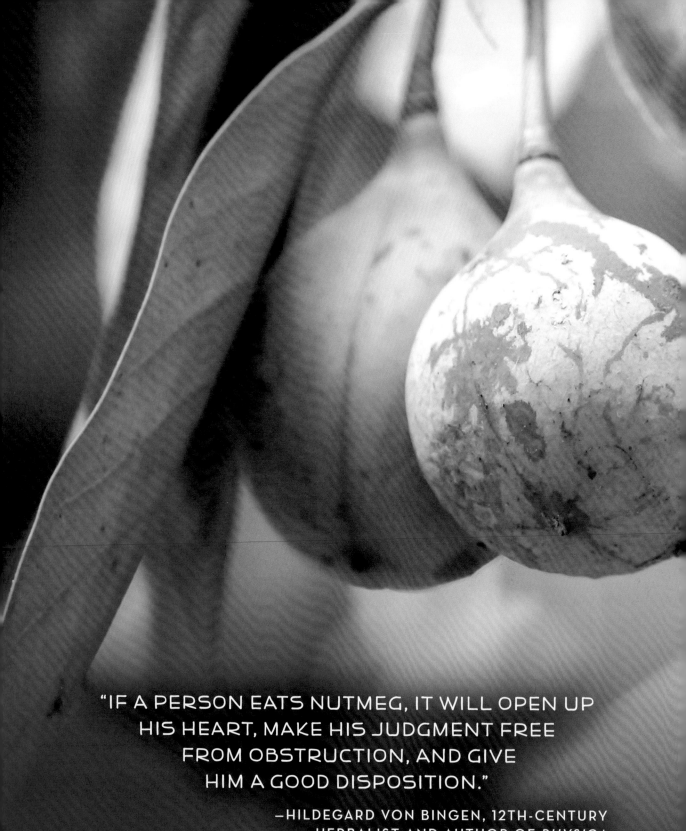

"IF A PERSON EATS NUTMEG, IT WILL OPEN UP
HIS HEART, MAKE HIS JUDGMENT FREE
FROM OBSTRUCTION, AND GIVE
HIM A GOOD DISPOSITION."

–HILDEGARD VON BINGEN, 12TH-CENTURY
HERBALIST AND AUTHOR OF *PHYSICA*

CHAPTER 14

Nutmeg

On a Far East island, once called a Spice Island, a pigeon devours a fleshy, cream-colored fruit along with the large seed inside it. This aromatic seed remains unharmed and is eventually deposited in the surrounding lush, tropical forest.

The seed germinates in the rich volcanic soil and a tree begins to emerge. If this seed is female, the tree will produce its first fruit within 9 to 12 years. When it reaches maturity in about 20 years, it will produce 2,000 fruits per year. Eventually the tree will reach to around 20 feet high and live for three-quarters of a century. This tree is the nutmeg.

Herbalists and culinary enthusiasts use both nutmeg seeds and nutmeg mace. Mace is a bright-red webbing that covers the nutmeg seed. This chapter is mainly about the seed.

When you hold nutmeg in your hand, you are holding a truly special treasure. That sweet and aromatic spice is often taken for granted as a "pumpkin spice" to be used occasionally in baking during the holidays. But the nutmeg tree and its fruit are a powerful medicinal herb.

Botanical name: *Myristica fragrans*

Family: Myristicaceae

Parts used: seed, mace

Energetics: warming, drying

Taste: pungent

Plant properties: relaxing, aromatic, antispasmodic, aphrodisiac, carminative, antimicrobial, antiemetic, hypotensive

Plant uses: insomnia, stress, common digestive problems such as gas/bloating and diarrhea

Plant preparations: freshly ground powder, essential oil

Nutmeg has a rich, although sometimes sad, history. The fruit, seed, and mace of the nutmeg have long been highly prized as both food and medicine. Nutmeg is native to the Banda Islands, north of Australia. For thousands of years the Banda people harvested the fruits of the nutmeg tree to use the flesh, the mace, and the nutmeg seed as food and medicine. They also traded nutmeg extensively with surrounding islands.

It's easy to love this sweet and aromatic spice, and when it arrived in Europe through the spice route, Europeans fell head over heels for it. Not only did it taste delicious, but it was believed to stop the plague and was used as a hallucinogen.

When the European spice trade over land was stopped in 1453, the race to win the spice trade over the seas began. Explorers braved the open sea to discover a route to the East Indies and the treasure of spices growing there. To get an idea of how lucrative this endeavor was, consider this: it is said that one small bag of nutmeg seeds in Europe could guarantee a comfortable retirement for a sailor.

MEDICINAL PROPERTIES AND ENERGETICS OF NUTMEG

Nutmeg is most commonly used as a culinary spice. The United States imports many tons and millions of dollars' worth of nutmeg from around the world. Most of this is ground and sold for use in baking, especially during the holidays. But nutmeg is also a powerful medicine that can be used for anxiety, sleep issues, digestion, colds, the flu, and more.

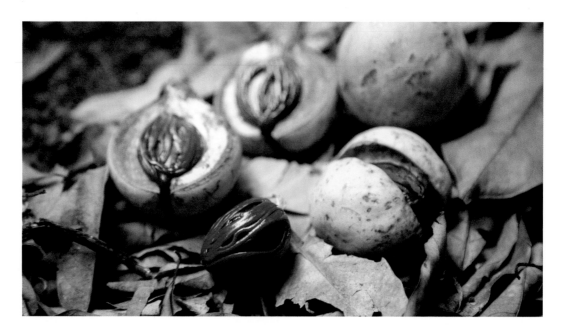

FOR INSOMNIA

A popular folk remedy for sleep is warmed milk with nutmeg. Yum!

However, when using nutmeg for serious insomnia, it can be a bit tricky. The dosage varies widely from person to person, it takes 4 to 6 hours to work, and then the effects last reliably for 8 hours. I recommend working with a trained herbalist to get the best benefits from nutmeg.

FOR DIGESTIVE ISSUES

Nutmeg is a warming and aromatic spice that can relieve many uncomfortable digestive symptoms. It's commonly used for bloating and gas. It can also relieve diarrhea and is popular for use with children.

Using aromatic culinary spices in food is a wonderful way to prevent common digestive problems. Nutmeg can be taken in an herbal chai (tea) blend and mixed with other spices like ginger, cinnamon, and cloves to relieve digestive discomfort. Vasant Lad, co-author of *The Yoga of Herbs*, states, "Nutmeg is one of the best spices for increasing absorption, particularly in the small intestine."[1]

FOR HYPERTENSION

Nutmeg has hypotensive abilities, meaning that it can reduce blood pressure. I don't know of any modern herbalists using nutmeg for that specific purpose. However, be cautious when using medicinal amounts of nutmeg in someone who tends to have low blood pressure.

AS AN APHRODISIAC

Nutmeg is often added in small amounts to herbal aphrodisiac formulas. But *aphrodisiac* is a troublesome term since it can give the illusion that someone takes it and suddenly becomes the plot of a cheesy '80s film where they fall helplessly in love with the first person they see. When it comes to herbalism, however, an aphrodisiac may influence a romantic evening in several different ways. For example, someone who is really stressed and unable to unwind might find a relaxing nervine to be an aphrodisiac because it relieves tension. Those who are suffering from chronic sleep debt and are tired all the time may find that an adaptogen helps them get the rest they need, which then leaves them more refreshed and open to expending energy in the bedroom. So don't expect nutmeg to be the magical secret ingredient in your love potion!

As Hildegard von Bingen pointed out in her 12th-century book, *Physica*, nutmeg can get rid of bitterness in your heart and make you more pleasant and cheerful. "Take some nutmeg and an equal weight of cinnamon and a bit of cloves, and pulverize them," she wrote. "Then make small cakes with this and fine whole wheat flour and water. Eat them often. It will calm all bitterness of the heart and mind, open your heart and impaired senses, and make your mind cheerful."[2]

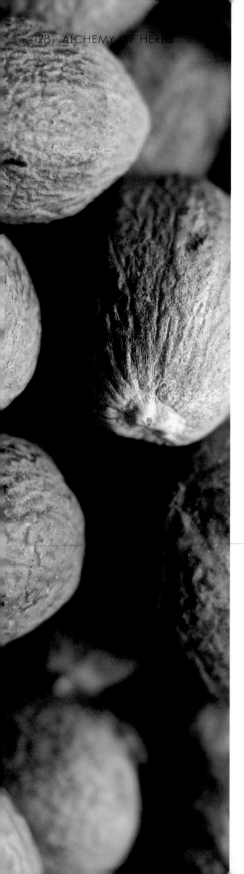

HOW TO USE NUTMEG

Walk into any grocery store and you'll find ground nutmeg powder in the spice aisle. While this nutmeg may give your apple pie a nice taste, it isn't always medicinally potent. If you want the best-quality nutmeg, then buy the whole nutmeg seed and grate it as needed. You can use a cheese grater or buy a specialty nutmeg grater.

Whole nutmeg seeds, when properly stored, can last for years. However, once grated, it quickly loses its potency, so try to use it immediately and keep any leftovers no more than a week.

RECOMMENDED AMOUNTS

Nutmeg can be used as a culinary spice to improve digestion and promote relaxation. The therapeutic range for nutmeg is 1 to 5 grams of the freshly grated seed.

SPECIAL CONSIDERATIONS

Large amounts of nutmeg can have adverse effects: 10 to 20 grams may leave a person feeling foggy-headed or groggy, and 30 grams (1 ounce) can bring on uncomfortable symptoms including vomiting, headache, and hallucinations. According to the *Botanical Safety Handbook*, the last reported death from nutmeg poisoning was in 1908.[3]

Medicinal dosages of nutmeg have not been proved safe for use during pregnancy or breastfeeding; however, normal culinary amounts in foods are fine.

SPICED EGGNOG

I look forward to the holiday eggnog season every year. This homemade version has more delicious spices and less sugar than what you would buy at the store. My husband and I make ours with fresh eggs from the neighbor's chickens, raw whole milk, and organic whipping cream. While we have never had a problem with raw eggs, they should be avoided during pregnancy and by those with weakened immune systems. In particular, avoid cheap conventional eggs to reduce the risk of salmonella.

Yield: approximately 3½ cups, 3 servings

---

1. In a bowl, whisk the eggs until they're very frothy (approximately 2 minutes).

2. Whisk in the honey until fully blended. Then add the vanilla, nutmeg, cinnamon, ginger, and cloves and continue whisking.

3. A little at a time, whisk in first the whipping cream, followed by the milk.

4. Finally, whisk in the rum, if desired. Store this in a quart-size mason jar.

5. Chill the eggnog for 1 to 2 hours. Stir before serving and serve with a sprinkle of nutmeg on top.

3 organic eggs

¼ cup raw local honey

2 tablespoons vanilla extract

1 tablespoon freshly grated nutmeg

¼ teaspoon cinnamon powder

¼ teaspoon ginger powder

⅛ teaspoon ground cloves

1 cup heavy whipping cream

1 cup whole milk

½ cup dark rum (optional)

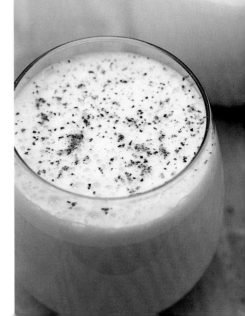

SPICED CARROT CAKE

For the cake:

6 tablespoons coconut flour, sifted

1 tablespoon ground cinnamon

1 teaspoon freshly grated nutmeg

1 teaspoon ginger powder

½ teaspoon ground cloves

½ teaspoon baking soda

½ teaspoon salt

5 eggs

1 tablespoon pure vanilla extract

½ cup maple syrup

½ cup organic coconut oil, melted

3 raw carrots, grated (peeled if desired)

½ cup raisins

For the frosting:

8 ounces softened cream cheese

½ cup softened butter

¼ cup maple syrup

1 tablespoon pure vanilla extract

1 tablespoon grated fresh ginger

1 cup chopped walnuts, for garnish

I am a sucker for carrot cake, but most recipes are full of sugar and tend to be fairly bland. This recipe is a dense coconut-flour cake with a generous amount of delicious aromatic spices. If you get invited to my birthday party, this is undoubtedly what we'll be serving! I recommend making it a day ahead as this cake tastes even better the next day.

Yield: 16 small servings

1. *To make the cake:* Preheat the oven to 325°F. In a small bowl, mix the coconut flour, cinnamon, nutmeg, ginger, cloves, baking soda, and salt.

2. In a large mixing bowl, beat the eggs, vanilla, maple syrup, and melted coconut oil.

3. Add dry ingredients to wet and mix well. Stir in the carrots and raisins.

4. Grease a 9 x 9-inch cake pan with coconut oil. Pour the batter into the pan and bake for 30 minutes. Test the center with a toothpick—if it comes out clean, the cake is done.

5. Remove the cake from the oven and allow to cool while you make the frosting.

6. *To make the frosting:* Cream together the cream cheese and butter. Mix in the maple syrup and vanilla extract. Stir in the fresh ginger.

7. Once the caked has cooled, frost it with the buttercream frosting. Garnish with walnuts and serve.

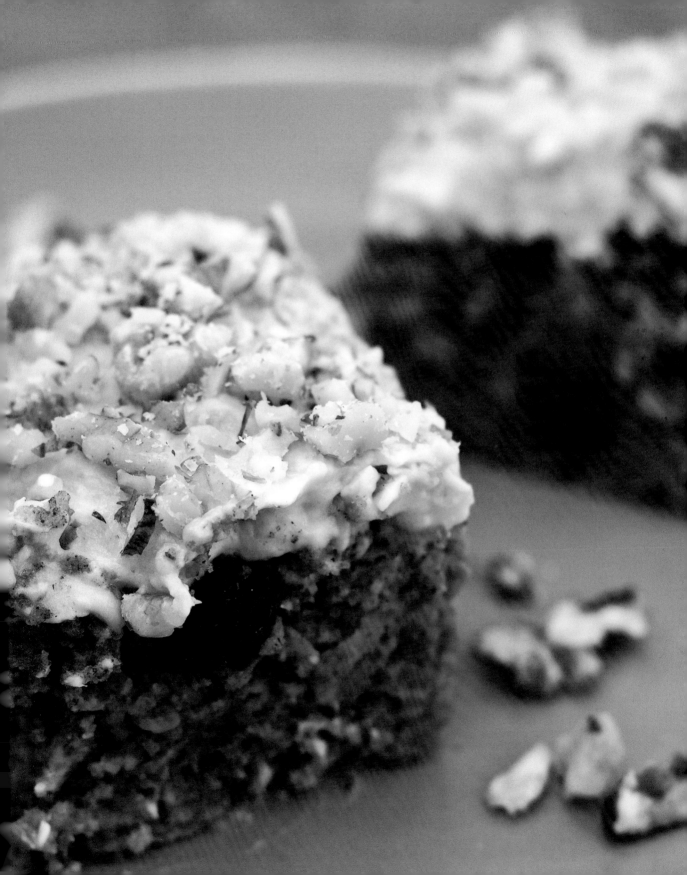

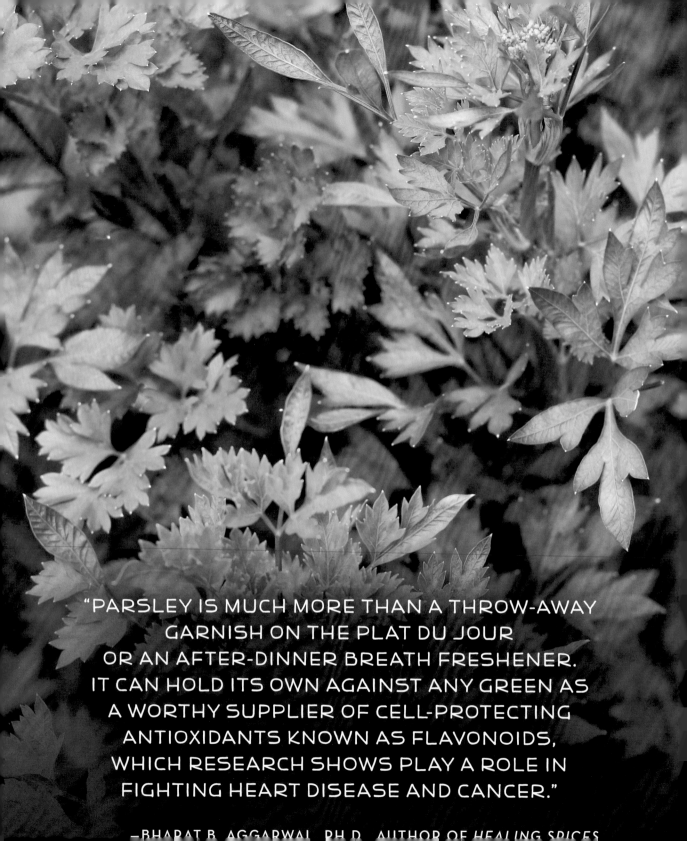

"PARSLEY IS MUCH MORE THAN A THROW-AWAY
GARNISH ON THE PLAT DU JOUR
OR AN AFTER-DINNER BREATH FRESHENER.
IT CAN HOLD ITS OWN AGAINST ANY GREEN AS
A WORTHY SUPPLIER OF CELL-PROTECTING
ANTIOXIDANTS KNOWN AS FLAVONOIDS,
WHICH RESEARCH SHOWS PLAY A ROLE IN
FIGHTING HEART DISEASE AND CANCER."

—BHARAT B. AGGARWAL, PH.D., AUTHOR OF *HEALING SPICES*

CHAPTER 15

Parsley

Unfortunately, many folks are so intent on finding the next exotic herb and spice in faraway lands that our common kitchen herbs rarely get the respect they deserve. Take parsley as an example. Oftentimes, it is thought of simply as a garnish to make a dish look more appealing. But few realize the power stored in a handful of leaves. Eaten frequently, it can freshen your breath, improve digestion, and decrease oxidative stress.

Botanical name: *Petroselinum crispum*

Family: Apiaceae (syn. Umbelliferae)

Parts used: roots, seeds, leaves

Energetics: warming, drying

Taste: sweet (root), pungent (leaves)

Plant properties: aromatic, diuretic, carminative, antioxidant, emmenagogue (especially the seeds), galactagogue

Plant uses: urinary tract infections, edema, kidney stones, cystitis, delayed menses, amenorrhea, digestive complaints, cancer prevention, heart disease

Plant preparations: tea, decoction, culinary, essential oil, fresh leaf poultice

Parsley most likely originated somewhere around the Mediterranean, but it has been used for so long it's hard to pinpoint its exact place of origin. Along with carrots and celery, it's a member of the Apiaceae family (which was previously known as the Umbelliferae family). It grows as a biennial herb in northern climates, meaning it takes two years for it to complete its life cycle. In the first year it puts out its leaves and grows a solid root. In the second year it flowers, goes to seed, and then dies.

Parsley was ceremonially used by the ancient Greeks and Romans and was associated with death. This reputation stuck through many ages, and there were numerous superstitions surrounding it in Europe well into the Middle Ages. Parsley has long had a prominent role in many different traditions of Middle Eastern cooking. It now grows all over the world and is frequently found in North American and Brazilian cuisine as well as Middle Eastern and European. Parsley is often featured in the Jewish holiday of Passover as part of the seder plate.

TYPES OF PARSLEY

If you know your parsley, you may be aware of the two distinct kinds commonly sold. One has really curly leaves while the other variety has a flat leaf.

You can tell a lot about herbs by their flavor, and this is a perfect example of letting your taste sensation be your guide. If you get a chance, try each kind. Do they taste the same? Does the stem taste the same as the leaves? (Hint: they don't! What's the difference?)

As you discover the different tastes of parsley for yourself, keep in mind that a stronger aromatic and pungent taste is going to be stronger herbal medicine for digestion and diuresis.

MEDICINAL PROPERTIES AND ENERGETICS OF PARSLEY

Parsley is high in nutrients, notably vitamin K1, vitamin C, and beta-carotene. However, if you want to get the most benefits of parsley as food, you'll need to do more than eat that sprig on your dinner plate. Instead, eat large amounts of fresh parsley in salads and sauces.

AS A DIURETIC

The best known of parsley's medicinal functions may be its effects on the urinary system. The leaves and roots are diuretics and have been used for a variety of ailments in which increased urination is beneficial, including urinary tract infections, kidney stones, cystitis, and edema. The roots have a stronger diuretic action than the leaves and are typically taken as a strong decoction or tea.

FOR DIGESTIVE ISSUES

One reason parsley so often spruces up a dinner plate could be its known connection with improving digestion and appetite. Have bad breath? Try fresh parsley. Have signs of stagnant digestion such as bloating, constipation, or gas? Try eating parsley. Maybe you have trouble finding a good appetite. Then try eating a few sprigs of parsley before the meal is served.

FOR HEART HEALTH

Vitamin K1 supplementation has been shown to decrease coronary artery calcification in adults already showing signs of this dysfunction, and a half-cup (roughly 30 grams) of parsley leaves has 554 percent of the recommended daily allowance of vitamin K1.[1,2] No human clinical trials have been done on parsley, but because it's so high in vitamin K1 it's easy to surmise its benefits.

Parsley is also an excellent source of folate. A diet rich in folate can help keep homocysteine levels low. High levels of homocysteine are related to an increased risk of heart attacks, stroke in people with atherosclerosis, and diabetic heart disease.

We have a growing awareness that chronic inflammation in the body is a root cause of many chronic diseases, including heart disease and cancer. Eating foods high in antioxidants, like parsley, is one way we can prevent oxidative stress.[3] Further, parsley has been shown to increase the benefits of other antioxidants. Dr. Bharat Aggarwal, in his book *Healing Spices*, describes parsley as an "antioxidant helper."[4]

Parsley is used for high blood pressure (most likely due to its diuretic effect). Extracts from parsley have been shown to reduce platelet aggregation, which could potentially reduce the risk of blood clots and cardiovascular disease.[5]

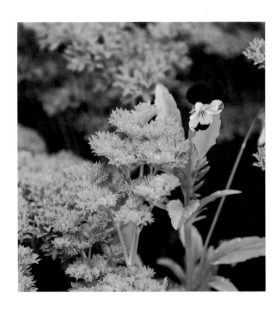

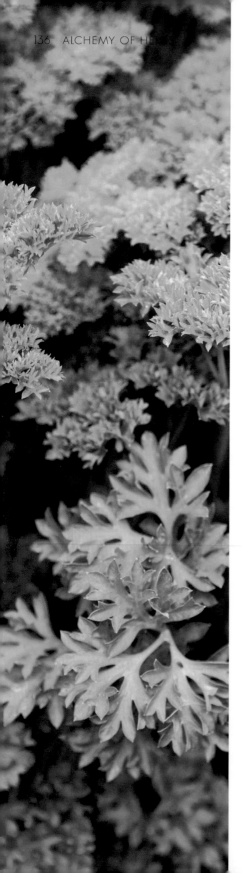

HOW TO USE PARSLEY

Parsley is best used fresh. It's easy to grow in your garden and can also be found in grocery stores all year round. When buying parsley, look for vibrant green bunches without any wilted or yellow leaves. If you aren't going to use the parsley right away, then cut ½ inch from the bottom of the stems and store it in a glass with a bit of water until ready to use.

In my home, we make an effort to get as much parsley in our diet as we can enjoy. During the hot summer months, we make salads that are at least half parsley leaves, and we regularly enjoy parsley pesto. We also like to include liberal parsley garnishes with all of our meals (think small handfuls rather than a sprig).

RECOMMENDED AMOUNTS

Parsley does not have a specific dosage. Unless you are pregnant, breastfeeding, or on blood-thinning medication, I recommend eating it in large amounts such as in a salad or pesto.

SPECIAL CONSIDERATIONS

The leaves, roots, seeds, and essential oil should be avoided in large amounts during pregnancy and lactation. (For example, avoid eating parsley pesto or salads made mostly of parsley.)

Rarely, parsley may cause a photosensitivity rash in some individuals.

Parsley is slightly blood-thinning. Avoid large amounts of parsley if you are taking blood-thinning medications.

PARSLEY AND CILANTRO PESTO

Bright, fresh, and delicious, this pesto is an easy way to get greens into your diet. I love this spread on top of meats and veggies, and it also goes well with fried or scrambled eggs. It can also be served as a dip.

Yield: approximately 1 cup

1. Place everything in a food processor and blend until smooth. Store in the refrigerator and eat within a couple of days.

2 cups lightly packed flat-leaf parsley leaves (approximately 2 ounces)

½ cup lightly packed cilantro leaves (approximately ½ ounce)

½ cup chopped walnuts

½ cup grated Parmesan cheese

2 large garlic cloves, crushed

½ teaspoon salt

1 teaspoon paprika powder

½ cup extra-virgin olive oil

1 tablespoon fresh lemon juice

1 teaspoon lemon zest

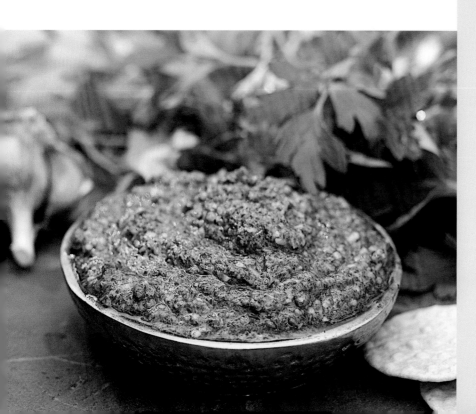

PARSLEY POTATOES

2 pounds potatoes, sliced
¼-inch thick

⅓ cup duck fat (or lard
or butter), melted

salt and pepper, to taste

2 cups finely minced
shiitake mushrooms

4 garlic cloves, minced

1 small bunch parsley, minced

This is a version of a traditional recipe that comes from central France, where it is called Pommes de Terre Sarladaises. While we were traveling through the area, a version of these potatoes was served at almost every meal. That's okay—they were delicious! What's not to love about lots of potatoes and fat seasoned with garlic and parsley?

Yield: 4 to 6 servings

1. Preheat the oven to 400°F.

2. Combine the potatoes in a large roasting pan with the melted duck fat. Add salt and pepper to taste.

3. Place the pan in the oven, and bake for 30 minutes, turning the potatoes halfway through.

4. When the potatoes are tender, add the shiitake mushrooms and garlic, then cook for another 5 minutes.

5. Remove the pan from the oven, and stir in the parsley. Serve immediately.

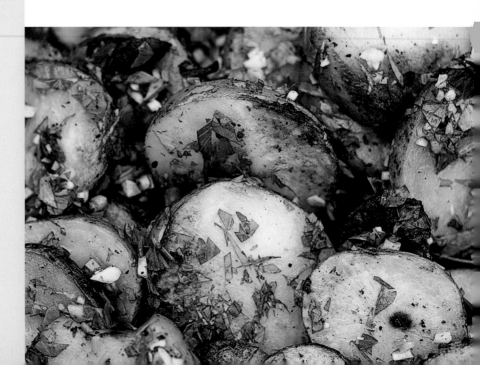

MUSTARD VINAIGRETTE SALAD DRESSING WITH PARSLEY

This is our family's favorite salad dressing. Besides loving the taste, we think it's a great way to enjoy the pungent flavors of mustard, garlic, and the blend of herbs. We especially love it on parsley salads, on salmon, and with artichokes. Try using an herbal-infused apple cider vinegar such as Fire Cider (page 56) or Hawthorn Vinegar (page 217).

Yield: ⅓ cup

1. Mix all the ingredients together, stirring until blended. Use immediately or store in the refrigerator for up to three days.

3 tablespoons olive oil

1 tablespoon apple cider vinegar (herb infused, if possible)

1 teaspoon prepared mustard (store-bought or Homemade Mustard, page 121)

1 teaspoon miso

1 garlic clove, smashed and minced

2 teaspoons dried parsley

1 teaspoon dried thyme

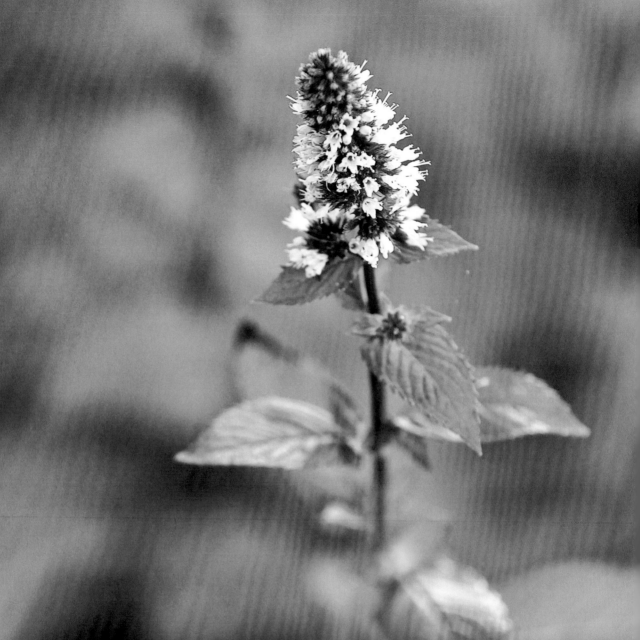

"EVER WONDER AT THE TRADITION OF A COMPLIMENTARY MINT AT THE END OF A MEAL? MINT STIMULATES DIGESTION AND RELIEVES NAUSEA—IT HELPS DISPEL THAT OVERFULL FEELING AND POSSIBLE INDIGESTION OR GAS."

—JOYCE WARDWELL, HERBALIST AND AUTHOR OF *THE HERBAL HOME REMEDY BOOK*

CHAPTER 16

Peppermint

Peppermint is popular! If someone has only one herbal tea in the house, it most often is peppermint. It's famous in candies such as peppermint drops and candy canes and is a frequent flavoring in chewing gum, liqueurs, and even over-the-counter medicine.

When is the last time you had a strong brew of peppermint tea? If it has been a while, I recommend trying some now. Drinking hot peppermint tea is a fun experience in herbal energetics. What you might notice is that even though you are drinking a hot tea, you'll feel a distinctly cooling feeling travel from your mouth to your esophagus and into your stomach. Go on, drink some more. You truly have to feel this sensation in order to fully appreciate it. This distinctly cooling action is due to the plant's high menthol content. This volatile oil is present in many mints and is one way this plant offers us powerful medicine.

Botanical name: *Mentha x piperita*

Family: Lamiaceae

Parts used: aerial portions (mainly leaves, flowers)

Energetics: variable: warming to cooling, drying

Taste: pungent

Plant properties: aromatic, carminative, analgesic, stimulating nervine, antispasmodic, stimulating diaphoretic, antiemetic

Plant uses: stomach upset, hiccups, bad breath, colds, flu, fever, sinus congestion, gas, nausea, spasms, headaches, externally to soothe itching and inflammation of the skin

Plant preparations: tea, tincture, wash, essential oil, culinary

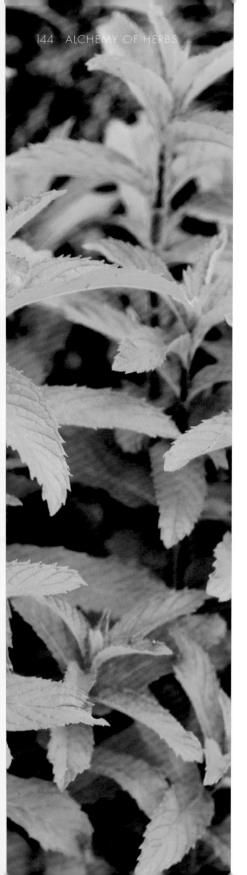

HOW TO USE PEPPERMINT

Both fresh and dried peppermint leaves work equally well for all purposes. If substituting one for the other in a recipe, use twice as much fresh herb than dried.

Peppermint makes a delicious tea, which can be enjoyed simply for taste or to improve digestion. Infuse 1 to 3 teaspoons or more of dried leaves into 1 cup of just-boiled water, and allow to steep for 3 to 5 minutes in a covered container to decrease the loss of volatile oils.

The peppermint leaves can also be used to create a poultice or fomentation.

The scent of peppermint essential oil can be inhaled to break up lung congestion, and the oil can be used externally in ointments or taken internally. (Consuming essential oil can cause serious problems if used incorrectly, so please use caution and work with an experienced practitioner.)

You can infuse peppermint leaves into oil to rub onto sore muscles for relief from pain and cramping.

RECOMMENDED AMOUNTS

The therapeutic amount for peppermint is:

As tea: 1 to 3 teaspoons (dried) or 2 to 6 teaspoons (fresh), 3 to 5 times per day

As tincture: 1:5, 30% alcohol, 3 to 6 mL, 2 or 3 times daily[10]

SPECIAL CONSIDERATIONS

Peppermint can cause or exacerbate heartburn in some sensitive individuals, so avoid it if you have active symptoms of GERD (gastroesophageal reflux disease).

Taken in excess, it could dry up breast milk.

MINT RAITA

This simple yogurt salad is a nice side dish to spicy entrées or hearty soups. I often make this in the summer when the garden is bursting with cucumbers and peppermint. (If peppermint is not available, spearmint [*Mentha spicata*] will do in a pinch.) I love that I can whip it up in just a few minutes, and it can also be made in advance for a gathering. The optional cayenne gives this a little bit of a spicy kick.

Yield: 3 cups

1. Combine all the ingredients except the paprika in a medium bowl. Mix well.

2. Store in the fridge and eat within 3 days. Sprinkle with paprika powder just before serving.

1 large unpeeled cucumber, seeded and chopped into cubes

2 cups plain whole-milk yogurt

½ cup (packed) chopped fresh peppermint

2 tablespoons fresh chopped chives (or green parts of scallions)

1 garlic clove, smashed and minced

1 teaspoon ground cumin

¼ teaspoon cayenne pepper (optional)

salt and pepper, to taste

paprika, for garnish

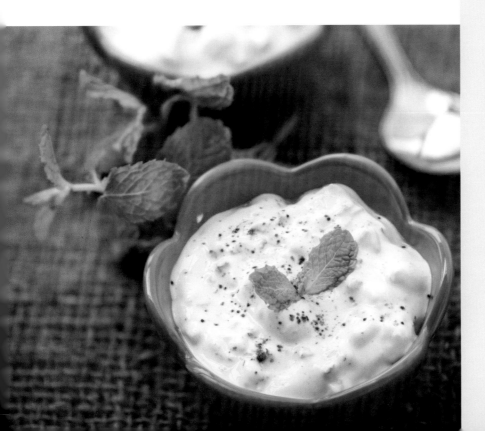

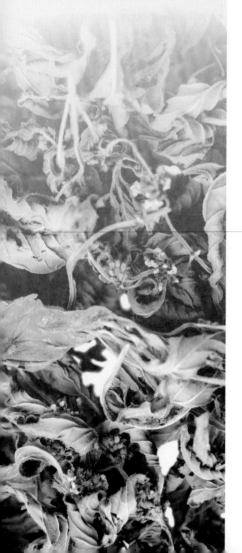

¼ cup dried peppermint
leaves (9 grams)

PEPPERMINT FOMENTATION
FOR HEADACHES

A fomentation is a simple preparation that helps you get herbs directly to the area that needs it most. Applying peppermint to the forehead or to the back of the neck can help relieve the pain of a headache.

Yield: 1 application

1. Bring 1 cup of water to a boil, then remove from the heat and add the peppermint. Stir well and then let steep, covered, for 10 minutes.

2. Strain the leaves out, and soak a cloth in the water once it is slightly cooled. (I like this to be as warm as possible without causing discomfort.) Wring out the cloth and apply it to your forehead or the back of your neck. If heat feels good, apply a hot water bottle over the cloth.

3. Keep the cloth on for 20 minutes, or as desired. An important part of this headache remedy is to lie down and rest with your eyes closed during this time.

PEPPERMINT AND HIBISCUS COOLER

One summer, temperatures regularly reached over 100°F, with humidity under 15 percent. In other words, it was extremely hot and dry. My husband and I survived with daily trips to our favorite mid-Alpine lake, bringing this iced tea with us. As soon as I created this recipe, I became obsessed with it! The cooling aromatics of peppermint and the slightly sour, tangy hibiscus will quench your thirst.

Yield: 8 cups

1. Bring 1½ quarts of water to a boil.

2. Place the peppermint, hibiscus, and lavender in a jar at least 2 quarts in size. (I like to use a large measuring glass to facilitate pouring later.)

3. Pour the boiling water over the herbs, then stir. Let this steep for 10 to 15 minutes, covered.

4. Strain into a large glass pitcher that gives you plenty of extra room to add ice later. (I use a strainer and a funnel.) While still warm, add the honey and stir until it is fully combined with the tea. Let cool on the counter or in the refrigerator.

5. About 10 to 20 minutes before serving, add ice to the top of the pitcher. Drink within 24 hours.

20 grams minced fresh peppermint, or ¼ cup dried peppermint (9 grams)

1 heaping tablespoon dried hibiscus (5 grams)

1 sprig of fresh lavender or a pinch of dried lavender flowers

1 tablespoon honey, or to taste

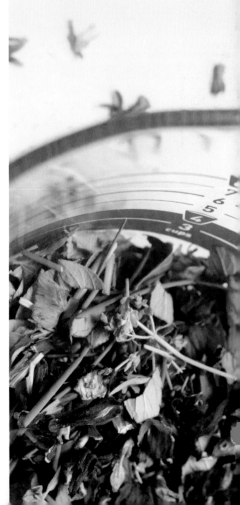

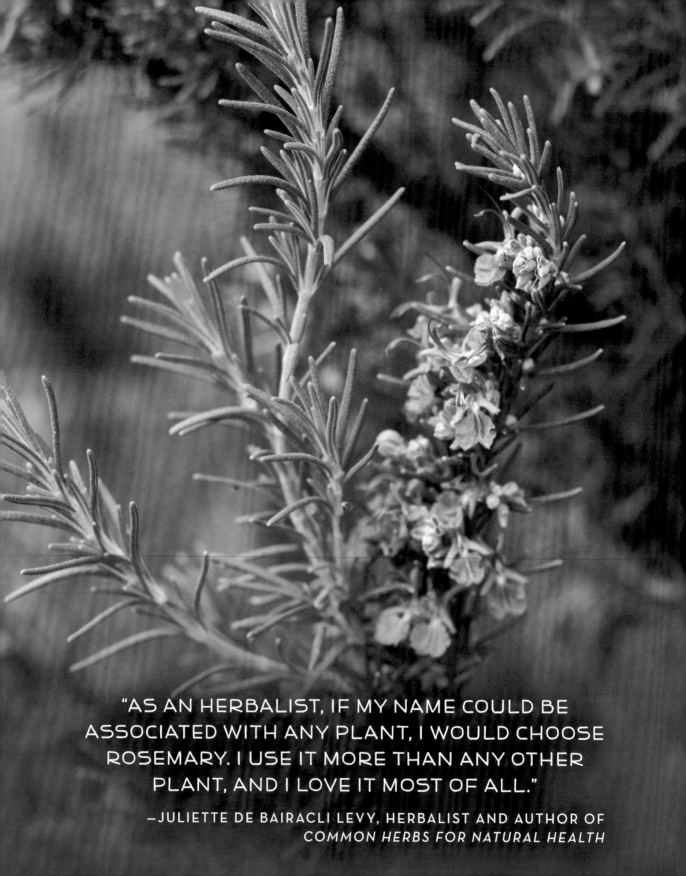

"AS AN HERBALIST, IF MY NAME COULD BE ASSOCIATED WITH ANY PLANT, I WOULD CHOOSE ROSEMARY. I USE IT MORE THAN ANY OTHER PLANT, AND I LOVE IT MOST OF ALL."

—JULIETTE DE BAIRACLI LEVY, HERBALIST AND AUTHOR OF *COMMON HERBS FOR NATURAL HEALTH*

CHAPTER 17

Rosemary

Right after teaching my first herbal intensive in southern France, I headed south to the famous Mediterranean coves, called calanques, near Marseilles. By the time I arrived, in early June, the rocky limestone soil was dry, with only the hardiest of plants peeking through. Undeterred by the sparse plant life, I set off on a short trail that steeply climbed up a hill. At the top, I was gifted a beautiful view of the deep-blue Mediterranean Sea.

After catching my breath, I quickly realized I had a treasure at my feet; rosemary was growing in dense patches all around me. I reached down and rubbed the leaves and was immediately rewarded with its powerful scent. Standing on a hillside on the coast of the Mediterranean, I was easily able to imagine what inspired its genus name, *Rosmarinus*, which means "dew of the sea."

Science has recently taken an interest in rosemary to boost cognition and as an antioxidant. In fact, we could easily call rosemary the "queen of antioxidants." But herbalists have long celebrated rosemary for its gently warming and dispersing effects, which bring benefits to the heart, digestion, liver, and mood.

Botanical name: *Salvia rosmarinus*

Family: Lamiaceae

Parts used: leaves

Energetics: warming, drying

Taste: pungent

Plant properties: aromatic, carminative, circulatory stimulant, hepatic, antimicrobial, stimulating/relaxing nervine, antioxidant

Plant uses: mental stimulation, digestion, colds/flu, fungal infections, hair wash, food preservation, skin protection

Plant preparations: culinary, tea, tincture, herbal steam

Rosemary is a small, woody evergreen shrub whose native habitat stretches across the Mediterranean region, where it thrives in harsh conditions and rocky soils. It's a member of the aromatic mint family (Lamiaceae), and its pleasing scent and taste have inspired humans through the ages. Besides being a common culinary ingredient, the plant was used as perfume and mentioned by Shakespeare in numerous plays.

The common English name, rosemary, is sometimes associated with the Virgin Mary. It's said that on her family's flight to Egypt, a rosemary bush sheltered and protected them. When Mary laid her cloak upon the bush, the white flowers turned blue and thus became the "rose of Mary."

MEDICINAL PROPERTIES AND ENERGETICS OF ROSEMARY

Rosemary blends really well with various meats. Before the widespread use of refrigerators, rosemary was rubbed into meats to prevent them from spoiling. Modern research has shown that rosemary does, in fact, prolong the quality and shelf life of meats through inhibiting the growth of bacteria.[1]

Rosemary also has the ability to reduce the risk of cancer from eating meats cooked on high heat. High-heat cooking methods, such as pan frying or grilling, creates compounds that have been shown to alter DNA and lead to cancer. In one study, researchers added rosemary extract to meats during cooking, and found that the high antioxidant content helped prevent the formation of these carcinogenic compounds.[2] While it would be best to avoid meats cooked at high temperatures, this illustrates rosemary's protective effects, which assuredly go far beyond charred meats.

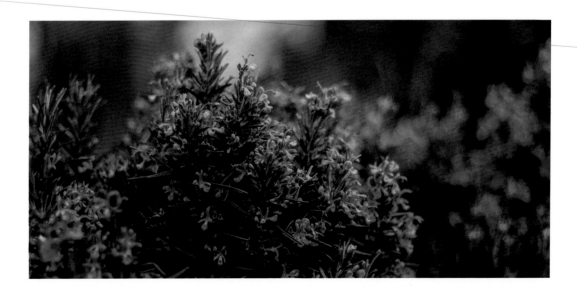

FOR SKIN PROTECTION

Rosemary extracts have also been shown to be helpful against the sun's UV damage. We all know about the importance of covering up or using safe sunscreens to protect against sunburn, but in one interesting study, researchers showed that taking an extract of rosemary and lemon internally decreased UV damage in humans. People taking these extracts saw good results after 8 weeks and even stronger results after 12 weeks.[3] (Rosemary is used in the Elderflower Facial Serum on page 208 and Green Tea and Rose Facial Cream on page 246.)

FOR HEART HEALTH

While not thought of as a primary herb for the heart, rosemary can be used to increase circulation and decrease inflammation in the cardiovascular system. British herbalist Jeremy Ross recommends rosemary combined with hawthorn for people with cardiac weakness alongside depression.[4]

FOR REDUCING PAIN

Like most herbs used for decreasing pain, rosemary seems to work in a variety of ways. As we've already discussed, rosemary is high in antioxidants, which can decrease oxidative stress and inflammation. It has long been used for inflammatory pain such as arthritis. Herbalists recommend both taking it internally and using it externally over the affected areas. One scientific study has validated this use and showed that a proprietary extract of rosemary decreased arthritic pain in human volunteers. It also decreased their levels of C-reactive protein, which is a marker for systemic inflammation that leads to pain.[5]

Another study looked at the effects of inhaling rosemary essential oil. The researchers concluded that while it didn't directly relieve pain, it improved the patient's experience of it.[6]

FOR MEMORY

Rosemary is famously called the herb of remembrance and has long been used as a symbolic way to remember a loved one or event, such as in weddings and funerals. It was traditionally used to improve memory, and herbalists often recommend that students smell a sprig while studying and then again while taking their exams. I've heard this tradition goes as far back as ancient Greece! Science has since validated that smelling rosemary essential oils reduces test anxiety and can significantly enhance memory.[7, 8, 9]

Not only does rosemary help with short-term memory, it may also have a role in preventing and addressing Alzheimer's, which affects an estimated 1 in 9 people in the United States over the age of 65 and nearly 44 million people worldwide.[10] In one short-term study, as little as 750 mg dose of dried rosemary had a significant beneficial effect on cognitive function in an elderly population.[11] Another study showed that

Alzheimer's patients experienced cognitive benefits by simply smelling the essential oil.[12] Rosemary, along with a holistic protocol, shows promising results for addressing this debilitating disease.

FOR DIGESTIVE ISSUES

Like other culinary herbs in the aromatic mint family, rosemary made into a tea can ease slow or cold digestion that is causing gas, nausea, cramping, or bloating. This herb is warming, and its milder energetic qualities allow it be enjoyed in moderate quantities with fewer adverse effects versus the hot energetics of ginger, garlic, and cayenne.

One reason that rosemary is often paired with fatty meats like lamb—along with the delicious taste combination—is for its ability to support the liver and help digest fats.

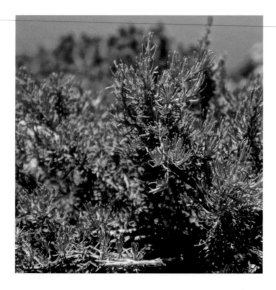

FOR COLDS AND THE FLU

Delicious and warming rosemary tea can bring welcome relief during cold and flu season. Relieve a sore throat with sips of rosemary tea or a spoonful of rosemary-infused honey. Drinking hot rosemary tea helps to warm you up during the first stages of a fever, when you feel cold and are shivering. It can also be a supportive herb in helping with stagnant congestion in the sinuses and lungs. (For this effect it combines well with ginger.)

FOR HAIR LOSS

One randomized, double-blind study split 86 patients with hair loss (alopecia areata) into two groups. One group was given a blend of essential oils that included rosemary to rub into the scalp. The other group was given an oil without essential oils. After seven weeks almost half of the people in the essential oil group showed improvement in hair growth, while only 6 percent showed improvement in the control group.[13]

To encourage hair growth, herbalist Lesley Tierra recommends a blend of 2 teaspoons of rosemary essential oil, 2 teaspoons of lavender essential oil, ½ ounce of cayenne tincture, and a pint of sesame oil. She suggests regularly massaging a bit into the scalp and letting it sit for a while.[14]

HOW TO USE ROSEMARY

Rosemary is often used as an essential oil, and the leaves can be enjoyed both fresh and dried. The most important thing is that it have strong aromatics. See the recipe on page 154 for the perfect cup of rosemary tea.

RECOMMENDED AMOUNTS

Using culinary amounts of rosemary is a great way to enjoy its flavor and improve digestion.

The therapeutic amount for rosemary is:

As tea (dried or fresh): 2 to 4 grams, up to 3 times per day

As tincture (dried herb): 1:5, 40% alcohol: 2 to 4 mL, 3 times per day[15]

SPECIAL CONSIDERATIONS

During pregnancy and breastfeeding, it is safest to avoid rosemary in large doses. Normal culinary amounts are fine. The essential oil should also be avoided.[16]

Rosemary may lower blood glucose. Those taking insulin should continue to monitor their blood glucose levels.[17]

A very small percentage of people have skin dermatitis when exposed to rosemary.[18]

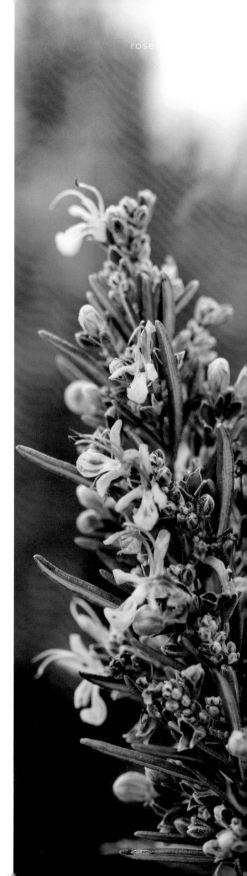

THE PERFECT CUP OF ROSEMARY TEA

1 tablespoon fresh rosemary leaves (twig removed)

This recipe comes from my friend and colleague Christophe Bernard. He's an herbalist and author who lives in the South of France, where rosemary grows in its native habitat. This perfect cup of rosemary tea features a very short steeping time, which will bring out the aromatics but not the tannins and bitters, which makes a lighter, more pleasant rosemary tea.

It's also important not to use water any hotter than 185°F or it will destroy some of the aromatic qualities. To do this easily, you can use a thermometer and a clock to figure out how long it takes for your boiled water to cool to this temperature. Then, the next times you boil water, you can set a timer to count down for this length of time. You can see more from Christophe at www.AltheaProvence.com.

Yield: 1 cup

1. Place your rosemary leaves in a tea mug. (Because the leaves are so thin, there is no need to chop them.)

2. Boil 1 cup water, then let the water cool to 185°F (85°C).

3. Pour the water over the rosemary and infuse, covered, for 3 or 4 minutes. Strain and enjoy.

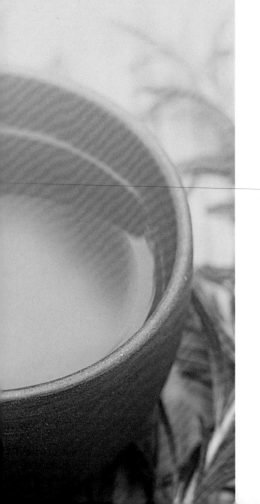

ROSEMARY TAPENADE

Tapenades are a traditional French preparation that combines a blend of olives and herbs to make a savory, salty spread. It's served before or alongside a meal. I love generously spreading some on a crusty baguette.

I suggest using pitted olives that have been stored in oil or dry cured. Choose high-quality olives for this recipe; I like to use 1 cup of niçoise olives and 1 cup of green olives.

Yield: 1½ cups

2 cups olives

1 tablespoon capers

2 anchovy filets preserved in olive oil

2 tablespoons lemon juice

2 tablespoons roasted tomatoes (I buy these in a jar)

3 garlic cloves

1½ tablespoons minced fresh rosemary

1½ tablespoons minced fresh thyme

2 tablespoons olive oil (approximately)

1. Assemble all of the ingredients with the exception of the olive oil and place them in a food processor or blender. Process until thoroughly mixed and the olives are broken into small but discernible chunks.

2. Slowly add the oil into the mix, continuing to process until the mixture forms a thick paste. Go slowly; it's easy to overdo it with the olive oil. (However, it won't be disastrous if you add too much; your mixture will just have excess oil around the edges.)

3. Serve this with bread or crackers or even on veggies or meats. It will keep in the fridge for about 1 week.

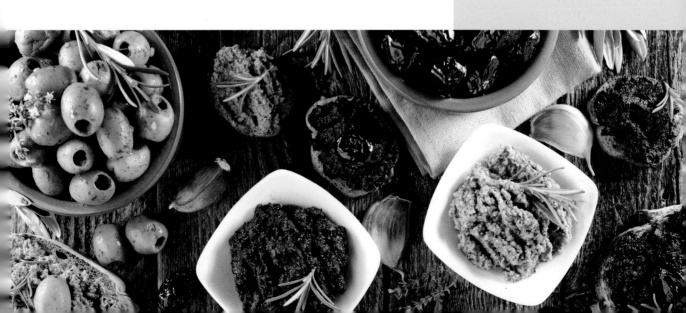

1 (3.5-oz.) jar anchovies preserved in olive oil

2 tablespoons olive oil

3 cloves garlic, minced

3 tablespoons minced fresh rosemary

4 lamb steaks (about 1½ pounds total)

ROSEMARY LAMB

I first ate a version of this dish at my bridal shower, and it's been a family favorite ever since. The aromatic and pungent flavors of the rosemary and garlic tame the strong taste of the lamb, while the anchovies give it a succulent, salty quality. The combined result is a delicious, hearty comfort food.

Yield: 4 servings

1.   Drain and mince the anchovies.

2.   In an 8 x 8-inch baking dish, combine the minced anchovies, olive oil, garlic, and rosemary. Crush everything together with a fork until it forms a thick paste.

3.   Make deep slits in the lamb with a sharp knife. Place the steaks in the baking dish and rub the marinade all over the meat, making sure it gets into the slits. Let marinate for about an hour at room temperature.

4.   Preheat the oven to 400°F. Drain the excess marinade from the baking dish, leaving the meat behind. Discard the marinade.

5.   Place the dish in the oven and bake for 35 minutes, or until a meat thermometer reads 125°F in the thickest part of the meat.

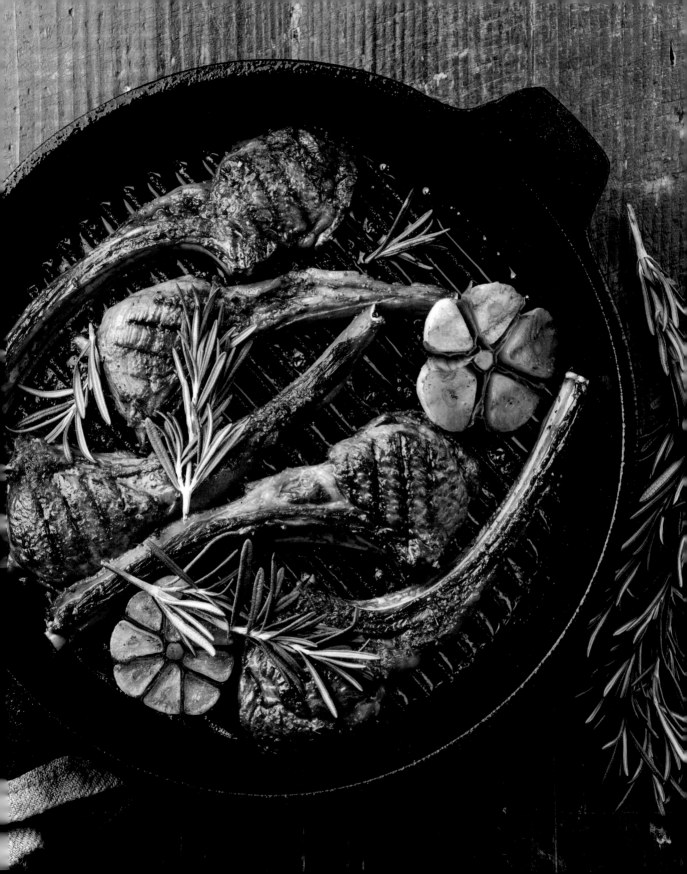

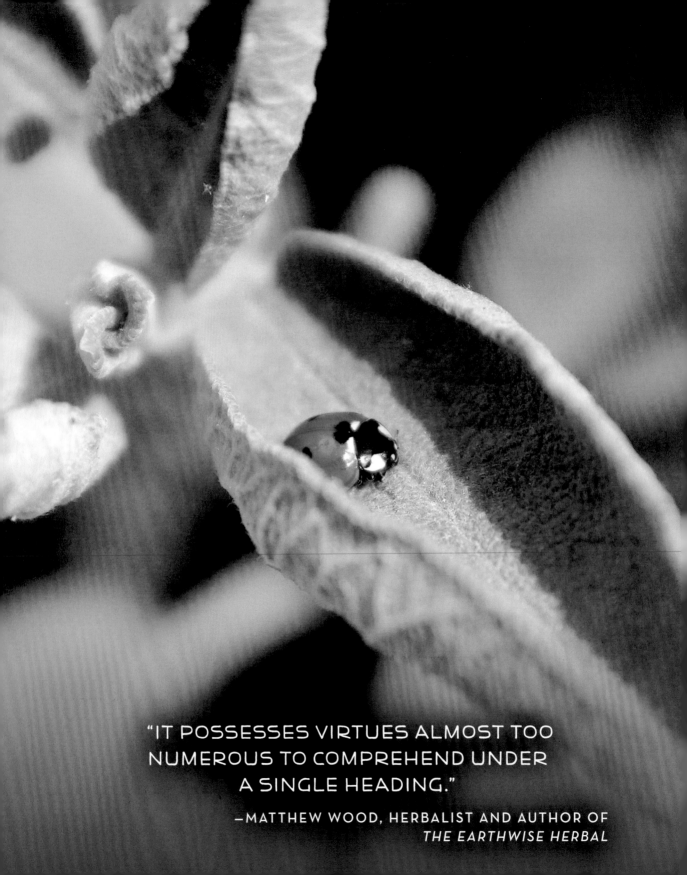

"IT POSSESSES VIRTUES ALMOST TOO
NUMEROUS TO COMPREHEND UNDER
A SINGLE HEADING."

—MATTHEW WOOD, HERBALIST AND AUTHOR OF
THE EARTHWISE HERBAL

CHAPTER 18

Sage

For most people in the United States, sage's usefulness begins and ends with Thanksgiving turkey stuffing. But while sage has been pigeonholed as a one-meal wonder in modern times, it has been revered for centuries for its wide range of abilities, from aiding digestion to healing wounds to stopping excessive secretions. New research is also showing that sage can be used to support a healthy mind and heart, two major concerns for our elder population. It's time to pull sage to the forefront of the spice cabinet and enjoy it regularly in foods as well as teas.

Botanical name: *Salvia officinalis*

Family: Lamiaceae

Parts used: aerial portions

Energetics: warming, drying

Taste: pungent, bitter

Plant properties: aromatic, astringent, carminative, diaphoretic, antiseptic, blood moving

Plant uses: sore throat, excessive sweating, infections, stagnant digestion, type 2 diabetes, hot flashes, toothache, sore muscles, high cholesterol, Alzheimer's

Plant preparations: tea, culinary, tincture, tooth powder, facial steam, essential oil

The genus name for sage is *Salvia*, which comes from the Latin root for "safe" or "healthy." Maud Grieve wrote in *A Modern Herbal* that sage was even sometimes known as *Salvia Salvatrix* or Sage the Savior.[1]

MEDICINAL PROPERTIES AND ENERGETICS OF SAGE

Sage is an astringent herb, and many of its beneficial effects are due to this plant action. Even if you are unfamiliar with the word, you've probably experienced astringency in your life. If you've ever bitten into an unripe banana or drunk a strong cup of black tea, then you've felt the astringent action. It is often described as a dry sensation in the mouth, but astringent herbs, like sage, actually tighten the mucosal tissues they come in contact with. This tightening and toning can be a valuable part of healing leaky or lax tissues. We'll explore this important herbal action more in the Sour section of this book, but it's important to be familiar with this as we explore the beneficial qualities of sage.

FOR IMPROVED COGNITION

In medieval times there was a saying, *"Cur moriatur homo cui salvia crescit in horto?"* which translates to "Why should a man die while sage grows in his garden?" Dr. Bharat Aggarwal, author of *Healing Spices*, points out that a 21st-century scientist might ask, "Why should he or she have memory loss when sage is available?"[2]

Indeed, sage has been shown to have beneficial effects on memory and attention in people with memory loss and Alzheimer's symptoms. One explanation for this is sage's anticholinesterase properties. I know that's a mouthful, so let's take a closer look. Acetylcholine is a chemical in the brain that supports both memory and cognition. In patients with Alzheimer's disease, acetylcholine breaks down, and less of it is produced over time. Both of these actions

result in a gradual loss of memory. An anticholinesterase is something that inhibits the breakdown of acetylcholine.

In one randomized, placebo-controlled, double-blind study, researchers showed that an extract of sage improves memory and attention in healthy older volunteers.[3] Another study gave sage extract to people with mild to moderate symptoms of Alzheimer's disease. After four months, those taking the sage extract showed a significant improvement in cognitive functions and less agitation as compared with the placebo group.[4] Sage has also been shown to improve both memory and mood in younger populations.[5]

John Gerard, an English herbalist who lived in the late 16th and early 17th centuries, wrote in his book, *The Herbal*, "Sage is singular good for the head and braine; it quickneth the sences and memory, strengthneth the sinewes, restoreth health to those that have the palsie upon a moist cause, takes away shaking or trembling of the members; and being put up into the nosthrils, it draweth thin flegme out of the head."[6]

FOR IMPROVING CHOLESTEROL AND DIABETES MARKERS

Even small amounts of sage extract have been shown to have positive effects on blood sugar, cholesterol, and triglyceride levels in people diagnosed with type 2 diabetes.[7] In one small study, healthy women drank sage tea (made with 300 milliliters of water and 4 grams of sage) twice daily. After four weeks they had a significant reduction in total cholesterol numbers and in LDL-C ("bad" cholesterol), while HDL-C ("good" cholesterol) increased. Beneficial effects were also shown in antioxidant defenses. All women completed the trial and reported no adverse effects. Because high cholesterol and inflammation are common aspects of insulin resistance, the researchers hypothesize that sage could be safe and beneficial for people with insulin resistance and diabetes.[8]

FOR SORE THROATS AND ORAL HEALTH

Sage has long been loved by herbalists for its ability to soothe a sore throat. While it may have many beneficial actions for doing this, one is that it tightens and tones swollen tissues, bringing relief. Science has since validated this old tradition.

In one randomized, double-blind trial, researchers compared the effects of a sage and echinacea extract on sore throats with the effects of a spray made up of the antiseptic chlorhexidine and the anesthetic lidocaine. For reducing sore throat symptoms, the sage/echinacea extract showed slightly better results after three days.[9] Another study showed that a fluid extract of sage worked better than a placebo in reducing pain due to viral pharyngitis (a throat infection).[10]

Another area that can often benefit from sage's tightening and toning of tissues is the mouth. Sage is a common ingredient in many herbal tooth powder and mouthwash recipes, and it can be used to relieve pain and heal mouth ulcers, canker sores, bleeding gums, spongy gums, and cold sores.

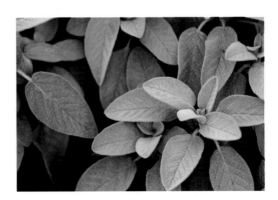

FOR MENOPAUSE

Sage is well known for stopping excessive sweating in women with common menopausal complaints such as night sweats and hot flashes. Herbalists recommend sage as a tea or tincture, either alone or combined with other herbs.

In 2011 researchers validated this tradition in a multicenter clinical trial in Switzerland. During this eight-week study, participants took a tablet of fresh sage leaves and reported a significant reduction in the intensity and frequency of their hot flashes. The researchers reported that "the mean total number of hot flushes per day decreased significantly each week from week 1 to 8. The mean number of mild, moderate, severe, and very severe flushes decreased by 46%, 62%, 79%, and 100% over 8 weeks, respectively."[11]

FOR DIGESTION

The taste of sage is both bitter and pungent. Often when we encounter these two tastes together in one plant, we know the plant can be used to promote digestion. Sage is a wonderful carminative for easing gas and bloating, moving stagnant digestion, and relieving painful cramping in the gut.

Sage is especially appropriate for people who cannot digest fats well. It can be taken as a tea before or after a meal, or simply used as a spice within the meal. Sage has long been paired with heavy meats such as duck and sausage in order to help digest them more easily.

FOR SKIN CONDITIONS

Sage is rich in compounds with high antioxidant and anti-inflammatory effects. Research has shown that sage extract, applied topically, has a similar effect to that of hydrocortisone and could be useful for treating inflammatory skin conditions.[12]

The appearance of varicose veins can be reduced through a topical spray of sage-infused witch hazel. To make this infusion, lightly pack a small jar with dried sage leaves, and then fill the jar with witch hazel distillate (commonly available at pharmacies). Stir well, let sit for 4 weeks, then strain. Spray onto affected areas as often as desired.

HOW TO USE SAGE

Sage works great as a dried or fresh herb. You can also purchase fresh herbs and dry the leaves yourself for later use. As with most aromatic herbs, the most important thing is that it both smell and taste vibrant. For culinary use, sage pairs well with poultry and makes a great tea. (I include a recipe for Sage-Lemon Tea in this chapter.)

Herbalists often use sage as a tea or tincture for internal use, but sage tea can also be strained and poured over the scalp as a treatment for dandruff.

Powdered sage leaves can be made into a tooth powder that is both astringent (great for weak or swollen gums) and antimicrobial. To make your own tooth powder, finely grind dried sage leaves and then dip your wet toothbrush into the powder. Brush as you would normally.

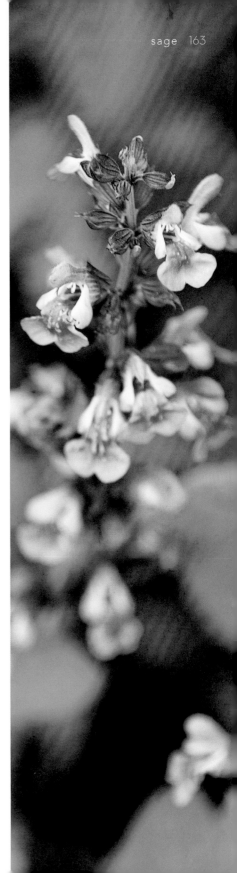

Sage can be infused into oil, which can relieve pain and increase circulation when massaged into achy and cold joints. To make sage oil, lightly pack a small jar with freshly dried sage leaves and then fill the jar with oil. Stir well. Let this sit for 4 weeks, then strain. Use as often as desired.

Sage has several uses as a vinegar infusion. Diluted with 50 percent water, this can be sprayed topically to reduce the pain of sunburns or used as a scalp rinse to treat dandruff. To make sage vinegar, lightly pack a small jar with freshly dried sage leaves, and then fill the jar with vinegar. Stir well and cover with a glass or plastic lid. If using a metal lid, place parchment or wax paper between the lid and the jar (vinegar will corrode metal). Let this mixture sit for 4 weeks, then strain. Use as often as desired.

RECOMMENDED AMOUNTS

Sage can be enjoyed in culinary amounts for its delicious taste and for improving minor digestive complaints.

The therapeutic amount for sage is:

As tea (dried): 1 to 2 grams, 2 to 3 times per day

As tincture: 1:5, 30% alcohol, 1.5 to 2 mL, 3 times per day[13]

SPECIAL CONSIDERATIONS

Sage is not recommended in large amounts in pregnancy.

Sage can dry up the flow of milk during lactation, so unless a mother wishes to wean, it is not recommended in large amounts while breastfeeding.

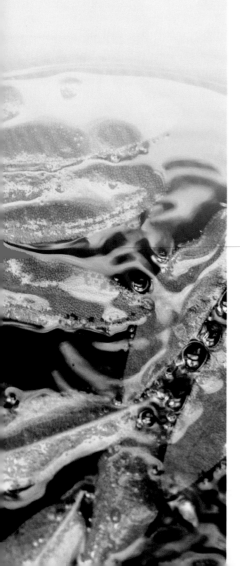

2 to 4 tablespoons
coconut oil

20 whole fresh
sage leaves

FRIED SAGE LEAVES

Fried sage leaves are crisp and delicious. They make a simple garnish that adds a unique taste to meals and cheese plates. I like to use coconut oil for frying, but any oil with a high heat tolerance will work well. If you are using fresh-picked sage leaves, let them wilt for a couple of hours before using.

Yield: 20 sage leaves

1. Heat the oil in a small frying pan on medium-high heat. (I use a small cast iron pan.) The amount of oil you use will depend on the size of your pan. Melt enough so that the leaves are submerged, but not much more than that. Keep an eye on the heat; if the oil smokes, reduce the temperature.

2. To determine if the oil is hot enough, drop a small leaf into the oil. If it sizzles, it's ready! To fry the leaves simply drop them in the oil for about 20 to 30 seconds and then, using a fork or tongs, flip them over for another 15 seconds or so.

3. Once fried, transfer them to a plate lined with paper towels or cloth to soak up excess oil. Eat when cool.

SAGE-LEMON TEA

Sage tea is a simple and delicious way to enjoy the many benefits of sage. Try this before or after a meal to support your digestion. I also like it iced in the summer.

Yield: 1¼ cups

1 tablespoon crumbled dried sage leaves

thin slice of lemon

honey, to taste (optional)

1.   Bring 1¼ cups of water to a boil. Place the lemon and sage leaves in a tea mug or large infuser. Avoid cramming the herbs into a small tea infuser; it's better for them to have room to expand and move around.

2.   Pour the just-boiled water over the sage and lemon. Steep, covered, for 5 minutes.

3.   Strain and add honey to taste.

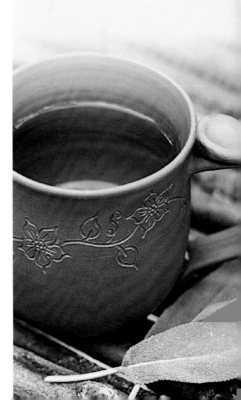

SAGE CHICKEN

1 onion, thinly sliced

2 tablespoons olive oil

salt and freshly ground
pepper, to taste

2 tablespoons minced fresh
sage leaves

2 garlic cloves, minced

¼ cup butter, softened

2 pounds chicken thighs,
with skin

1 lemon, thinly sliced
into rounds

I learned this sage butter technique from one of my favorite
authors and bloggers, Jenny McGruther of NourishedKitchen
.com. Sage pairs very nicely with poultry and gives this dish a
fresh and succulent flavor.

Yield: 4 servings

1. Preheat the oven to 350°F.

2. Place the onion in a small casserole baking dish and toss
    with olive oil, salt, and pepper.

3. In a separate bowl, combine the sage leaves, garlic, and
    butter. Use a knife to gently separate the chicken skin from
    the meat without detaching it. Spread the sage and garlic
    butter evenly on all the chicken thighs, between the meat
    and the skin.

4. Place the chicken on top of the onion in the baking dish.
    Sprinkle the chicken with more salt and pepper, to taste.
    Cover the chicken with thin slices of lemon.

5. Place the dish in the oven and bake for approximately 40
    minutes, or until the chicken is cooked through (when the
    center of the chicken reads 165°F on a meat thermometer).

6. Remove the lemons from the chicken and set aside. Broil the
    chicken for 2 minutes, or until the skin is golden and crisp.

7. Remove the dish from the oven, and serve the chicken with
    the reserved lemon slices.

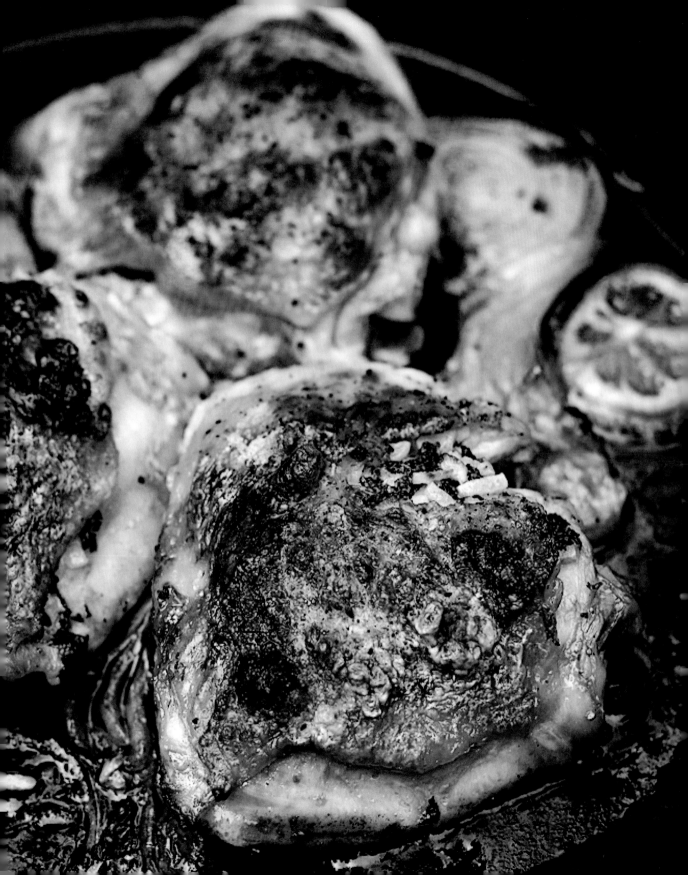

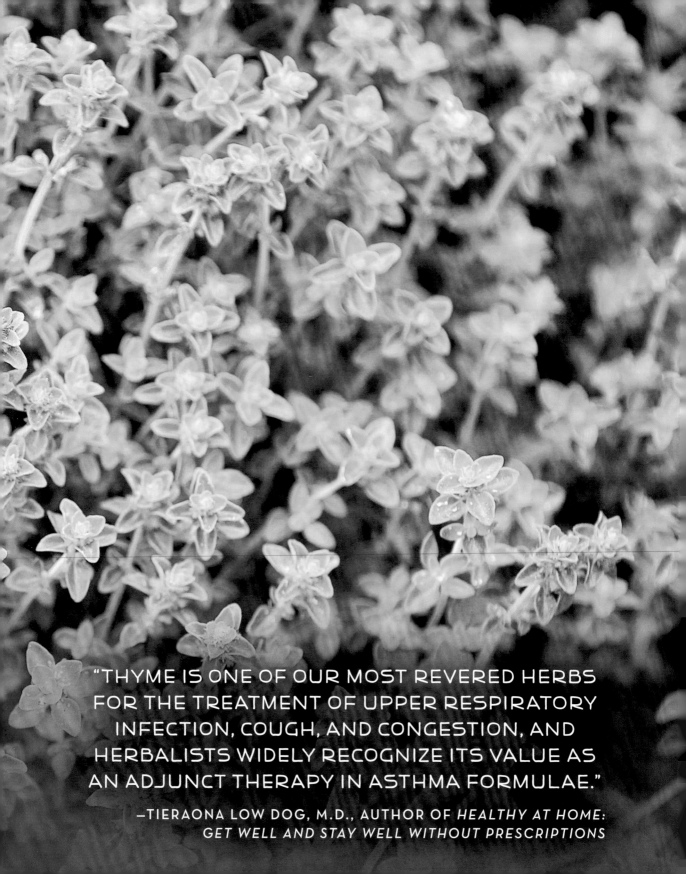

"THYME IS ONE OF OUR MOST REVERED HERBS FOR THE TREATMENT OF UPPER RESPIRATORY INFECTION, COUGH, AND CONGESTION, AND HERBALISTS WIDELY RECOGNIZE ITS VALUE AS AN ADJUNCT THERAPY IN ASTHMA FORMULAE."

—TIERAONA LOW DOG, M.D., AUTHOR OF *HEALTHY AT HOME: GET WELL AND STAY WELL WITHOUT PRESCRIPTIONS*

CHAPTER 19

Thyme

Several years ago I was hiking in southern Provence with a friend and fellow herbalist, Christophe Bernard. When Christophe, who's always about 10 steps ahead on the trail, suddenly and excitedly called out to me, I hurried to catch up and see what he had found. Growing about six inches off the ground, with lots of tiny leaves, was wild thyme. We both crouched down to get a better view.

After meeting this little plant, I finally understood why many herbalists differentiate between using wild thyme and garden thyme: the aroma of those tiny leaves was incredibly strong, and the flavor was a lot spicier and hotter than the garden variety. With just one taste, I knew there was a lot of potent medicine in this small and unassuming plant.

Botanical name: *Thymus vulgaris*

Family: Lamiaceae

Parts used: leaves

Energetics: warming, drying

Taste: pungent

Plant properties: aromatic, antimicrobial, carminative, stimulating/relaxing diaphoretic, antispasmodic, expectorant, emmenagogue, vermifuge

Plant uses: infections, symptoms of colds and flu (fever, sore throat, cough), urinary tract infections, yeast infections, topical fungal infections, dyspepsia, wounds, burns, toothaches, congested sinuses, mouthwash, inflammation, whooping cough, digestive spasms, menstrual cramps, amenorrhea

Plant preparations: infused honey, infused vinegar, tincture, steam inhalation, infused oil and salve, culinary spice, cough syrup, douche

Thyme's native habitat is southern Europe and the Mediterranean, where it grows wild in hard, rocky soil. This well-loved plant was domesticated and now grows in gardens around the world.

There are hundreds of different varieties of thyme, and most of them can be used as medicine. Use your sense of taste as your guide. Is it spicy and hot tasting? If so, it's most likely good medicine. Varieties of thyme with a milder taste won't have as potent an effect as their spicier cousins.

MEDICINAL PROPERTIES AND ENERGETICS OF THYME

Thyme has hot and drying energetics. Along with tasting great, it helps with digestion, immune system support, and pain relief. It has a strong scent and flavor, so it is normally used in smaller quantities in foods rather than in large, therapeutic doses.

FOR INFECTIONS

Traditionally, thyme been used for many types of bacterial infections. It can be used as a tea or tincture in mouthwashes to treat sore or inflamed gums and minor mouth infections. A gargle made with thyme tea or fresh thyme infused into honey can soothe a sore throat. A topical application can be used to treat yeast and fungal infections like ringworm or vaginal yeast infections. Herbalist Aviva Romm recommends thyme, as well as other herbs, as a vaginal suppository to address group B streptococcus in the late stages of pregnancy.[1]

Modern research supports thyme's strongly antimicrobial properties. Furthermore, in his book *Herbal Antibiotics*, Stephen Buhner says thyme has been shown to inhibit the mechanisms that can make bacterial cells resistant to antibiotics.[2] Numerous in vitro studies on thyme essential oil have shown thyme's ability to inhibit pathogens like *Candida albicans*, *Staphylococcus*

aureus, *Enterococcus fecalis*, *Escherichia colia*, and nosocomial infections.[3,4,5,6,7] The Centers for Disease Control and Prevention estimates that 2 million people in the United States get antibiotic-resistant infections resulting in as many as 23,000 deaths every year.[8] Thyme, as well as many other herbs with similar effects, may be a ray of hope for the growing threat of antibiotic-resistant bacteria.

Many herbalists feel that thyme also broadly supports the immune system. In his book *Combining Western Herbs and Chinese Medicine*, British herbalist Jeremy Ross says, "Thyme may be especially appropriate for those who have had repeated antibiotic therapy, for example, for respiratory or urinary infection, with the result that the immune system and digestive system have been weakened. This, in turn, can result in an accumulation of pathogens that are not cleared from the body."[9]

FOR COLDS, FLUS, AND COUGHS

Thyme has been used for a variety of symptoms related to colds and flu for thousands of years. Even the first-century physician Dioscorides wrote, "Everyone knows thyme."[10] He recommended a drink of thyme with salt and vinegar for driving out phlegmy matter through the bowels.

Thyme's hot and drying energetics make it a great match for cold and stagnant conditions, which are indicated by a thick white coating on the tongue and congested mucus in the lungs. It is widely employed as an antitussive; it can stop coughing spasms and even dry coughs like whooping cough.

Science has begun to further confirm herbalists' traditional use of thyme for acute bronchitis. In one double-blind, placebo-controlled clinical trial, researchers found that patients with acute bronchitis who were given dry extracts of thyme and evening primrose had significantly better healing times than those given the placebo.[11] Another double-blind, placebo-controlled clinical trial found that an extract of thyme and ivy leaves given to patients with acute bronchitis resulted in a 50 percent reduction in coughing fits two days sooner than in those taking the placebo.[12] The combination of thyme and ivy leaves has also been shown to be effective and safe for children aged 2 to 17 with acute bronchitis.[13]

FOR DIGESTION

Thyme can be enjoyed in meals to support already healthy digestion, or it can be taken in larger quantities to treat symptoms of stagnant digestion like bloating, belching, and flatulence. It can also calm digestive spasms and could be helpful for those with diarrhea or irritable bowel syndrome (IBS).

Have unwanted guests in your digestive system? Thyme has long been used as a vermifuge to help the body get rid of parasites and worms. According to herbalist Anne McIntyre, "A teaspoonful of tincture half an hour before breakfast has been used traditionally with castor oil for worms. In France, thyme is used particularly as a cleansing liver tonic, stimulating the digestive system and liver function, and to treat indigestion, poor appetite, anaemia, liver and gall-bladder complaints, skin complaints and lethargy."[14]

FOR REDUCING PAIN

While thyme is known primarily for its ability to address digestive issues, infection, and upper respiratory symptoms, it has also been long used for pain. Maud Grieve recommends using thyme externally on painful joints as a counter-irritant or rubefacient. (A rubefacient is something that works by irritating tissues, thus bringing circulation and heat to the affected area.) Many historical herbalists recommend thyme for delayed menses and painful menstrual cramps.

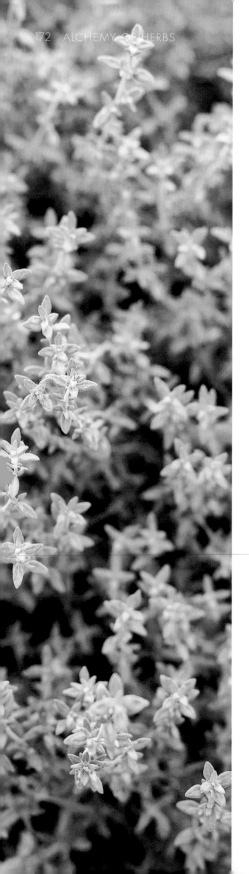

HOW TO USE THYME

Thyme is easy to grow in the garden. Just before the plant flowers, I harvest it by cutting the thin, woody stems a few inches above the ground. I am able to harvest two or three times each growing season, which supplies our household with plenty of thyme for the season. I will warn you that patience is required for removing those small leaves from the thin stems. Once they are well dried, they can be stored in a tightly sealed glass container.

Thyme can be used in a variety of different herbal preparations. It works well as a tea or tincture, or infused into oil, vinegar, or honey.

Many of the antimicrobial qualities of thyme have been shown by using thyme essential oil. There are at least seven different chemotypes (chemically distinct types) of thyme essential oil. Work with a professional when choosing thyme essential oil, as knowledge about the different qualities of these chemotypes is important for both safety and effectiveness.

RECOMMENDED AMOUNTS

Thyme is a delicious culinary herb. Because it has such a potent scent and taste, it is normally used in smaller quantities in foods.

The therapeutic amount for thyme is:

As tea (dried): 2 to 6 grams per day[15]

As tincture (dried): 1:5, 35% alcohol: 2 to 4 mL, 3 times per day[16]

As essential oil: dilutions of 1% or less (1 drop of essential oil in 100 drops of carrier oil)[17]

SPECIAL CONSIDERATIONS

Women who are pregnant should not use medicinal amounts of thyme, nor should they use thyme essential oil. Thyme may stimulate uterine contractions and menstrual flow.

Large amounts of thyme and thyme essential oil are not recommended when a woman is breastfeeding.

Thyme essential oil should be chosen for its chemotype and used diluted and in very small amounts. Working with a clinical aromatherapist trained in the internal use of essential oils will ensure safety with this potent extraction.

Thyme has been associated with a few rare allergic reactions.[18]

THYME OXYMEL

Dating back as far as the ancient Greeks, oxymels are herbal preparations made by combining herbs with honey and vinegar. These sweet-and-sour preparations are specific to the treatment of respiratory symptoms and can be used for bronchial complaints, especially when there is a lot of mucus present, as in congested coughs.

A simple spoonful of honey can soothe a sore throat, but it also offers a wide range of benefits. It's antimicrobial, which means it inhibits the growth of pathogens, as well as slightly expectorant.

While I've included specific amounts of thyme in the ingredient list, you can also just eyeball the amount if you're using a 1-pint jar. If using fresh thyme, you'll want enough minced leaves and small stems to fill the jar ¾ full. If using dried thyme, fill the jar ⅓ full with leaves.

Yield: 1½ cups

4 handfuls fresh thyme, or ⅔ cup dried thyme

¼ cup local raw honey

1½ cups organic apple cider vinegar (approximately)

1. Add thyme to a 1-pint jar, then add the honey. Fill the jar the rest of the way with apple cider vinegar, and stir well.

2. Cover the jar with a glass or plastic lid (or, if using a metal lid, place parchment or wax paper between the metal and the liquid; otherwise, the vinegar will corrode the lid).

3. Shake the mixture gently once a day for 2 weeks. Strain, then store the oxymel in the fridge or another cool place. It should last for a year, possibly longer.

4. *To use:* Adults can use 1 tablespoon every hour for a sore throat or congested cough. (This recipe also combines well with olive oil to create a salad dressing.)

TOMATOES PROVENÇAL

My *belle-mère* (mother-in-law) first cooked these up for me while we were visiting southern France. I was instantly smitten with this simple and delicious way to enjoy the heirloom tomatoes of late summer. Many traditional recipes call for bread crumbs, but I've opted for a simpler version to highlight the aromatic herbs like thyme and basil.

Yield: 6 servings

3 medium heirloom tomatoes, sliced in half crosswise

2 garlic cloves, minced

1 tablespoon chopped fresh parsley

1 tablespoon chopped fresh basil

2 teaspoons fresh thyme, or 1 teaspoon dried thyme

¼ teaspoon freshly ground black pepper

¼ teaspoon salt, or to taste

3 tablespoons olive oil

¼ cup Parmesan cheese

1. Preheat the oven to 350°F. Arrange the 6 tomato halves in a baking dish.

2. Mix together the garlic, parsley, basil, thyme, black pepper, and salt with the olive oil. Sprinkle this mixture on the tomato halves.

3. Bake for 20 minutes or until tomatoes are tender.

4. Sprinkle with Parmesan cheese and broil for 1 to 2 minutes or until the cheese is golden. Cool slightly and eat while still warm.

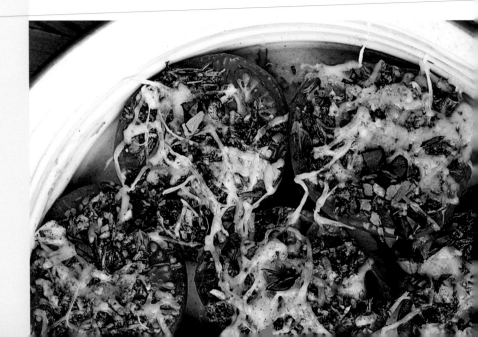

THYME AND CHERRY BARK COUGH SYRUP

This recipe is a variation of a syrup I developed for my Herbal Cold Care online course (www.HerbalColdCare.com). It helps to stop those dry, hacking, and unproductive coughs. The marshmallow root and honey help to moisten dry tissues, and the wild cherry bark and thyme relieve the coughing reflex. Because many of the herbs in this recipe are oddly shaped, it's best to measure them by weight rather than volume.

Yield: approximately 1¾ cups

30 grams dried wild cherry bark (*Prunus serotina*)

10 grams dried marshmallow root (*Althaea officinalis*)

7 grams dried thyme leaves

½ cup honey

¼ cup tart cherry juice concentrate

1. Combine the wild cherry bark, marshmallow root, and 2 cups water in a pan. Bring to a boil, then simmer, uncovered, for 20 minutes. The water should be reduced by roughly a half.

2. Remove from heat. Add the thyme and steep, covered, for 5 minutes.

3. Strain off the herbs and measure the remaining liquid. Add a half part honey and a quarter part tart cherry juice concentrate (e.g., if you have 1 cup of liquid, you would add ½ cup honey and ¼ cup tart cherry concentrate).

4. Stored in the fridge, it should last for a month. It can also be frozen for later use. If it develops mold, throw it out.

5. *To use:* Adults take 1 teaspoon every 30 minutes, or as needed. Another option for this recipe is to add a lot less honey and sip it frequently as a tea, but don't drink it all in one day; this recipe should last at least two days as a tea.

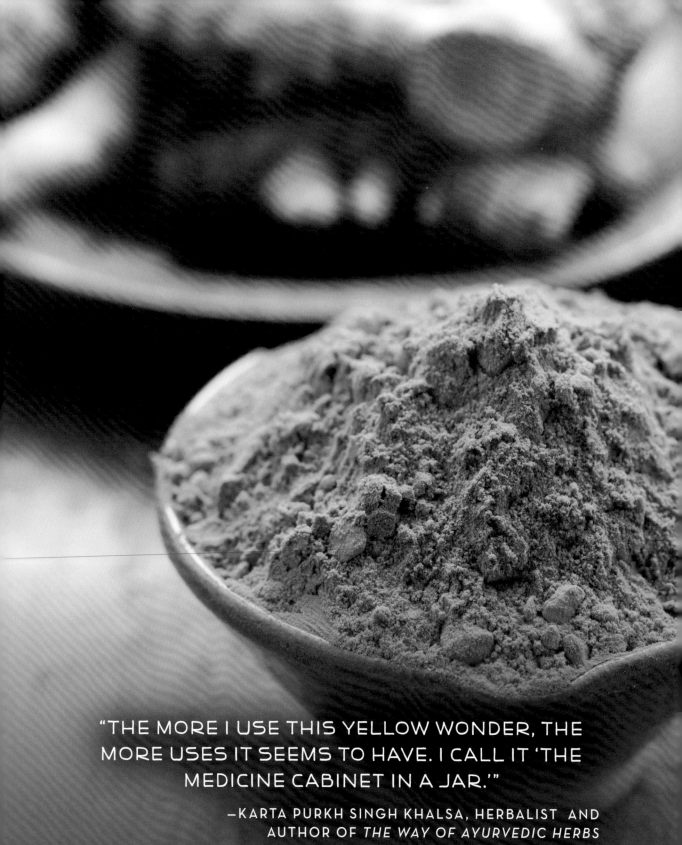

"THE MORE I USE THIS YELLOW WONDER, THE MORE USES IT SEEMS TO HAVE. I CALL IT 'THE MEDICINE CABINET IN A JAR.'"

—KARTA PURKH SINGH KHALSA, HERBALIST AND AUTHOR OF *THE WAY OF AYURVEDIC HERBS*

CHAPTER 20

Turmeric

If you saw a list of all the ways herbalists use turmeric to help improve people's health, it would be so extensive you might think it unbelievable. How can one herb do so much? It may be due to turmeric's incredible ability to modulate inflammation. Inflammation plays a significant role in cancer, type 2 diabetes, autoimmune disorders, asthma, arthritis, ulcerative colitis, periodontitis, eczema, psoriasis, and many other ailments. In fact, many of the major diseases plaguing the Western world can be linked to chronic systemic inflammation.[1]

Botanical name: *Curcuma longa*

Family: Zingiberaceae

Parts used: rhizome (root)

Energetics: warming, drying

Taste: pungent, bitter

Plant properties: analgesic, blood mover, cholagogue, antioxidant, astringent, carminative, anti-inflammatory, hemostatic, vulnerary, antispasmodic

Plant uses: arthritis, digestion, eczema, bleeding, wounds, ulcers, diarrhea, liver problems, pain, Alzheimer's, colds/flu, cancer, heart health, type 2 diabetes

Plant preparations: culinary, powder, tincture, tea

Turmeric is closely related to ginger. As with ginger, it is the rhizome, or root, of the plant that is most frequently used as a culinary spice and as herbal medicine. Turmeric is originally from Southeast Asia but now grows in tropical locations all over the world. It has been a beloved spice in India for thousands of years, frequently found in Indian cuisine and in Ayurvedic medicine. India currently grows most of the world's turmeric and consumes 80 percent of it.[2] In the Western world, turmeric and its constituents, like curcumin, have been extensively studied and applauded for their beneficial effects.

MEDICINAL PROPERTIES AND ENERGETICS OF TURMERIC

We often hear about the negative effects of inflammation, but what we don't hear as often is that not all inflammation is bad. Acute inflammation is a very important process the immune system employs to heal broken bones, sprains, bruises, scratches, etc. However, problems arise when acute inflammation evolves into chronic inflammation.

Nonsteroidal anti-inflammatory drugs (NSAIDs) are commonly prescribed to reduce both chronic and acute inflammation. NSAIDs dramatically decrease all inflammation, whether good or bad, and in the process they also block important fatty acids that are responsible for maintaining the integrity of the stomach lining. NSAIDs have repeatedly been shown to adversely affect healing time for soft-tissue injuries, especially when taken long-term.[3,4] And while many people think of these over-the-counter medications as being safe, the reality is that every year thousands of people die from taking them.[5]

Turmeric is an equally effective and *safer* alternative to NSAIDs for chronic inflammation. While turmeric is referred to as an anti-inflammatory, it doesn't suppress inflammation in the same indiscriminate way that NSAIDs do. It supports the body's ability to address inflammation, so it's more accurate to say that turmeric *modulates* inflammation than to say it is "anti-inflammatory." Instead of inhibiting fatty acids like prostaglandins, and thereby blocking the beneficial aspects of inflammation, turmeric assists the body's healing abilities in numerous ways: it increases glutathione production (important for detoxification), decreases free-radical damage, and blocks specific inflammatory enzymes.[6]

FOR DIGESTION AND LIVER HEALTH

Turmeric can effectively and safely support the health of your liver, especially when consumed regularly. Your liver is an amazing organ, responsible for filtering your blood; breaking down and removing metabolic waste; storing glycogen, which is important for energy; and making bile, which helps you digest fats. Herbalists correlate poor liver function to many digestive problems, hormone imbalance, poor nutrient absorption, and inflammatory rashes like eczema.

Extreme detox diets and liver cleanses are common practices in the natural health community, the idea being that strongly "cleansing" your liver a couple of times a year can improve your health all year long. In the context of holistic health, this approach just doesn't make sense. Since detoxification is something that naturally happens in your cells every moment of the day, it is more beneficial to support the health of your detoxification systems every day. In this way, you can ensure your body's systems are working well all the time, not just a couple of times a year!

In one randomized controlled study, researchers showed that turmeric is able to dramatically improve liver function by significantly reducing levels of the enzyme ALT over a 12-week period.[7] (Elevated ALT levels are associated with inflamed or injured liver cells.)

FOR HEALING WOUNDS

Turmeric's ability to heal wounds and modulate inflammation make it a perfect herb for many inflammatory digestive problems. Herbalists successfully use turmeric for acute digestive problems such as diverticulitis, colitis, and ulcers. From an herbal energetic perspective, turmeric tones the surface of the ulceration, decreases inflammation, stops bleeding, and helps to prevent infection. ("Toning" here means to close the gaping wound of an ulcer and shrink the cells, reducing rates of infection.)

FOR ULCERS

Researchers have confirmed turmeric's ability to address peptic ulcers. In one study, patients with ulcers were given turmeric capsules. After 12 weeks, 76 percent of the people in the study no longer had ulcers.[8] Another study showed that taking curcumin extracts was an effective way to avoid relapse in patients who previously had ulcerative colitis.[9]

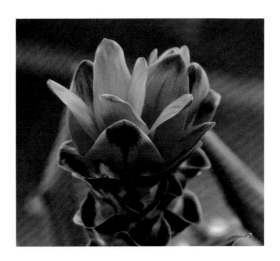

FOR INSULIN RESISTANCE AND TYPE 2 DIABETES

Insulin resistance, metabolic syndrome, and type 2 diabetes constitute a growing epidemic in the Western world. Effectively addressing these metabolic disorders requires a holistic approach that includes healthy sleep habits, exercise, and a whole-foods diet low in carbohydrates. Turmeric, when used alongside these measures, has repeatedly been shown to be a powerful herb for decreasing inflammation associated with type 2 diabetes and for lowering fasting insulin.[10]

Type 2 diabetes is the most common cause of kidney failure, with 44 percent of new cases being attributed to this chronic inflammatory disease.[11] Research has shown that people taking turmeric had significant improvements in biomarkers that are risk factors for developing end-stage kidney disease.[12]

FOR HEART HEALTH

Turmeric supports heart health by modulating inflammation. (There is also a growing understanding that inflammation is the cause of many heart problems, including atherosclerosis and imbalanced cholesterol levels.) It may also modulate cholesterol levels, but more human clinical trials are needed to confirm this.

Turmeric even helps people who already have heart disease. In one study, researchers showed that a curcumin extract reduced the risk of heart attack in people who had undergone coronary artery bypass grafting.[13]

Turmeric can help you maintain heart health too. A low-dose of curcumin extract was given to healthy middle-aged adults and was shown to reduce triglyceride levels and other inflammatory markers associated with heart disease.[14] Another study looked at cardiovascular improvements in postmenopausal women taking curcumin and doing regular aerobic exercise. The results showed that these two interventions together can improve the age-related decline in endothelial function.[15] (The endothelium is the lining of the blood vessels, and decreased endothelial function is associated with an increased risk of cardiovascular disease.)

FOR IMPROVED MEMORY AND ALZHEIMER'S

Alzheimer's, like any chronic disease, is complex, and I don't want to give the impression that taking one herb is going to cure it. However, in one human trial, turmeric was shown to improve the working memory of people who had prediabetes and biomarkers for Alzheimer's disease.[16] (Alzheimer's has recently been dubbed type 3 diabetes because of its strong correlation to this metabolic syndrome.)

FOR CANCER

"Can we eat to starve cancer?" asked William Li in a TED talk. Li is the cofounder of the Angiogenesis Foundation. His work centers on the relationship between angiogenesis (the growth of blood vessels) and the growth of cancer. Angiogenesis is normally a beneficial effect that is necessary for healing wounds, but in some cases, excessive angiogenesis can supply cancer cells with blood and nutrients that can dramatically increase their growth as well as their ability to spread. In his interesting TED talk, Li highlighted turmeric as a substance that stops blood vessel growth to cancers.[17]

FOR PAIN AND INFLAMMATION

Turmeric can be taken preventively to keep the musculoskeletal system healthy. In fact, yogis take turmeric to support tendons and ligaments and promote flexibility. Furthermore, several double-blind, placebo-controlled studies have shown that turmeric is as effective as NSAIDs for relieving arthritic pain without the common gastric side effects associated with these drugs.[18,19]

I have personally witnessed the amazing power of this spice. The results I've seen with two of my clients, Judy and Susan, are typical of what I see with those starting to take turmeric for inflammatory pain. Every time, I feel a bit of amazement and a bit of sadness—amazement that this root has dramatically helped again, and sadness that more people don't know of its powerful benefits.

When Judy first came to see me, she had severe pain in her fingers from both osteoarthritis and rheumatoid arthritis. She had a lot of difficulty performing normal activities like chopping vegetables. She was taking two pharmaceutical drugs that had serious side effects, including a weakened immune system and risk of sudden blindness.

Judy and I worked together to create a customized plan to support her health. One of the herbs she started taking was turmeric. After only a week, I got an elated e-mail from her—the debilitating pain in her hands was gone! Judy worked closely with her endocrinologist to slowly reduce her medications, and within six months she was off them completely while still maintaining a pain-free life.

Susan had been experiencing knee pain for almost a decade by the time I started working with her. Simple things like stepping from a road onto the curb caused extreme discomfort. She regularly took NSAIDs just to make it through her normal life activities. Within two weeks of starting to take turmeric, all of her knee pain was gone for the first time in years and she no longer needed to take over-the-counter pills for pain.

HOW TO USE TURMERIC

You can most easily find turmeric in powdered form. The best-quality turmeric will be a very bright orange. If it has turned to a browner shade, then you know it is not very fresh.

Turmeric is full of amazing antioxidants and constituents, but it is not easily absorbed by the digestive system. Here are two important tips for dramatically increasing the bioavailability of turmeric. The first is to add a small amount, roughly 3 percent, of freshly ground black pepper to your turmeric. This has long been the practice in Ayurveda, and science has proved that piperine, an extract of black pepper, increases the bioavailability of curcumin by as much as 2,000 percent.[20] Another tip is to take your turmeric heated in oil. The heat and oil help to better extract its constituents, making them more available in your body.

If you walk into any health food store, you will see many different options for taking curcumin, a constituent of turmeric. In fact, it's impossible to read about the plant turmeric without also hearing about curcumin. However, I am skeptical anytime science reduces a complex herb down to one component. The fact that herbs have hundreds if not thousands of constituents that work on a variety of pathways in the body is what makes them so uniquely powerful. Although studies have shown that curcumin extracts may have certain benefits, I recommend reaping the rewards of the whole root.

RECOMMENDED AMOUNTS

When you enjoy turmeric in culinary dishes for preventive care, the amount of turmeric you use isn't very high—perhaps 1 gram a day. However, if you are using turmeric for more specific conditions, then higher dosages may be necessary to get the results you would like, and taking capsules may be the easiest choice.

The therapeutic amount for turmeric is as follows:

As powder: 1 to 10 grams per day

As tincture: 1:2, 60% alcohol, 2 to 4 mL, 2 to 3 times per day[21]

SPECIAL CONSIDERATIONS

Turmeric will stain everything it touches a golden yellow, including your hands, cutting board, counters, and so on.

Turmeric is mildly warming and drying and may exacerbate hot and dry conditions. If you take too much, you might feel unusually thirsty or experience hot flashes or night sweats. Turmeric is often combined with ghee or demulcent herbs to offset this effect.

The following people should avoid large amounts of turmeric: those who are currently taking blood thinners, people with blood-clotting disorders, people who have known gallstones (although this is controversial), and women who are pregnant or breastfeeding (also controversial).

WARMED GOLDEN MILK

Combining turmeric with milk has a long tradition in India. I first learned how to make a version of golden milk from my mentor, Karta Purkh Singh Khalsa, and since then I've experimented with many variations. This is my current favorite and is a wonderful way to enjoy the many benefits of turmeric. As you become more familiar with these tastes, try to increase the amount of spices so you can get a lot of turmeric in each serving.

If you are sensitive to dairy, any type of dairy alternative—including almond, rice, or coconut milk—will work well as a substitute for the milk. In place of the ghee (clarified butter), you can use butter or coconut oil instead.

Yield: 2 cups, 2 servings

2 tablespoons ghee

1 teaspoon turmeric powder

½ teaspoon ginger powder

pinch of finely ground black pepper

2 cups milk

1 teaspoon honey, or to taste (optional)

1.   Melt the ghee in a small saucepan over medium-high heat. Add the spices, and stir continuously for 30 seconds or until fragrant.

2.   Add the milk and stir constantly until steaming hot.

3.   Remove from heat and add honey. Stir to dissolve the honey.

4.   Place the liquid in a blender. Blend on high, allowing the steam to escape, for 30 seconds. The mixture should now be blended with the oils from the ghee and be golden and frothy. (Blending it is necessary to get the right consistency.)

5.   Pour and enjoy immediately.

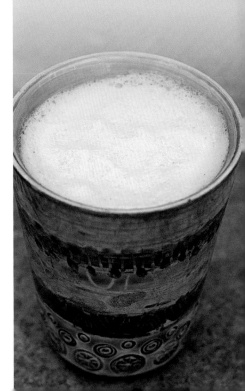

1½ cups pumpkin seeds, soaked in water overnight and drained

2 tablespoons kelp flakes

2 tablespoons tamari or soy sauce

2 garlic cloves, minced

1 tablespoon turmeric powder

1 teaspoon cumin powder

2 teaspoons paprika powder

½ teaspoon freshly ground black pepper

1 cup chicken or vegetable broth

¼ cup olive oil

salt, to taste

TURMERIC AND PUMPKIN SEED PATÉ

This high-protein snack is a delicious way to enjoy turmeric. By soaking the pumpkin seeds first, you help break down the phytic acid they contain, making them easier to digest. (To soak your seeds, place them in a container, cover them with water, add a pinch of salt, and stir. Cover and let sit for 6 to 8 hours or overnight.)

Yield: 1¼ cups

1. Place the soaked pumpkin seeds, kelp flakes, tamari, garlic, turmeric, cumin, paprika, and black pepper into a food processor.

2. With the motor running, drizzle the broth and the oil into the mixture and process until it is smooth and spreadable.

3. Use this as a dip with veggies or crackers, or spread it on a sandwich.

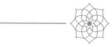

2 tablespoons cumin powder

2 tablespoons coriander powder

1 tablespoon turmeric powder

1½ teaspoons cinnamon powder

¾ teaspoon clove powder

¾ teaspoon cardamom powder

GARAM MASALA

This traditional Indian spiced blend works well in curries and on meats and veggies. We cook a lot of Indian-inspired cuisine, and this mix goes in practically every dish. For the freshest and most vibrant mix, I recommend grinding the spices fresh and using the mixture within 1 week.

Yield: 6 tablespoons

1. Combine all the ingredients in a small bowl and mix thoroughly. Store in an airtight container in a cool and dark location. Use liberally on veggies and meats.

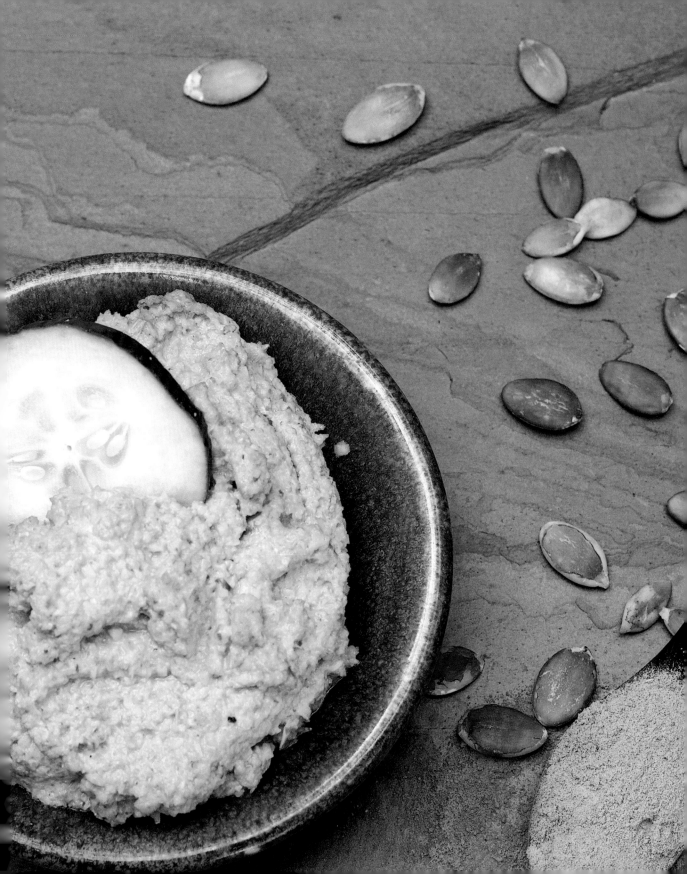

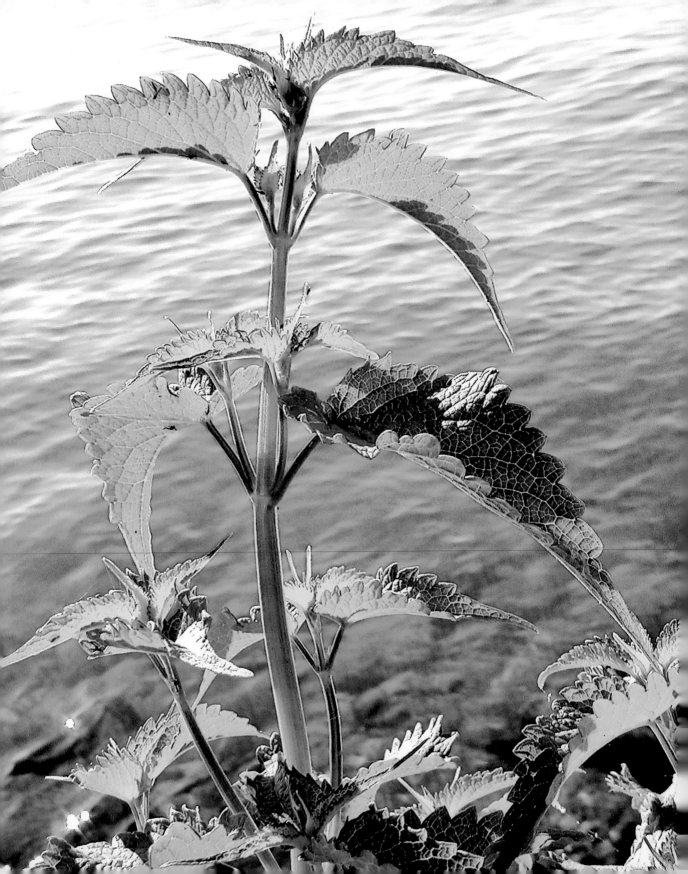

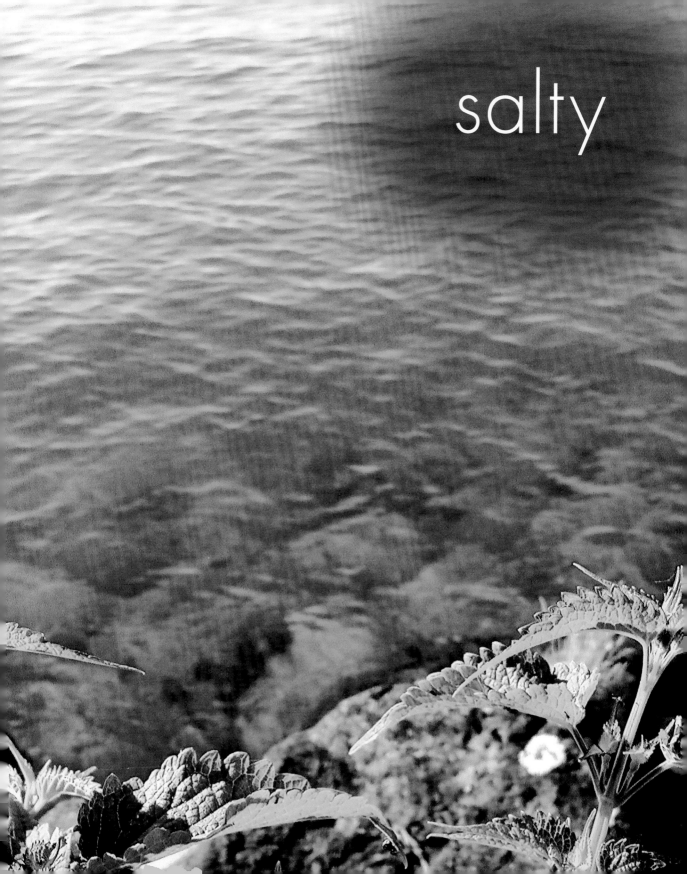

salty

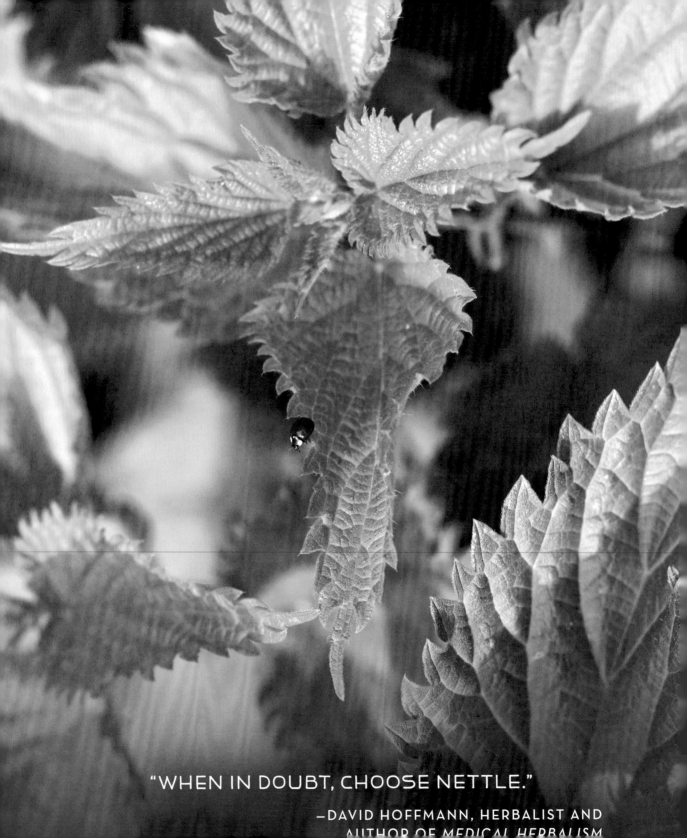

"WHEN IN DOUBT, CHOOSE NETTLE."

—DAVID HOFFMANN, HERBALIST AND
AUTHOR OF *MEDICAL HERBALISM*

CHAPTER 21

Nettle

In the age of exotic miracle herbs imported from all over the globe, stinging nettle remains an unsung champion for improving health in many powerful ways. According to herbalist Susun Weed, nettle infusions are "recommended for those wanting to stabilize blood sugar, reset metabolic circuits to normalize weight, reduce fatigue and exhaustion, restore adrenal potency to lessen allergic and menopausal problems and eliminate chronic headaches."[1] And she's not exaggerating! Nettle's nutrient-dense qualities, as well as a myriad of other beneficial constituents, make it a powerful ally for a variety of health challenges.

Other common names: stinging nettle, common nettle

Botanical name: *Urtica dioica*

Family: Urticaceae

Parts used: young leaves (before the plant flowers), seeds, roots

Energetics: cooling, drying

Taste: salty

Plant properties: nutritive, kidney/adrenal trophorestorative, adaptogen, diuretic, astringent, hemostatic

Plant uses: arthritis, eczema, low metabolism, hypothyroid, weak hair/teeth/bones, fatigue, low lactation, building blood, seasonal allergies, urinary tract infections, asthma, menstrual cramps, amenorrhea, insulin resistance, type 2 diabetes

Plant preparations: nourishing herbal infusion, tea, tincture, culinary, freeze-dried product

Nettle grows abundantly in protein-rich soils all over the Northern Hemisphere and has been used for food and medicine for countless generations. The fibers that can be harvested from nettle stalks have been a historically important source for ropes, nets, and clothing. When I was visiting ancient cave dwellings in central France, I found many abundant patches of nettle, making me wonder how many tens of thousands of years we've been utilizing this important plant.

Perhaps you've already become acquainted with nettle while out hiking. Absentmindedly brushing your skin against this plant will quickly bring your awareness back to the present moment! The leaves and stems are covered in tiny spikes that, when brushed against, release formic acid, which causes a mild but annoying skin reaction. It's no surprise that this plant is also commonly referred to as "stinging nettle."

I can imagine that the plant must have developed its form of protection in an attempt to ward off those who would make frequent use of its nutrient-dense gifts. Cooking and drying the plant removes these stinging hairs, but as you'll see, these can also be an important part of its medicine. Herbalists regularly use nettle leaves, roots, and seeds in remedies.

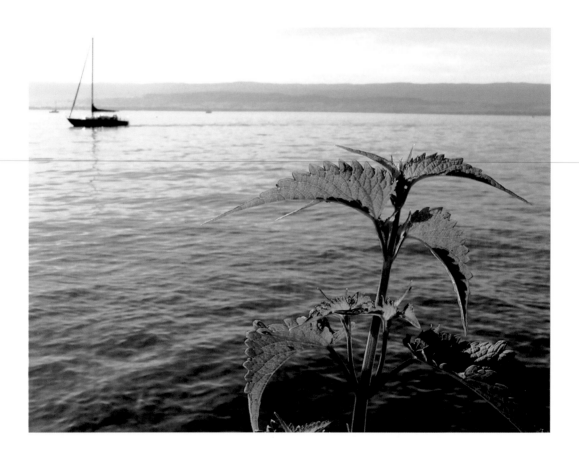

MEDICINAL PROPERTIES AND ENERGETICS OF NETTLE

Nettle is effective for such a wide variety of ailments that herbalists recommend it for supporting general good health. Taken internally, it relieves pain by relieving muscle spasms caused by nutrient deficiencies.

Feeling sluggish? Herbalists often recommend taking nettle regularly to help increase energy levels. While nettle assuredly works in many ways, I surmise that its high nutrient level is what helps create more energy.

FOR HEALTHY BONES, TEETH, AND HAIR

Nettle is full of nutrients that are important for healthy bones, teeth, and hair. Many women have improved their bone density levels after drinking nourishing herbal infusions made with nettle (see the recipe in this chapter).

Nettle has approximately 2,900 mg of calcium for each 100 grams of the dried leaf.[2] The naturally occurring calcium found in nettle is easily absorbed by our bodies (which is not the case when it comes to calcium supplements). Nettle is also high in magnesium, another critical nutrient for bone health.[3]

FOR WOMEN'S HEALTH ISSUES

Iron deficiency is a common problem during pregnancy, but iron supplements can be hard to digest and may result in constipation. Nettle to the rescue! Many women have told me that they were able to improve their iron levels during pregnancy by drinking a daily infusion of nettle.

Nettle can also support healthy menstruation. It is commonly used by herbalists for amenorrhea, or lack of menstrual cycles. Regular nettle infusions can help decrease menstrual cramping; this is probably due in part to this herb's high magnesium content.

FOR DECREASING SEASONAL ALLERGIES

Another common effect of drinking nettle regularly is a reduction in seasonal allergy symptoms. Researchers aren't entirely sure of the mechanism behind this, but they surmise it may be due to the plant's histamine content, which reduces an inflammatory response.[4,5] For best results, start drinking nettle infusions daily at least a month before the allergy season starts. To alleviate acute seasonal allergy symptoms, I prefer freeze-dried nettle.

FOR INSULIN RESISTANCE AND TYPE 2 DIABETES

Nettle is yet another herb with a myriad of positive effects on metabolism and blood glucose. Numerous studies have shown the beneficial effects of nettle on inflammation and hyperglycemia, both of which are complications of insulin resistance and diabetes.[6,7,8]

Clinical trials using nettle in people diagnosed with insulin resistance and type 2 diabetes showed significant improvements in levels of fasting blood glucose, HA1c (a marker that shows average blood glucose levels over time), and inflammation.[9]

FOR DETOXING

Many people think of detoxing as something you do on rare occasions, perhaps with the aid of green smoothies and a restrictive diet. In truth, detoxing is a critical function that happens every moment of every day in the cells of your body. The best way to promote healthy detoxing is to give regular support to your major detox organs to do their job well.

Nettle supports many detox organ systems, including the liver, lungs, and urinary tract. Herbalists often use it to treat signs of poor elimination, such as eczema or constipation. It is also used to strengthen the lungs and is beneficial for people with asthma or shortness of breath.

Nettle is a diuretic, and seems to strengthen the urinary system in general. I often recommend daily nettle infusions for people who have recurring urinary tract infections.

FOR PROSTATE HEALTH

Nettle root has long been used by herbalists to support prostate health.[10] In one study using nettle root and saw palmetto, researchers concluded that the herbs were more effective and safer than the conventional drugs prescribed for benign prostatic hyperplasia (BPH), an enlarged prostate.[11]

FOR REDUCING PAIN

The sting of nettle has long been known. Herbalist Nicholas Culpeper, from the 17th century, romantically described them in his book, *Culpeper's Complete Herbal*. "Nettles are so well known, that they need no description; they may be found by feeling, in the darkest night."[12]

The tiny hairs of fresh nettle release formic acid when brushed against the skin, causing a slightly uncomfortable rash—which can be used therapeutically! The use of fresh nettle topically, known as urtication, can reduce musculoskeletal pain. I've done this myself and was amazed at how well it relieved my severely stiff neck. I've also heard many stories of urtication being helpful for painful joints caused by arthritis. Researchers have taken this to the lab and shown beneficial results using fresh nettle stings for knee pain and thumb pain.[13]

Taken internally, nettle relieves pain by easing muscle spasms and inflammation.

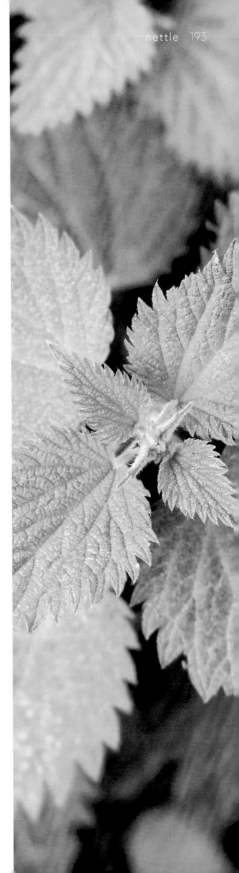

HOW TO USE NETTLE

The recipes in this book use dried nettle leaves, which can be purchased from online herbal retailers.

Wild fresh nettle can be carefully harvested in the spring when the leaves are still young and tender. Because the leaves are lined with stinging hairs, they need to be cooked before being eaten. Ethical wildcrafting (the identifying and harvesting of wild medicinal herbs) is beyond the scope of this book; however, you can find lots of resources about this topic on HerbMentor.com.

RECOMMENDED AMOUNTS

Nettle is a nourishing herb and can be consumed in larger quantities like a food, such as ounces at a time.

The therapeutic amount for nettle leaf is as follows:

As tea (dried): 28 grams or 1 ounce (approximately 2 cups of finely crumbled leaves) per day

As tincture (fresh): 3 to 5 mL, 75-95% alcohol, 3 to 5 times per day

SPECIAL CONSIDERATIONS

It is not recommended that nettle leaves be eaten after the plant has gone to flower/seed.

Use nettle with caution in people with dry constitutions.

For some, nettle can be a strong diuretic.

Very occasionally I've heard from people that nettle gives them a headache.

NETTLE LEAF DUKKAH

1 cup raw hazelnuts

2 tablespoons sesame seeds

⅓ cup whole coriander seeds

3 tablespoons whole
cumin seeds

½ cup dried nettle leaf

¼ cup dried parsley leaves

1 teaspoon fine sea salt

¼ teaspoon freshly ground
black pepper

Years ago a friend gave us a delicious blend of spices that he bought at a Middle Eastern market. All the ingredients were listed in another language so we had no idea what was in the mix, but we knew we loved it! Years later I discovered it was a traditional Egyptian blend of nuts, seeds, and spices called *dukkah*. My own interpretation of the mix adds nutritious nettle and parsley. We combine this with olive oil until it forms a slightly runny paste, and then we use it as a spread on bread, meats, eggs, or even veggies.

Yield: 2 cups

1. In a shallow pan on low heat, dry-toast the hazelnuts until they are fragrant and the skins start to fall off (approximately 10 minutes). Stir frequently to prevent burning. Put aside.

2. Dry-toast the sesame seeds on low heat until they turn golden and are fragrant (approximately 5 minutes). Stir frequently to prevent burning. Set aside with the hazelnuts.

3. Dry-toast the coriander and cumin seeds until fragrant (2 to 3 minutes). Set aside with the hazelnuts and sesame seeds, and allow the mixture cool completely.

4. In a food processor, combine all ingredients. Pulse until the mixture is ground quite finely but before it turns into a butter.

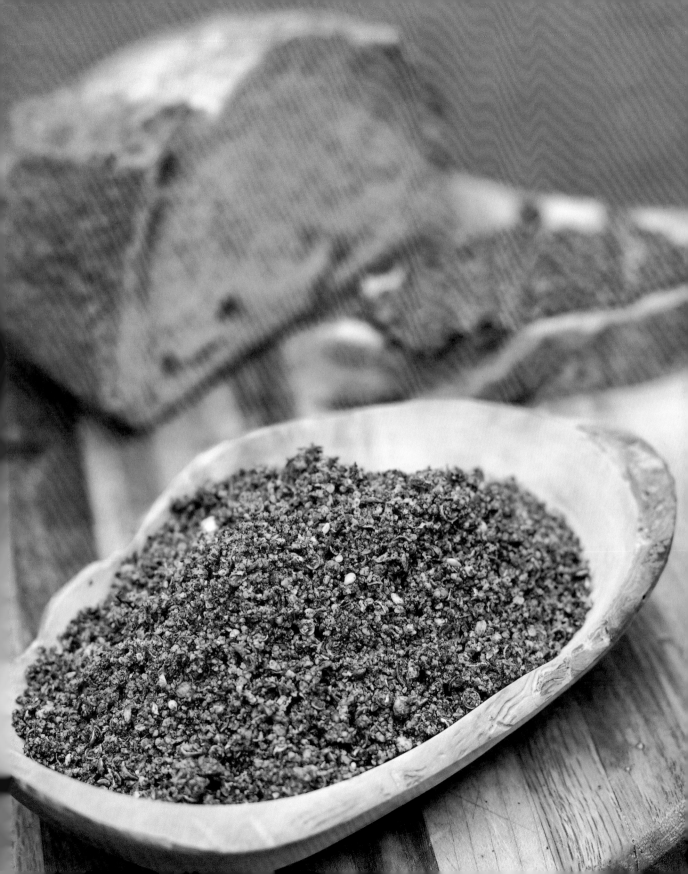

NOURISHING NETTLE INFUSION

28 grams dried nettle leaves (approximately 2 cups finely crumbled leaves)

large pinch of lemongrass for flavor (optional)

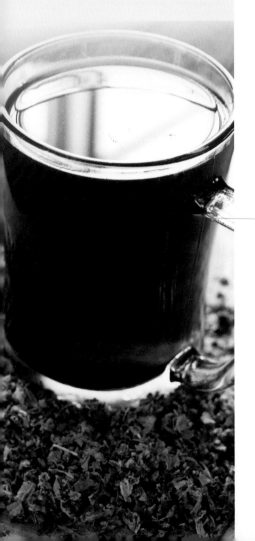

While most of us are familiar with making a cup of tea with a small amount of herbs and a short steeping time, nourishing herbal infusions use a lot of herbs and an extended period of steeping. Nettle infusions were made popular by herbalist Susun S. Weed, who writes, "My daily cup of nourishing herbal infusion is my safeguard against cancer, my longevity tonic, and my beauty treatment—all in one cup."[14] Consider drinking this daily for general health, as it contains an amazing amount of nutrients that can support your energy level as well as the health of your bones, hair, and teeth.

Susun recommends creating nettle infusions without any additional herbs. However, if you find these flavors to be too strong, use half the amount of nettle at first, then slowly increase as your taste for the herb develops. You can also add a flavor, as I do in this recipe, such as lemongrass, peppermint, or ginger.

Yield: approximately 3 cups, 1 serving

1. Bring 4 cups of water to a boil. Place all the herbs in a 1-quart jar or French coffee press.

2. Pour the just-boiled water over the herbs, stir well, and then cover with a lid. Allow herbs to infuse for 4 hours or overnight. (If using a French press, do not press the plunger down until it is done infusing.)

3. Strain when done. You can drink the infusion warm or cold, but do so within 36 hours.

NETTLE AND EGGPLANT SAUTÉ

Nettle is a nutritious plant that can be added to your diet long past its short growing season. This recipe hydrates dried nettle and adds it to a spicy eggplant dish. This recipe is full of flavor and is nutrient dense. It was inspired by a recipe in one of my favorite cookbooks, *The Three Sisters Indian Cookbook* by Sereena, Alexa, and Priya Kaul.

Yield: 6 servings as a side dish

1. Place the nettle leaves in a small bowl and cover with the broth for approximately 15 minutes. The broth should cover the nettle; if necessary, add more broth as the nettle rehydrates. It is okay if the nettle leaves don't absorb all of the broth. Set aside.

2. Heat the oil on medium heat in a large skillet. Add the onion, cumin seeds, and salt and sauté for 3 minutes.

3. Add the garlic and the eggplant. Cook, covered, until the eggplant turns translucent, stirring occasionally so it doesn't stick.

4. Add the tomatoes, hydrated nettle leaves and broth, chili powder, coriander powder, ginger powder, and turmeric powder.

5. Stir everything together and cook, partially covered, until the eggplant is soft and translucent and the sauce has thickened, approximately 10 minutes.

1 cup dried nettle leaf flakes

¾ cup chicken or vegetable broth

¼ cup olive oil

1 medium onion, thinly sliced

½ teaspoon whole cumin seeds

½ teaspoon salt

3 garlic cloves, minced

1 pound eggplant, cut in ½-inch slices

1 pound tomatoes, cubed

1 teaspoon chili powder

½ teaspoon coriander powder

1 teaspoon ginger powder

1 teaspoon turmeric powder

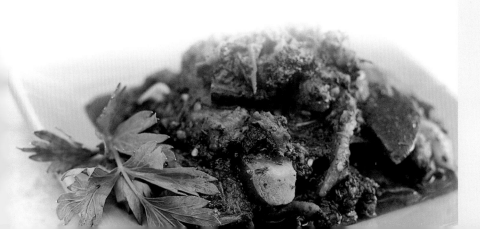

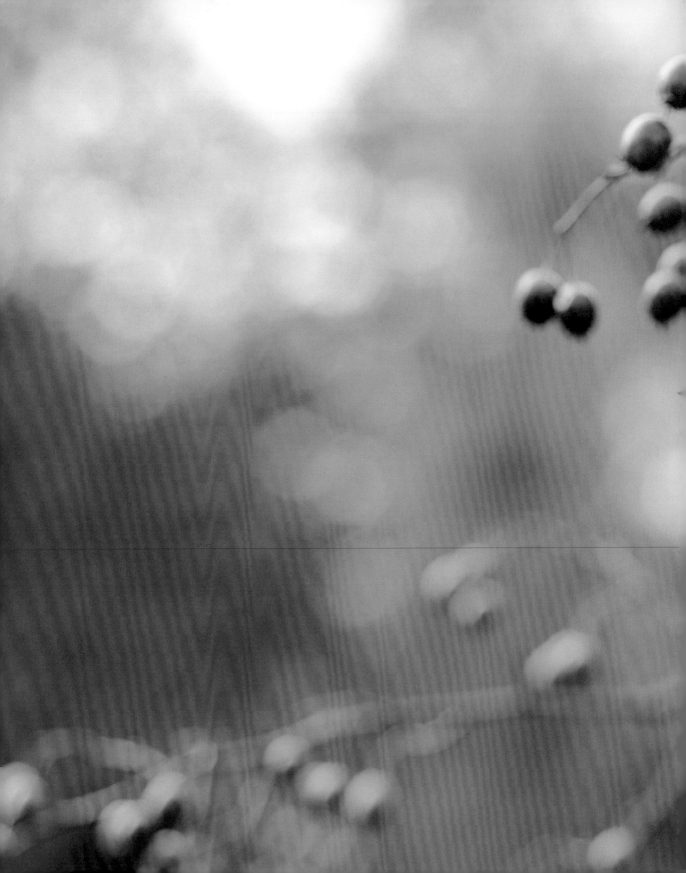

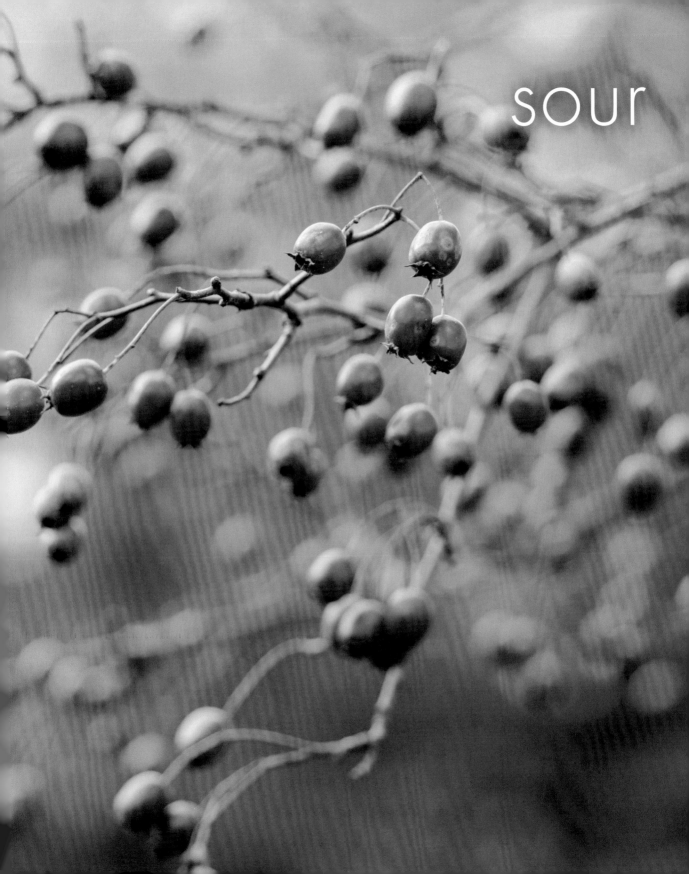

sour

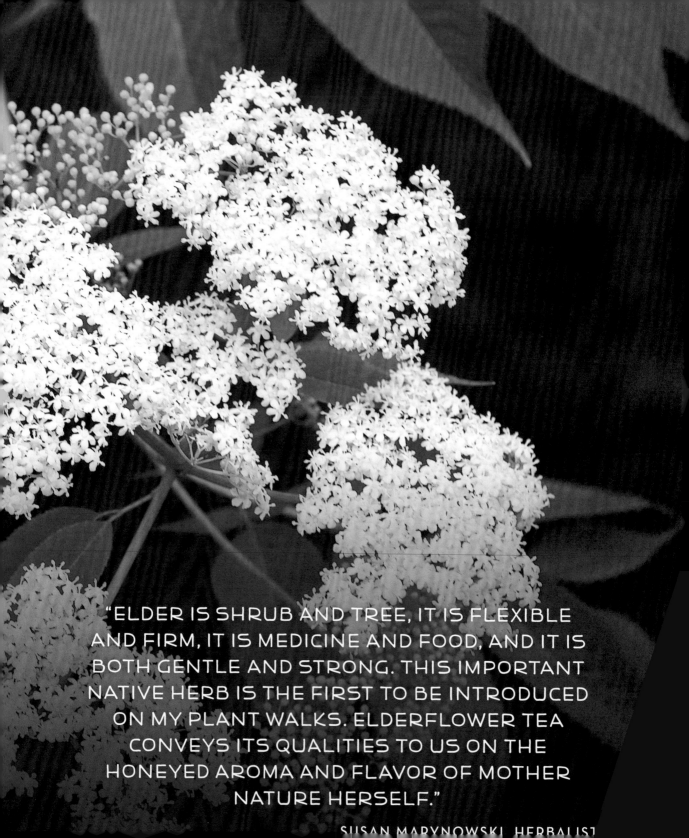

"ELDER IS SHRUB AND TREE, IT IS FLEXIBLE AND FIRM, IT IS MEDICINE AND FOOD, AND IT IS BOTH GENTLE AND STRONG. THIS IMPORTANT NATIVE HERB IS THE FIRST TO BE INTRODUCED ON MY PLANT WALKS. ELDERFLOWER TEA CONVEYS ITS QUALITIES TO US ON THE HONEYED AROMA AND FLAVOR OF MOTHER NATURE HERSELF."

SUSAN MARYNOWSKI, HERBALIST

CHAPTER 22

Elder

In Washington's Methow Valley, where I live, elder shrubs tend to quietly blend in with their surroundings for most of the year. But just after the summer equinox, the shrubs burst out of hiding. First I'll see one bloom here, then another there. Pretty soon, large white blooms dot the landscape to announce the elder plants' presence in the grandest of fashions. Then, in the fall, flowers will give way to large purple clumps of elderberries.

Both the flowers and the berries are incredible herbs for preventing and addressing upper respiratory infections like colds and especially the flu. I can't imagine going through a winter without a good supply of either of these powerful herbs. In fact, herbal preparations with elderberry have been shown to be as effective as modern antiviral drugs for the flu, but without the risk of adverse effects. This is yet another example that, despite the many advances of modern science, herbs continue to offer us powerful medicinal tools.

Other common names: black elder, European elder

Botanical name: *Sambucus nigra, Sambucus nigra ssp. cerulea; Sambucus nigra ssp. canadensis*

Family: Adoxaceae

Parts used: berries, flowers

Energetics: cooling, drying

Taste: sour (berries), bitter (flowers)

Properties (berries): antiviral, immunomodulating, antioxidant rich, inflammatory modulating

Properties (flowers): antiviral, relaxing nervine, relaxing diaphoretic, diuretic, skin protectant, antioxidant rich

Plant uses: colds and the flu, herpes, strengthening eyes, fevers, ear infections

Preparations (berries): food, syrup, tincture, tea, dye

Preparations (flowers): tea, infused oil, salve, cream, tincture, syrup

Elder has a long history of use in Europe. Archaeological excavations have unearthed large numbers of seeds at prehistoric sites, indicating that elders were consumed during the Magdalenian era (9,000 to 17,000 years ago). Excavations have also exhumed ceremonial flint spearheads that were modeled after elder leaves, giving us the insight that the elder was probably revered then as it is now.[1]

Elderberry shrubs continued to be an important source of food, medicine, and material for tools for people in Europe, and many areas have stories and myths associated with the plant. One folkloric belief was that it was bad luck to cut down an elder shrub. Given that elders provide such important medicine, I can see how removing it would bring ill favor.

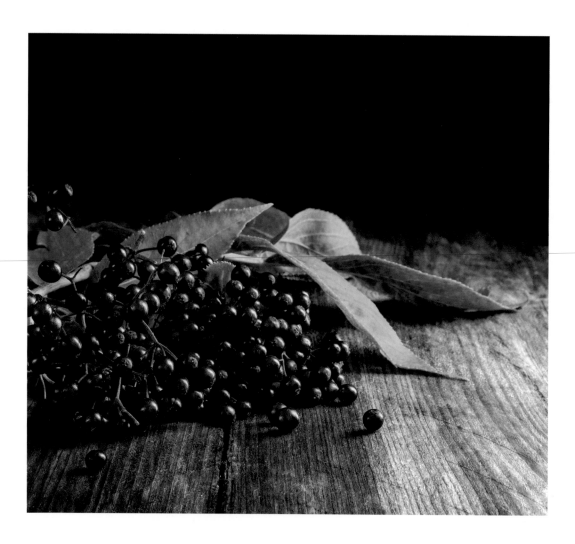

MEDICINAL PROPERTIES AND ENERGETICS OF ELDERBERRIES

Elderberries are powerful medicine. For more than 1,000 years, herbalists have revered elder's abilities, and mentions of the shrub are included in many important historical texts. While they are most famous for their ability to shorten the duration of the flu, they have many other uses, too.

These flavonoid-rich berries can modulate inflammation and decrease oxidative stress. Herbalists recommend elderberries to strengthen the eyes, decrease arthritic pain, and even as treatment to shorten the duration of a herpes breakout. Elderberries may also be an important herb for type 2 diabetes, but human clinical trials are needed to verify this.

Considering the long-standing traditional use of elderberries, the personal experience of many herbalists, and the positive clinical trials, more research into elderberries' effects against infections is warranted.

FOR RESPIRATORY INFECTIONS AND THE FLU

Long referred to as "the people's medicine chest," elderberries have a strong history of use against upper respiratory infections. In fact, one study found that elderberry has specific immunomodulating constituents that aid in treating respiratory illnesses.[2]

An herbal preparation of elderberry extract was shown to be effective against a number of influenza viruses in both human clinical trials and in vitro studies.[3] In one placebo-controlled, double-blind study, 93.3 percent of those taking the elderberry preparation saw a significant improvement in symptoms within two days; by comparison, it took six days for 91.7 percent of those taking the placebo to see improvement.[4] These results were so outstanding that it propelled elderberry syrup into one of the most popular herbal remedies for the flu.

Another clinical study has further validated those results. In this randomized, double-blind, placebo-controlled study in Norway, researchers gave 60 patients who had been suffering from influenza-like symptoms for less than 48 hours either 15 mL of elderberry syrup or a placebo four times per day. On average, those receiving the elderberry syrup reported that their symptoms were relieved four days earlier than those taking the placebo. As an additional benefit, those taking the elderberry syrup reported using significantly less over-the-counter medications to relieve their symptoms.[5]

In vitro studies have shown elderberry to be effective against many different strains of the influenza virus as well as human pathogenic bacteria.[6] This is particularly important, as bacterial infection during an influenza infection can lead to severe pneumonia. During the H1N1 scare of 2009, in vitro studies of elderberries were found to be effective against the virus. Researchers further discovered that it was the flavonoid content of the berries that can block a virus from entering a host cell.[7]

MEDICINAL PROPERTIES AND ENERGETICS OF ELDERFLOWERS

In the past, elderflowers were more commonly used externally for problems with the skin. They can be used as a tea wash or infused in oil for a cream or salve. They are said to soften and rejuvenate the skin, and elderflower water used to be a very common toiletry for women. In vitro studies have shown that elderflowers are useful additions to cosmetic formulations because they "fulfill the official requirements for sunscreen products due to their broad spectrum of UV protection combined with their high photostability and remarkable antioxidant properties".[8]

While elderflowers are also used for upper respiratory infections, they are used differently than elderberries. Judging from my own experience as well as the reports of countless herbalists, the flowers (like the berries) undoubtedly have some immunomodulating or antiviral activity that can help to shorten a cold or flu. Elderflowers, like elderberries, have also been used to support eye health. Further, in vitro studies have confirmed that the potent anti-inflammatory ability of elderflower extract is particularly effective against periodontitis.[9]

FOR FEVERS

Until very recently, fevers were feared by most folks, and the best defense was believed to be an immediate reduction in the fever using over-the-counter medications like acetaminophen. However, we now know that fevers are an important and beneficial immune system response. By immediately decreasing a fever, we are essentially cutting off the legs of our immune system!

Elderflowers are often used to support a healthy fever process. As we saw in the Pungent section, some spicy herbs can aid a person's ability to warm up. These are used during the stage of fever when someone feels chilled and is shivering. Later in the fever process the patient may feel restless and hot but not have any sweating. This is when elderflowers are used.

Elderflowers let the heat out of the body by dilating the capillaries close to the skin. Herbalist jim mcdonald likens this to opening the window in a hot and stuffy room. While using elderflowers doesn't artificially lower a fever, it can bring relief during this hot and restless phase.

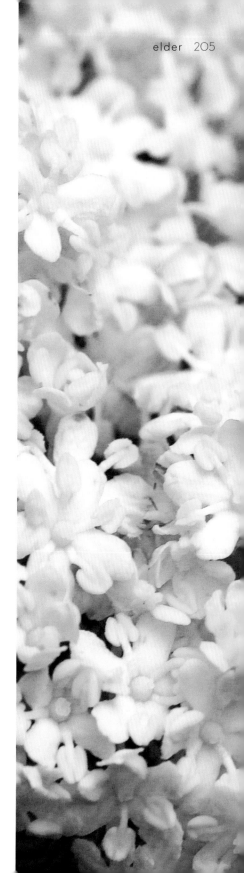

HOW TO USE ELDER

Elderberries and elderflowers can be bought commercially, and both work well when dried.

When using them for acute conditions like the flu or a fever, it is better to take smaller dosages frequently, rather than larger dosages a couple of times per day.

My favorite preparations for elderberries are a syrup, oxymel, or decoction. Many herbalists also like making a tincture (alcohol extract) from the berries. Elderberries can be made into a variety of yummy treats including wine, jelly, or my favorite: a chocolate elder syrup that is great on pancakes.

RECOMMENDED AMOUNTS

Elderberries are a foodlike herb and can be consumed in larger quantities, as you would any other food.

The therapeutic amount for elder is as follows:

As syrup (elderberries): 1 teaspoon to 1 tablespoon every hour

As tincture (dried elderberries): 1:4, 30% alcohol, 4 to 6 mL, 4 to 8 times per day

As tincture (dried elderflowers): 1:5, 30% alcohol, 3 to 5 mL, 4 to 6 times per day

As tea (elderflowers): 15 grams, taken in small doses throughout the day

SPECIAL CONSIDERATIONS

Eating the raw seeds of the berries may cause nausea, but cooking them diminishes this effect.

I have heard from people that commercially bought elderberry powder can cause vomiting (presumably due to the seeds in the powdered product).

1 cup dried elderberries
(115 grams)

1 cup apple juice

9 grams licorice root

½ teaspoon freshly ground
black pepper

1 tablespoon dried thyme
(3 grams)

2 tablespoons dried rosemary
(5 grams)

honey, to taste (optional)

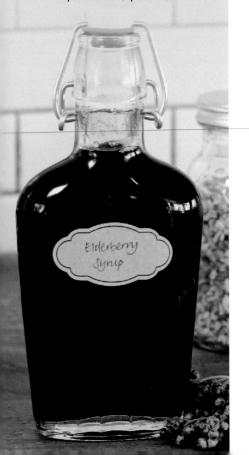

ELDERBERRY SYRUP

For years I have used a version of this recipe as my go-to remedy for avoiding a cold or flu. It works best when you start to take it at the very onset of symptoms. You know that feeling. Maybe it starts with an itchy throat or a sudden onset of fatigue with a bit of chills—those early warning signs you are about to come down with something.

Frequent doses will also be more effective than simply taking it a couple of times per day. It's not unusual for me to take a spoonful every 30 to 60 minutes.

If you taste the mixture before adding the honey, you will probably find that this recipe is already quite sweet. However, the amount of honey you add will determine how long this will last. If you add an amount of honey equal to the amount of juice, and it will probably last for a year. Generally, I add only a little honey and then use the mixture within a few days.

Yield: approximately 2 cups

1. Place the elderberries, apple juice, licorice, black pepper, and 2 cups water into a medium saucepan. Turn the heat to high to bring the mixture to a boil, then reduce the heat and simmer for 20 minutes, covered.

2. Remove the pan from the heat. Add the thyme and rosemary. Stir well and let steep, covered, for 5 minutes.

3. Strain well. I like to strain the herbs through a jelly bag or cheesecloth so I can really squeeze out all the juice.

4. Add honey to taste. Store in the refrigerator until needed.

ELDERFLOWER TEA

Versions of this recipe have been passed down for centuries and are often attributed to 20th-century herbalist Juliette de Bairacli Levy, who spent time learning about herbs with the gypsies of Europe. I have repeatedly heard back from people who swear by this as their number one choice for relieving cold and flu symptoms. For best results, put the hot tea in a thermos and drink throughout the day.

Yield: roughly 2½ cups

1. Bring 3½ cups water to a boil.

2. Place all the herbs in a 1-quart jar. Cover with the just-boiled water and stir.

3. Steep, covered, for 30 minutes. Strain well.

4. Add honey, if desired, and drink warm.

½ cup dried elderflowers (20 grams)

¼ cup dried yarrow leaves and flowers (9 grams)

2 tablespoons dried rose hips (15 grams)

2 tablespoons dried peppermint (4 grams)

honey, to taste (optional)

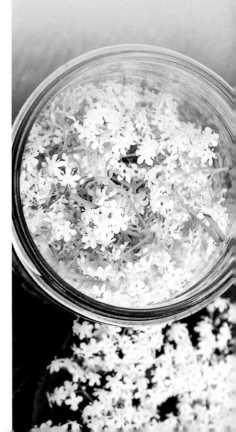

ELDERFLOWER FACIAL SERUM

½ cup jojoba oil

¼ cup dried elderflowers
(10 grams)

6 grams dried calendula
flowers

1 teaspoon rosemary anti-
oxidant extract

10 to 15 drops lavender
essential oil

This is a luxurious recipe that can potentially protect the skin from sun damage. It's not a sunscreen, but it can protect your skin from oxidation and UVA damage. It has a soft and silky feel to it, without being oily. Use it daily in the morning and at night. To use, simply place a small amount of serum on your fingertips and rub into your face, neck, chest, and anywhere else that receives a lot of sun. You don't need to use a lot; this recipe may last two people an entire sunny season.

This serum can also be used to hydrate and rejuvenate your skin. I use jojoba oil in the recipe because I love its silky texture—but it is expensive. If you wish, you can substitute grapeseed oil, apricot kernel oil, or almond oil.

Because calendula is a light and oddly shaped herb, I recommend using a scale to accurately measure it.

Yield: just under ½ cup

1. The first step is to infuse your oil. You can do this with a double boiler or slow cooker. Take care not to let the oil get too hot and "fry" the herbal material. An ideal temperature for the oil is 100°F.

2. *Double boiler method:* Put 1 to 2 inches of water in the bottom pan of a double boiler. (Alternatively, fill a pot with 1 to 2 inches of water and place a tight-fitting bowl on top.) Place the jojoba oil, elderflowers, and calendula into the top. Heat over low until the oil is warm to the touch, then turn off the heat and cover with a lid. Repeat this warming and cooling process every hour or two for 24 to 48 hours. (However, you don't need to tend to the pot overnight—you can let it rest while you sleep!)

3. *Slow cooker method:* Place the jojoba oil, elderflowers, and calendula in a slow cooker, yogurt incubator, or other low-temperature appliance that can maintain the oil temperature at 100°F. Allow to infuse for 24 to 48 hours.

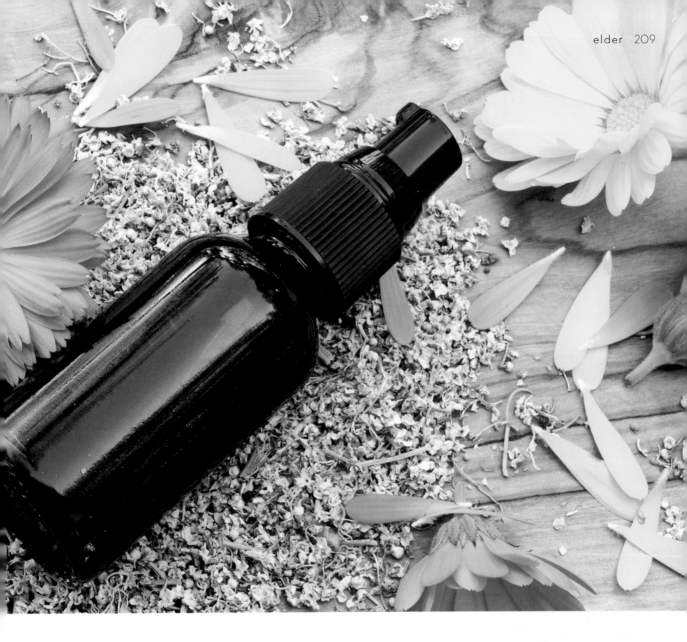

4. Strain off the herbs from the oil through several layers of cheesecloth. Add the rosemary extract and the essential oil, and stir well.

5. Put the oil into bottles with a treatment pump. You could also put it in a traditional tincture bottle with a dropper or any other small, decorative bottle that seals well.

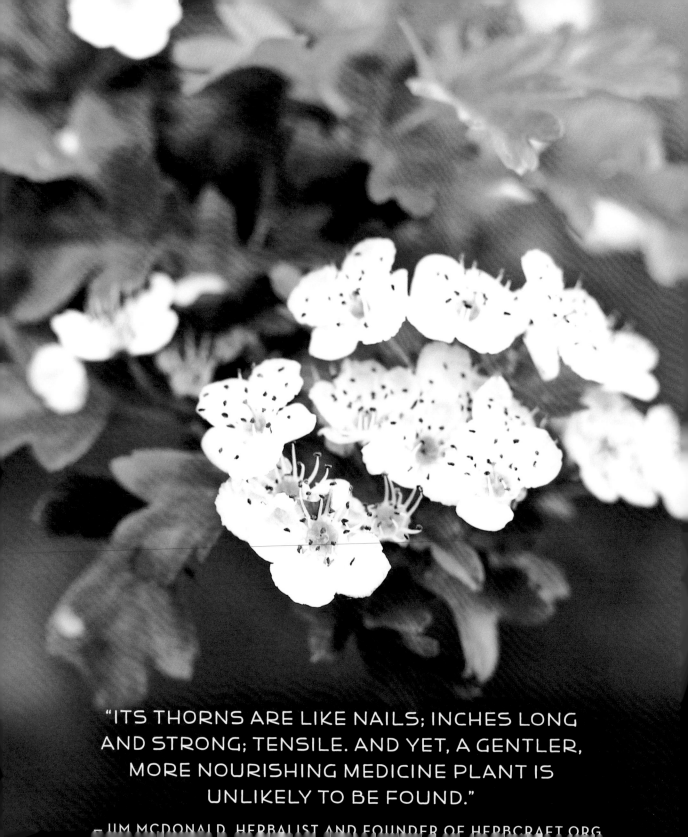

"ITS THORNS ARE LIKE NAILS; INCHES LONG
AND STRONG; TENSILE. AND YET, A GENTLER,
MORE NOURISHING MEDICINE PLANT IS
UNLIKELY TO BE FOUND."

— JIM MCDONALD, HERBALIST AND FOUNDER OF HERBCRAFT.ORG

CHAPTER 23

Hawthorn

I recently asked a group of herbalists to tell me the first herb they thought of for the heart. Out of the 153 people who responded, 93 chose hawthorn. In fact, hawthorn leaves, flowers, and berries have been used by herbalists for centuries to support heart health. In the past handful of decades, scientists have studied hawthorn's ability to decrease blood pressure, reduce cholesterol, and improve quality of life for those with heart disease. Most of these studies have shown significant benefits.

With heart disease being the number one cause of death in the United States, it's surprising to me that more people don't know about hawthorn. Before I start sounding like a snake-oil salesman, I should note that people get heart disease for numerous reasons, and hawthorn is no silver-bullet cure to be taken while ignoring major foundations of wellness such as a healthy diet and an active lifestyle. However, hawthorn can strongly support heart health, both in preventing cardiovascular disease as well as providing benefits to people already dealing with cardiovascular problems.

Botanical name: *Crataegus spp.*

Family: Rosaceae

Parts used: leaves and flowers, berries

Energetics: slightly cooling, neutral

Taste: sour

Plant properties: cardiac trophorestorative, relaxing nervine, digestant, astringent, diuretic, antioxidant

Plant uses: heart-related illness, cardiac weakness, stagnant digestion, regulating blood pressure

Plant preparations: tea, tincture, vinegar, food

European culture has long been fascinated with hawthorn, and many myths and bits of folklore surround this thorny tree. Besides being used for medicine, the hard wood of the tree was made into tools and the thick, thorny nature of the tree made it a popular choice as a natural hedge or fence. Various species of hawthorn are native to North America, where it was used by many First Nations to treat a variety of ailments, including wounds and digestive problems. People in China also have a well-developed relationship with hawthorn, often using it for stagnant digestion.

In the spring, hawthorn trees produce a plethora of lovely white to pink flowers. Following pollination, the tree begins to form many bunches of berries that ripen in late summer. These red berries are dry and mealy and can range from bitter to sweet, depending on species.

TYPES OF HAWTHORN

Hawthorn is a tree in the rose family that grows all over the Northern Hemisphere. There are more than 280 species, and herbalists use them all similarly. The species most studied in science have been *Crataegus monogyna*, *C. oxyacantha*, and *C. laevigata*.

MEDICINAL PROPERTIES AND ENERGETICS OF HAWTHORN

Herbalist David Hoffmann says, "A tonic in the true sense, *Crataegus* [hawthorn] can be considered a specific remedy for most cardiovascular disease."[1]

The current Western medicine paradigm for treating chronic disease relies heavily on suppressing symptoms rather than addressing the factors causing the problem. For instance, if you have seasonal allergies you might be given something to block your body's attempt to create histamine, but you often aren't given anything to modulate your immune system and prevent the allergy symptoms in the first place. This paradigm can be seen in the range of pharmaceuticals that Western medicine uses to address the symptoms of heart disease. While this Band-Aid attempt can save lives in the short term, it doesn't address why the person has heart disease in the first place.

In fact, many commonly prescribed medications actually deplete the body of nutrients necessary for heart health. Statins, commonly prescribed to lower cholesterol, deplete the body of CQ10, an important enzyme for a healthy heart. Diuretics, commonly prescribed for high blood pressure, deplete the body of potassium. Potassium deficiency leads to an irregular heartbeat. Hawthorn, in nourishing and strengthening the heart, does something that no other pharmaceutical can lay claim to.

How does hawthorn work? Like most herbs, hawthorn works in numerous and complex ways, many of which we don't understand yet. However, one important factor is hawthorn's high flavonoid content. Heart disease is often related to inflammation, and regularly eating herbs and foods high in flavonoids has been shown to decrease the inflammation and oxidative stress.

FOR OPTIMIZING CHOLESTEROL

From the 1950s to fairly recently we mistakenly believed that high levels of cholesterol were caused by eating foods that were themselves high in cholesterol. An updated perspective on high cholesterol levels is its relationship to systemic inflammation, which hawthorn, with its high flavonoid content, helps to reduce.

Research scientists have been studying hawthorn in relationship to various symptoms of heart disease for decades. In one study researchers gave people who were diagnosed with diabetes and coronary heart disease 1,200 mg of hawthorn leaf and flower every day for six months. After that time, those taking the hawthorn showed a greater trend toward lower LDL cholesterol ("bad" cholesterol) and decreased neutrophil elastase (an enzyme that, when elevated, is related to heart disease) than those taking a placebo.[2] The dose used in this study was relatively low compared with herbalist standards, and it would be interesting to see the effects of the larger doses more commonly used by herbalists.

FOR HIGH BLOOD PRESSURE

For herbalists, one of the most common indications for hawthorn is high blood pressure. Some herbalists use hawthorn singly, others combine it with other herbs, and it is commonly suggested alongside a healthy diet and regular exercise. After centuries of use, it remains a favorite for decreasing hypertension.

Clinical trials have supported this traditional use. In a double-blind, placebo-controlled study done in Iran, 92 men and women with mild hypertension were given an extract of a local species of hawthorn for four months. Blood pressure was measured every month, and the results showed a significant decrease in both systolic and diastolic blood pressure after three months.[3] Another study gave hawthorn to patients diagnosed with type 2 diabetes and showed that the herb reduced diastolic blood pressure.[4]

FOR HEART HEALTH

Herbalist Charles Kane says, "As a heart medicine there is no other herb with such a positive, yet gentle influence than Hawthorn."[5] Besides helping to reduce particular heart problems such as high blood pressure and hyperlipidemia, hawthorn has been shown to improve general heart function in people with mild to moderate heart disease.

One study looked at 1,011 people diagnosed with stage 2 heart disease who were taking a high dose of a patented hawthorn product. After 24 weeks, a significant improvement in symptoms was observed, including decreased ankle edema, improved cardiac performance, and reduced blood pressure.[6]

Another trial used the same hawthorn product but studied patients for two years. After that time, those taking the hawthorn had significant improvements in the three main symptoms of heart disease—including fatigue, pain with increased exertion, and palpitations—as compared with the control group. The researchers concluded that hawthorn had a clear benefit for patients with mild to moderate heart failure.[7]

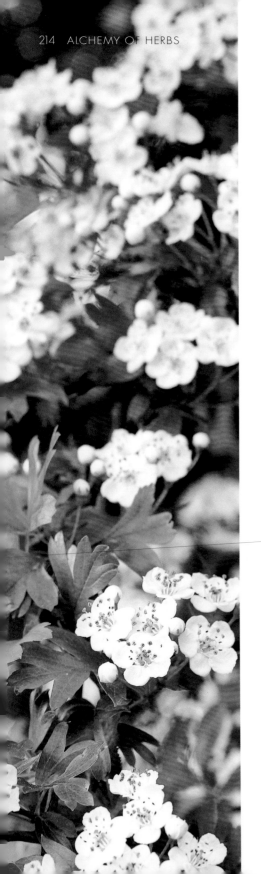

HOW TO USE HAWTHORN

Western herbalists tend to use the berries more frequently; however, the flower and leaf have gotten more attention in research studies in recent years.

The berries can be eaten like food and enjoyed in a variety of ways, including infused into alcohol or vinegar or made into honeys, jams, or even ketchup. I recommend regularly enjoying hawthorn in large quantities; taking it daily keeps hearts nourished and strong!

The leaves and flowers make a delicious, slightly tannic tea that is reminiscent of black tea.

RECOMMENDED AMOUNTS

Hawthorn berries are a foodlike herb that can be consumed in larger amounts, as you would a food. For best results with the berries, leaves, or flowers, use it daily and long-term.

The therapeutic amount for hawthorn is as follows:

As tea: up to 30 grams of berries, and up to 30 grams of leaves and flowers, per day

As tincture (fresh berries): 1:1, 40–60% alcohol, 5 mL, 3 to 5 times per day

As tincture (dried leaf and flowers): 1:5, 30% alcohol, 5 mL, 3 times per day

SPECIAL CONSIDERATIONS

People taking heart medications such as digitalis and beta blockers should consult with an experienced practitioner before taking hawthorn.

Large dosages of the leaf and flower may cause stomach upset in some individuals. If this happens, decrease the amount.

Hawthorn should not be used with people who have diastolic congestive heart failure.[8]

HAWTHORN NOURISHING INFUSION

This recipe blends together the nourishing properties of hawthorn leaves, flowers, and berries, making this a delicious way to support your heart health. The taste is slightly astringent, with the delicate perfume of the flowers and leaves complementing the sweetness of the berries. I love to drink this as an iced tea on a hot summer day.

Yield: approximately 3½ cups, 1 serving

1. Bring 4 cups of water to a boil. Place all the herbs in a 1-quart jar or French coffee press.

2. Pour the just-boiled water over the herbs, stir well, and then cover with a lid. Allow to infuse for 4 to 8 hours or overnight. (If using a French press, do not press the plunger down until it is done infusing.)

3. Strain off the herbs. Add the honey or stevia, to taste, and drink the tea within 24 hours.

¼ cup dried hawthorn berries (20 grams)

½ cup dried hawthorn flowers and leaves (15 grams)

pinch of stevia or honey, to taste

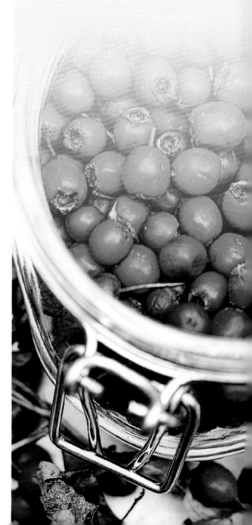

HAWTHORN CORDIAL

1 cup dried hawthorn berries
(80 grams)

1 apple, chopped, seeds
removed

1 teaspoon minced fresh
ginger

3 cardamom pods, crushed

1 vanilla bean, cut in half
lengthwise

1 cinnamon stick

zest of 1 lemon

2 tablespoons dried hibiscus

⅓ cup unsweetened 100%
pomegranate juice

½ cup honey, or to taste

2 cups brandy

This recipe combines the nourishing qualities of haw-thorn with delicious spices that help digestion. Enjoy in small amounts after an evening meal. (I find that it helps me wind down from the day.)

I recently brought this to a potluck and served 1 to 3 tea-spoons of the cordial in approximately 1 cup of sparkling water for a low-alcohol cocktail. It was a hit, and several people asked to buy a bottle from me (I gave them the recipe instead).

Yield: approximately 1½ cups

1. Place all of the herbs, spices, and fruit in a 1-quart jar.

2. Add the pomegranate juice and honey, then fill the jar the rest of the way with brandy (approximately 2 cups).

3. Infuse this for 4 weeks, shaking often.

4. Strain. This can be stored in a dark, cool location and is best consumed within 1 year.

HAWTHORN VINEGAR

Hawthorn berries make a delicious herbal vinegar that is a beautiful shade of red. I use this on many of my homemade salad blends. It can also be taken by the teaspoon prior to eating to help with digestion. I've left the exact measurements out of this recipe so you can decide how much to make. If you choose to make a pint, you would need roughly 2 cups of fresh berries or 1 cup of dried berries, plus approximately 1½ cups of vinegar.

Yield: variable

fresh or dried
    hawthorn berries

apple cider vinegar

jar with glass or plastic lid

1.   If using fresh berries, fill the jar with berries. If using dried berries, fill the jar halfway (to leave room for them to expand).

2.   Fill the jar with apple cider vinegar. Cover with a glass or plastic lid. If using a metal lid, place parchment or wax paper between the lid and the jar (vinegar will corrode metal).

3.   Allow the vinegar to infuse for 2 weeks, shaking once a day. Strain when ready. This does not need to be refrigerated (although it can be). Use within 1 year.

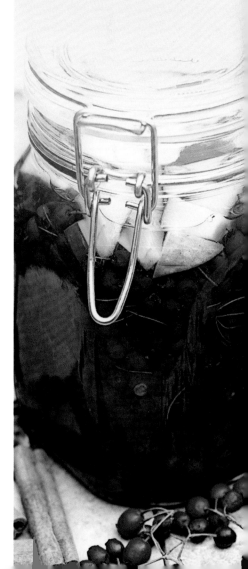

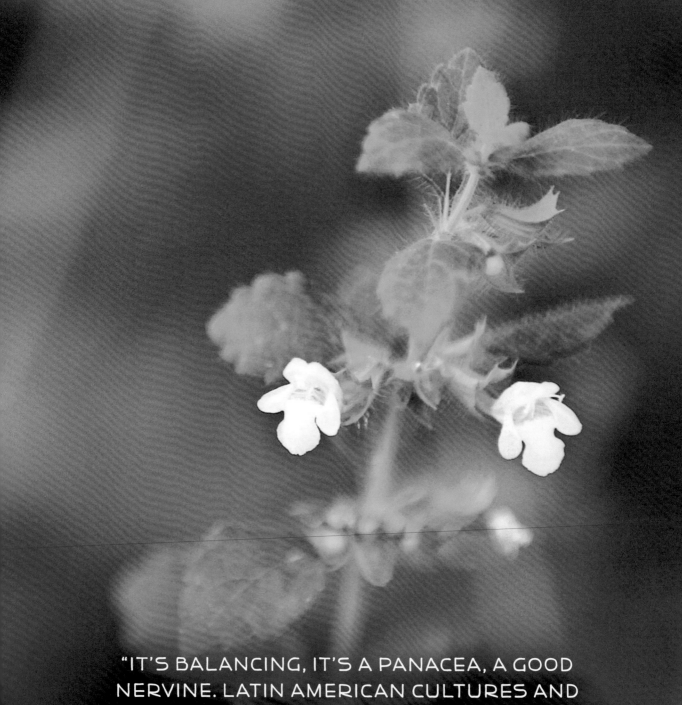

"IT'S BALANCING, IT'S A PANACEA, A GOOD NERVINE. LATIN AMERICAN CULTURES AND PEOPLE IN THE MEDITERRANEAN CONSIDER IT A POWERFUL RELAXING HERB, GOOD FOR THE HEART, FOR THE SOUL, FOR BABIES, FOR THE ELDERLY AND EVERYONE IN BETWEEN."

—CASCADE ANDERSON GELLER, HERBALIST AND ACTIVIST

CHAPTER 24

Lemon Balm

A couple of years ago I was hiking with a group of people in an old-growth forest in the Pacific Northwest. We were following an overgrown trail covered with giant ferns and other undergrowth. While gazing at the massive trees towering above us, someone stepped on a wasp's nest, and we were quickly surrounded by an angry mob of stinging insects. I ran to safety, but not before getting a handful of throbbing stings. As I looked for something to relieve the pain, I saw feral lemon balm growing freely along the trail. I chewed some of the leaves into a paste, applied it on the stings, and watched in amazement as the pain and swelling disappeared.

Since that adventure in the old-growth forest, I've used fresh lemon balm leaves to soothe bee stings on children numerous times. Parents are always amazed by how well their screaming child is calmed. Besides being a fantastic first-aid plant for insect bites, lemon balm is profoundly relaxing. It is also used against viral infections and has even been shown to protect against the negative effects of radiation.

Other common names: common balm, balm mint

Botanical name: *Melissa officinalis*

Family: Lamiaceae

Parts used: aerial portions; leaves, just before flowering

Energetics: cooling, drying

Taste: sour

Plant properties: aromatic, relaxing nervine, antiviral, relaxing diaphoretic, aromatic digestant, antispasmodic

Plant uses: anxiety, nervousness, stress, viral infections, bug bites, nervous digestion, fevers, coughs

Plant preparations: tea, infusion, tincture, essential oil, infused oil, strewing herb, culinary

Lemon balm gets its common name from the fresh, lemony scent and taste. Most people will drink this lovely tasting herbal medicine gladly.

Lemon balm originally comes to us from the Mediterranean. It's been used for medicine for thousands of years. Pliny, Hippocrates, Galen, Culpeper, and even Shakespeare all spoke of its attributes. There are also records of Thomas Jefferson growing lemon balm at Monticello.

The genus name for lemon balm is *Melissa*, which comes from Greek meaning "honey bee" or simply "honey." In Greek mythology Melissa was a nymph who shared the wisdom and honey of the bees. Lemon balm is a favorite plant of bees. Not only does it produce lots of nectar, but it has also been used by beekeepers to prevent bees from swarming.

MEDICINAL PROPERTIES AND ENERGETICS OF LEMON BALM

Lemon balm has long been treasured for its calming and relaxing properties. Herbalists classify it as a relaxing nervine, an herb that relaxes, soothes, and supports the nervous system.

As a mild antispasmodic, it can help relieve pain due to tension, including headaches, back pain, and stomach cramps. Since it tastes good and is very safe, it is a great choice for soothing teething children.

FOR IMPROVING MOOD AND RELIEVING STRESS

Human clinical trials have shown that lemon balm can relieve agitation in people with dementia and improve the mood and stress levels of healthy adults.[1,2,3,4] It can also be used for anxiety, frayed nerves, stress, insomnia, seasonal affective disorder, and nervous tension.

FOR PROMOTING SLEEP

Lemon balm can be used as a gentle sedative to promote sleep. In one study a combination of valerian and lemon balm was shown to support healthy sleep cycles in menopausal women.[5] In another study the same combination was shown to benefit children who suffered from restlessness and dyssomnia (irregular sleeping patterns).[6]

AS AN ANTIVIRAL

Lemon balm can relieve painful cold sores and other herpes outbreaks. I've seen it lessen the severity and duration of an acute attack and, and when taken regularly, reduce future outbreaks.

In recent years, lemon balm has been researched for its antiviral properties, especially in relation to herpes simplex 1 and 2. In one study a cream made with lemon balm was shown to relieve common symptoms of genital herpes such as itching, tingling, burning, stabbing pain, and swelling. The cream also shortened healing time of the sores.[7]

Herbalist Karta Purkh Singh Khalsa recommends lemon balm applied externally to the eruptions of chicken pox, a virus closely related to herpes simplex.[8]

FOR PREVENTING DNA DAMAGE

With its high antioxidant levels, lemon balm has been shown to markedly improve oxidative stress and DNA damage. In one study, 55 radiology staff members were asked to drink lemon balm tea twice a day for 30 days. (The radiation from X-rays can damage DNA and induce oxidative stress.) Oxidative stress markers were recorded before they began drinking the tea and again after the 30 days. Researchers recorded numerous improvements in oxidative stress markers, including a "marked reduction in plasma DNA damage."[9] Now that I've read this study, I'll be drinking lemon balm tea before and after any X-rays I may need.

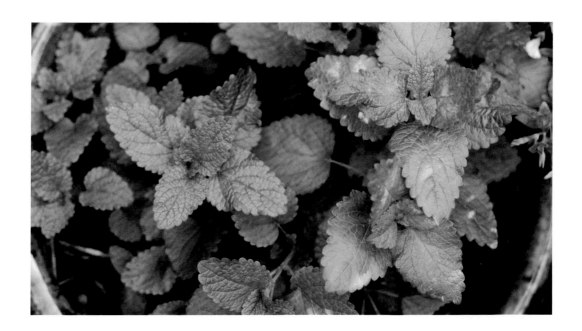

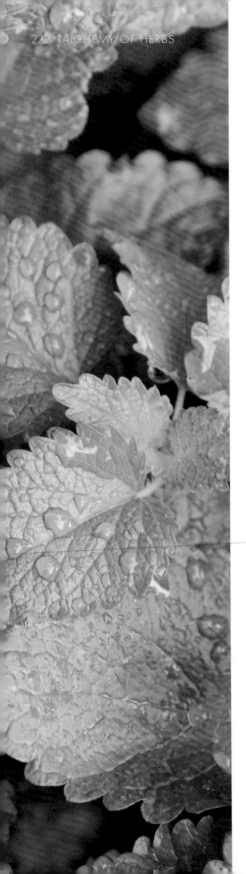

HOW TO USE LEMON BALM

For the most benefit, I recommend using fresh lemon balm. This mint is easy to grow and does well in containers. Freshly dried lemon balm retains its virtues, but you'll most likely find that the older it gets, the more it loses its pizzazz. Lemon balm's wonderful taste means there are many ways we can enjoy this herb, such as in a delicious tea or extracted into alcohol.

Lemon balm can be infused into oil for use as a salve, lip balm, or treatment for herpes sores. (This can be an affordable substitute for lemon balm essential oil.) To make an infused oil with lemon balm, lightly pack a jar with freshly dried lemon balm that has been crushed and crumbled. Then fill the jar with your oil of choice. (I recommend using shelf-stable oils such as olive or jojoba.) Stir the lemon balm and oil mixture well. Keep it in a cool, dark place and stir it daily for 2 weeks. Strain and use the oil as desired.

Don't forget to use lemon balm in the kitchen! It goes well with meats, fish, and vegetables or sprinkled into sauces, green salads, fruit salads, and herb butters.

RECOMMENDED AMOUNTS

Lemon balm, whether fresh or dried, can be consumed regularly in varying quantities. You can make a simple, light tea using 1 teaspoon of the plant or make a strong brew using up to 1 ounce (approximately 2 cups). (Larger quantities are more accurately measured by weight; however, a teaspoon of herbs is too light to measure accurately on the average kitchen scale.)

The therapeutic amount for lemon balm is as follows:

As tea: 1 teaspoon to 1 ounce per day

As tincture (fresh herb): 1:2, 45% alcohol, 3 to 5 mL, 3 to 5 times per day

SPECIAL CONSIDERATIONS

In vitro studies show that lemon balm may inhibit thyroid function. This effect has not been shown in humans; however, if you have an underactive thyroid, avoid consuming this plant in excess.

LEMON BALM NOURISHING INFUSION

This recipe uses a lot of lemon balm and an extended steeping time so you can really feel the calming and relaxing properties of this minty plant. It's combined with oatstraw (*Avena sativa*), which is also commonly used as a calming and restoring herb. This tea is also lovely iced.

Yield: approximately 3 cups, 1 to 2 servings

1. Bring 3½ cups of water to a boil.

2. Place the herbs in a 1-quart jar. Fill the jar with just-boiled water.

3. Let steep, covered, for 4 hours or overnight. Strain. Add stevia or honey if desired, for sweetness.

4. Drink within 24 hours.

½ cup dried lemon balm

½ cup dried oatstraw (*Avena sativa*)

2 tablespoons dried rosebuds or rose petals

pinch of stevia or honey, to taste

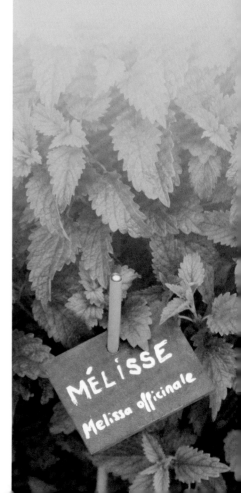

1½ pounds boneless chicken breasts, cut into 1-inch pieces

3 tablespoons olive oil

½ red onion, thinly sliced

½ pound green beans, cut into 1-inch pieces

1 large carrot, cut into matchstick-size pieces

½ cup fresh lemon balm leaves, stems removed

2 teaspoons toasted sesame seeds

For the marinade:

1 tablespoon cornstarch

¾ cup orange juice

1 tablespoon finely grated organic orange peel

¼ cup tamari or soy sauce

1 tablespoon toasted sesame oil

1 tablespoon grated fresh ginger

1 tablespoon honey

3 teaspoons five-spice blend

LEMON BALM AND ORANGE CHICKEN

I love making this dish at the height of summer, when the veggies can come straight from the garden to the table. The fresh lemon balm gives this a lemon-mint taste that combines well with the orange flavors. If you don't have lemon balm, you can even substitute another aromatic mint. The five-spice blend can be bought in many grocery stores, or you can make your own using the recipe on page 46.

Yield: 6 servings

1. *To make the marinade:* Whisk ¼ cup cold water and the cornstarch together in a bowl. Then whisk in the orange juice, orange peel, tamari, sesame oil, ginger, honey, and five-spice blend.

2. In another small bowl, mix the chicken and ¼ of the marinade. Let this stand for 15 to 30 minutes. (You can prep the veggies during this time.)

3. Heat the olive oil in a large skillet over medium-high heat. Add onion and stir-fry 30 seconds.

4. Add the marinated chicken to the pan, stir frequently, and cook for 5 minutes or until the chicken is no longer pink on the outside.

5. Add the green beans and carrot to the pan. Cook until crisp-tender, stirring frequently.

6. Add the rest of the marinade to the pan. Continue to cook for 3 to 5 minutes or until the sauce thickens and the chicken is cooked through.

7. Remove from heat. Stir in half of the lemon balm leaves and all of the sesame seeds.

8. Sprinkle on the rest of the lemon balm leaves just before serving.

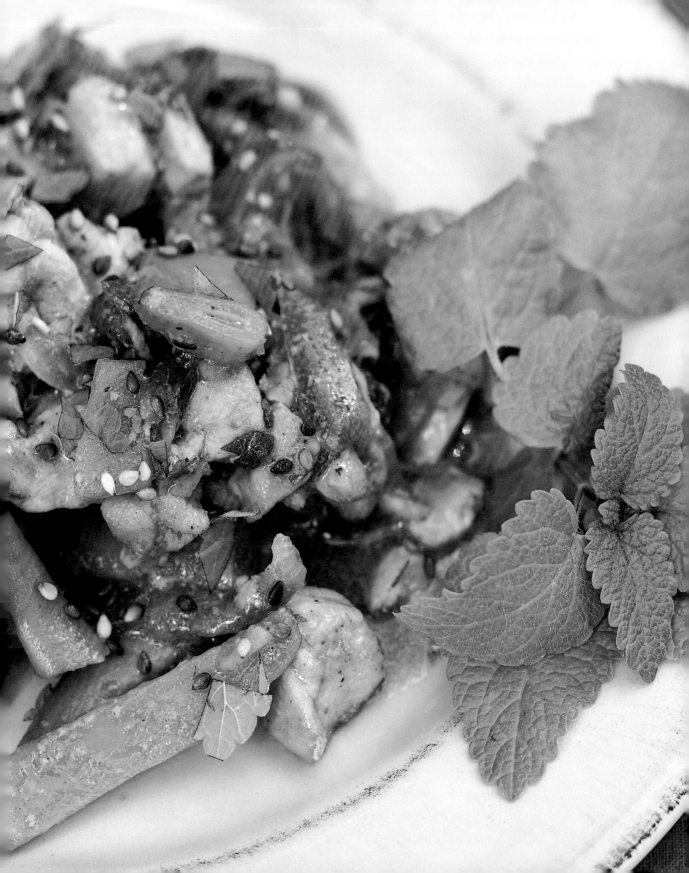

LEMON BALM WATER

1 sprig fresh lemon balm
(approximately 10 leaves),
or 1 tablespoon dried
lemon balm

1 thin slice of lemon

2 thin slices of cucumber

This is a simple way to lightly flavor your water and make a delicious and refreshing drink on a hot summer day. I especially like to make this when traveling. If using fresh lemon balm, slightly crush the lemon balm sprig between your palms to release its aromatic properties.

Yield: 4 cups

1.   Place the fresh or dried lemon balm, lemon slice, and cucumber slices in a 1-quart jar.

2.   Fill the jar with 4 cups of lukewarm water and let sit for 2 to 4 hours so the flavors can infuse. (If you've used dried lemon balm, you may want to strain this to avoid drinking the tiny leaves, or use a straw with a strainer.)

3.   Drink within 24 hours, as is or iced.

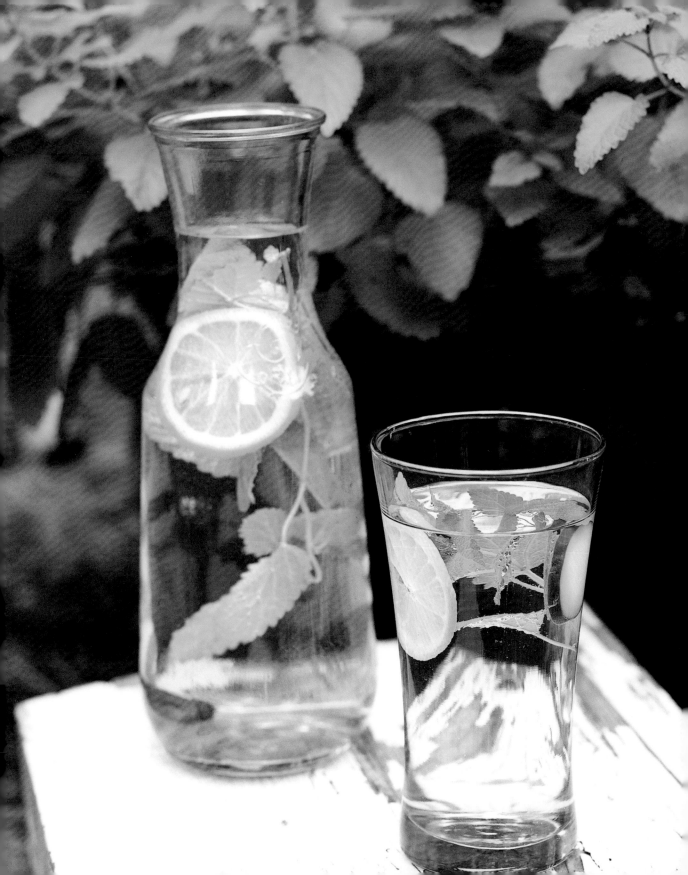

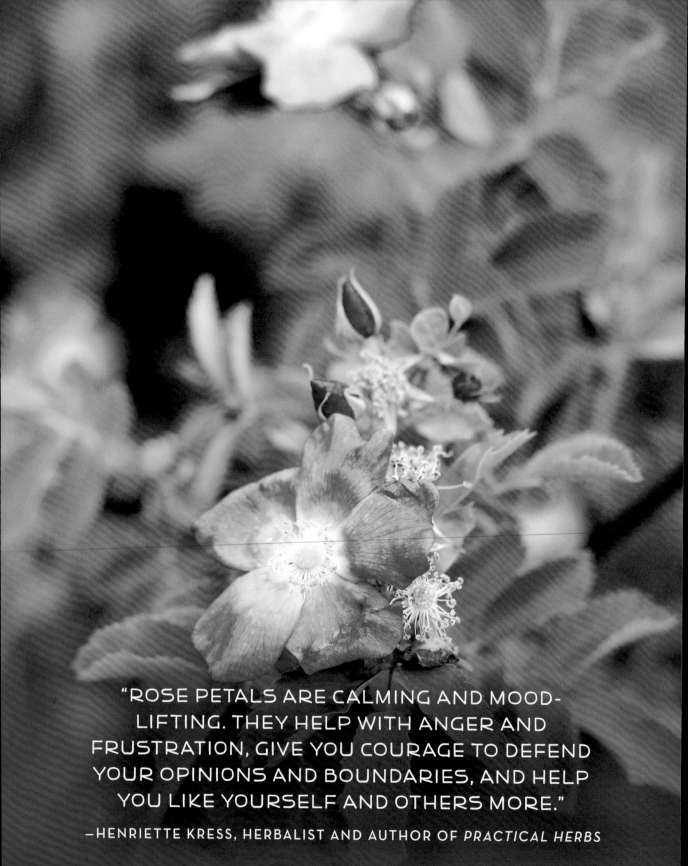

"ROSE PETALS ARE CALMING AND MOOD-LIFTING. THEY HELP WITH ANGER AND FRUSTRATION, GIVE YOU COURAGE TO DEFEND YOUR OPINIONS AND BOUNDARIES, AND HELP YOU LIKE YOURSELF AND OTHERS MORE."

—HENRIETTE KRESS, HERBALIST AND AUTHOR OF *PRACTICAL HERBS*

CHAPTER 25

Rose

The valley where I live explodes with wild roses every June. Modest, anonymous green bushes suddenly jump out in the landscape with their pink blossoms. When walking along a trail, I often smell and hear the signs of a rose bramble long before I see it. The heady scent of wild roses follows the breeze and the steady buzz of busy bees vibrates the air. Each year, I savor this season.

Together my husband and I have done a fair bit of wildcrafting, or harvesting wild plants. And without a doubt, out of all that we've gathered, wild rose petals are my favorite. Feeling the silky texture of the petals on my fingers and being enveloped in their perfume is a luxurious and joyful experience.

While roses have been adored for their beauty for thousands of years, they are more than a pretty face and scent. They offer us powerful medicine for relieving both emotional and physical pain, for healing wounds, and for decreasing systemic inflammation.

Botanical name: *Rosa spp.*

Family: Rosaceae

Parts used: petals, inner bark, leaves, fruit (hips)

Energetics: cooling, drying

Taste: sour (astringent)

Plant properties: astringent, analgesic, nervine, aphrodisiac, anti-inflammatory, antioxidant

Plant uses: bladder infections, pain, colds, flu, grief, depression, inflammation, wounds

Plant preparations: tea, tincture, honey, syrup, vinegar, food

f there were a flower popularity contest, my guess is that roses would win. Entire gardens, books, decoration themes, and even professions are devoted to this single flower. Roses are native to many parts of the Northern Hemisphere. It's speculated that cultivation began in China, and that subsequent hybrids were eventually taken to Europe, where the obsession with this flower continued to grow.

Marie-Josèphe-Rose Tascher de La Pagerie, more commonly known as Joséphine Bonaparte, the first empress of France, is credited with financing and supporting the first intentional hybrids of roses. Her home, Château de Malmaison, is said to have had hundreds of different rose hybrids, earning her the title of "Godmother of modern rosomaniacs."[1]

Roses have long been used to symbolize and celebrate love and friendship. And in modern times we have brought that to a whole new level. The National Retail Federation says that in 2015 American consumers spent more than $2.1 billion on roses for their loved ones on Valentine's Day![2]

TYPES OF ROSE

True wild roses are beautiful yet simple, with only five petals and a starburst of stamens in the center. They range in color from pure white to a deep pink and are almost always aromatic. How then did we end up with the thousands of variations of rose species today?

Our obsession with the rose has led to breeding countless changes, so now roses can have numerous petals and come in a multitude of colors: white, yellow, pink, orange, red, blue, and everything in between. Unfortunately, as many roses have been bred for beauty, much of their scent and medicinal properties have been lost along the way.

When choosing roses for your health, look for aromatic wild roses as your best source. If you don't have access to wild roses, then domesticated roses could be used, although there are a couple of considerations. Only use roses that you know have not been sprayed with pesticides. Never use roses from florists, since these are almost always sprayed. (Besides wanting to avoid consuming roses that have been sprayed, you also might consider avoiding even handling them in a decorative bouquet.) Second, I recommend using rose petals from flowers that are aromatic. If your roses don't have any scent, then look for another source.

MEDICINAL PROPERTIES AND ENERGETICS OF ROSE

Our culture commonly focuses on the physical aspects of illness. We use objective physical measures to diagnose and treat disease, while relegating a person's spiritual and emotional well-being to another branch of medicine, a church, or a spiritual teacher. Roses can remind us that this separation is only a recently created reality. Their scent, their physical beauty, and their medicine fluidly address our physical and emotional health, making it a wonderful medicine for our whole heart.

FOR YOUR HEART

Roses have a positive effect on the physical heart. In one study people were given 40 grams of rose hip powder daily for six weeks. At the end of the six weeks, there was a significant improvement in blood pressure and plasma cholesterol in the people taking the rose hip powder as compared with the control group.[3]

Researchers wanted to investigate the physiological effect of rose oil on humans by applying it on the skin. Those receiving the rose oil had decreases in breathing rate, blood oxygen saturation, and systolic blood pressure, which indicated there was an overall decrease of autonomic nervous system arousal. They also self-rated themselves as being more calm and relaxed than those in the control group.[4] This study is a wonderful example of the rose's effect on multiple dimensions of health.

Besides being a symbolic gift of the heart, roses can be used to gladden the heart. They are commonly used for mending a broken heart and supporting someone going through grief, sadness, and depression. Herbalist David Winston recommends a tincture of rose petals in combination with hawthorn leaves and mimosa bark for grief and post-traumatic stress syndrome.[5] Furthermore, a four-week study that looked at the combination of rose oil and lavender essential oil for women at high risk for postpartum depression found that those receiving the aromatherapy treatments had significant improvements in both anxiety and depression without any adverse effects.[6]

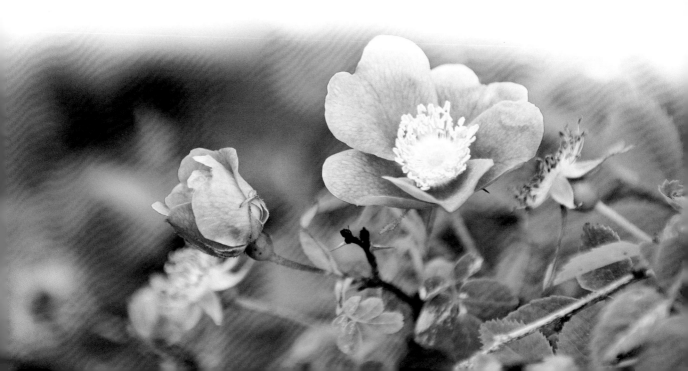

FOR HEALING WOUNDS

All parts of the rose plant have long been used to heal both external and internal wounds. In his book *Native American Ethnobotany*, Daniel Moerman recorded numerous uses of roses by America's indigenous people. One common wild rose species, *Rosa woodsii*, was used extensively by the Paiute in topical applications for boils, sunburns, sores, cuts, swellings, and wounds. The Okanogan-Colville used chewed leaves as a poultice for bee stings.[7]

One of the most common reported uses of roses across North America was for diarrhea. Herbalists commonly use plants that are astringent for helping to heal wounds, and the rose is a reliably astringent plant. This tissue-toning property helps to mend skin or address tissues that have become too lax, such as when teeth become loose in the gums or when excessive diarrhea has made intestinal tissues lax.

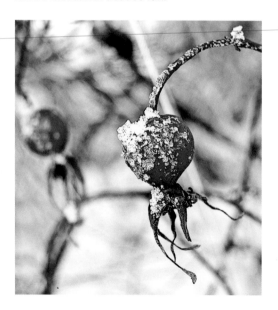

FOR INFLAMMATION AND PAIN

Another application for the astringent properties of roses is ulcerated tissues, as the tightening of the tissues helps with healing. In one double-blind, placebo-controlled study a mouthwash made with rose extract was shown to be effective at relieving pain, decreasing inflammation, and reducing the size and number of ulcers in those suffering from recurrent canker sores (aphthous stomatitis).[8]

Rose seeds and rose hips have been the focus of several studies demonstrating their ability to modulate inflammation and decrease pain.[9] To date, several studies have shown that the daily consumption of rose hips can reduce pain and improve general well-being in patients with osteoarthritis in the hips and knees and also benefit patients with rheumatoid arthritis.[10,11,12] One study showed that rose hips reduced inflammatory markers like serum C-reactive protein in patients with osteoarthritis.[13]

Rose does more than address inflammatory pain. Another study demonstrated rose tea's ability to improve the symptoms of premenstrual syndrome (PMS) in adolescent girls. In this study 130 adolescents were randomly assigned to two groups. One group received rose tea and the other a placebo. Those drinking the rose tea had less menstrual pain, distress, and anxiety than the control group.[14]

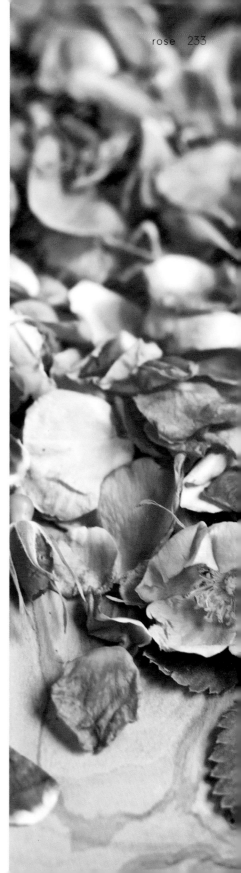

HOW TO USE ROSE

While many parts of the rose can be used as medicine, including the leaves, bark, and root, I am most familiar with using the petals and rose hips. (Rose hips are the fruits of the rose, which ripen to a deep-red color in the late summer and fall.)

Both rose petals and hips are high in bioflavonoids, and rose hips are famously high in vitamin C. Drying and cooking decreases vitamin C content, so to get the most benefit from rose hips, eat them straight off the bush. However, the hips can also be made into a variety of condiments including jelly, honey, vinegars, and preserves. Fresh rose petals can be made into jams, wines, honeys, and vinegars, sprinkled on salads, and enjoyed in tea.

If you live in the Northern Hemisphere, a trusted field guide will help you identify the wild roses in your region. (You can also check out the "Learning Your Plants" course that I created on HerbMentor.com.)

RECOMMENDED AMOUNTS

Rose petals and rose hips are a food and can be eaten in foodlike quantities. Studies showing medicinal benefits of rose hips have used dosages anywhere from 5 grams to 45 grams per day.

SPECIAL CONSIDERATIONS

Avoid using roses that have been sprayed with pesticides. (Almost all that come from florists will contain traces of pesticides, as they are not meant for consumption.)

Rose essential oil boasts an intoxicating scent and a steep price. It takes an amazing amount of roses to make a single ounce of the essential oil. If you find cheap rose essential oil, then it has most likely been adulterated with some other plant.

ROSEBUD TEA

2 heaping tablespoons dried rosebuds or petals (approximately 6 grams)

1 teaspoon dried lemon verbena

1 teaspoon dried cornflower (optional)

honey, to taste (optional)

This is a lovely way to enjoy the sweet tastes of rose and lemon verbena and a great way to unwind at the end of your day. The cornflower (*Centaurea cyanus*) gives a slightly bitter and nuanced flavor; it can be omitted if you can't easily find it.

Yield: 1¼ cup

1. Bring 1¼ cups of water to a boil. Mix the herbs together and place them in a tea cup or large tea infuser. Avoid cramming the herbs into a small infuser; it's better for them to have room to expand and move around.

2. Pour the just-boiled water over the herbs. Cover and steep for 7 to 10 minutes. Occasionally stir or dip the infuser while steeping. Strain.

3. Add honey if desired. Sip while warm.

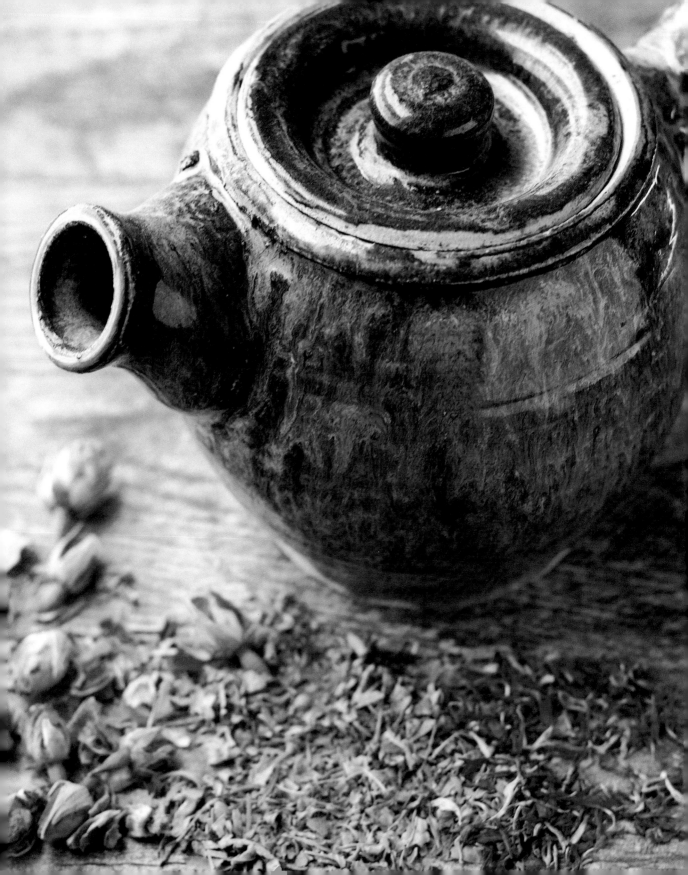

ROSE HIP–CRANBERRY COMPOTE

3 cups chopped apples
   (about 3 medium apples)

2 cups fresh cranberries

⅓ cup dried rose hips,
   with seeds removed

1 tablespoon lemon juice

1 tablespoon lemon zest

1 cup apple juice

½ cup pomegranate juice

2 tablespoons grated
   fresh ginger

2 teaspoons cinnamon
   powder

½ teaspoon freshly
   grated nutmeg

¼ teaspoon ground cloves

¼ cup honey or sugar,
   or to taste

freshly whipped cream
   (optional)

Compotes are stewed fruit with spices and are a simple and delicious way to create a fruit-based dessert. This particular recipe is a favorite in our house and often signifies the coming of winter and the holiday season. Cranberries are a wonderful source of antioxidants and deserve to be eaten in more than one meal a year. The apples may be peeled or not—it's up to you.

Yield: 4 cups, 8 servings

1. Place the fruits, rose hips, lemon juice, lemon zest, apple juice, pomegranate juice, and ginger into a pan and bring to a boil. Reduce the heat so the mixture is at a low simmer.

2. Continue to simmer for 20 minutes, stirring occasionally to prevent burning. After 20 minutes the fruit should be soft and the mixture will looked jelled and cooked down.

3. Add the spices and the honey. Taste and add more honey if desired. Stir for another 2 minutes, then remove from heat.

4. Serve warm with whipped cream, if desired.

ROSE HIP AND APPLE MUESLI

Muesli is an oat-based breakfast that often includes nuts and dried fruits. Soaking the mixture overnight makes the oats and nuts more easily digestible and allows the rose hips to rehydrate. With a little prep the night before, you can have a quick and delicious breakfast in the morning.

Yield: 4 servings

1. Mix the oats, rose hips, almonds, cinnamon, and nutmeg in a bowl with a lid. Stir in the milk, yogurt, juice, vanilla extract, and honey. Leave in the fridge overnight to soak.

2. In the morning, add the apple. Serve with additional milk if desired. It's fine to eat as is, but if you prefer warm breakfasts, feel free to heat this up.

1¼ cups oats

⅓ cup dried rose hips with
   seeds removed

½ cup chopped raw almonds

1 teaspoon cinnamon powder

pinch of freshly grated
   nutmeg

⅔ cup whole milk

⅓ cup plain yogurt

½ cup apple juice

1 teaspoon vanilla extract

2 teaspoons honey, or to taste

1 cup diced apple
   (about 1 medium apple)

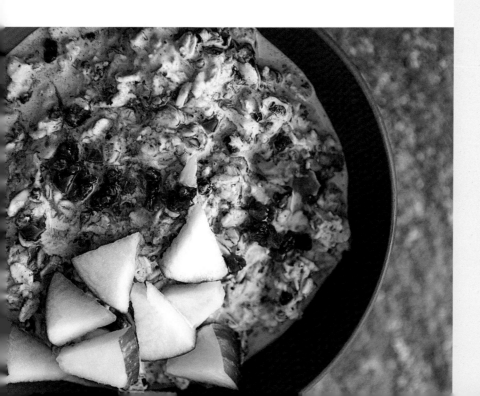

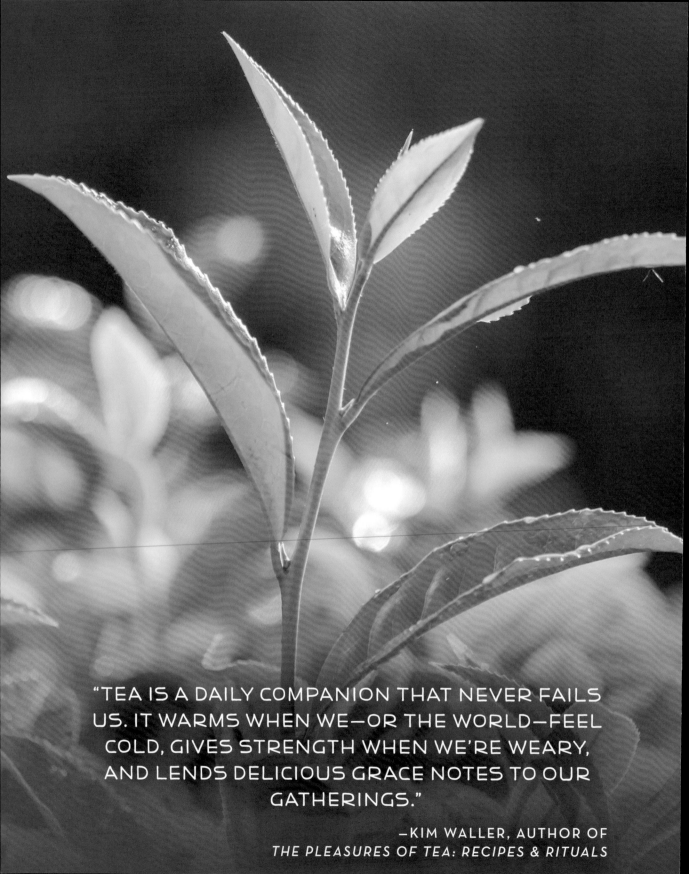

"TEA IS A DAILY COMPANION THAT NEVER FAILS US. IT WARMS WHEN WE—OR THE WORLD—FEEL COLD, GIVES STRENGTH WHEN WE'RE WEARY, AND LENDS DELICIOUS GRACE NOTES TO OUR GATHERINGS."

—KIM WALLER, AUTHOR OF
THE PLEASURES OF TEA: RECIPES & RITUALS

CHAPTER 26

Tea

If you were to award one herb as having the most influence on humans, honors would undoubtedly go to the humble tea plant. This shrub has shaped entire cultures and inspired wars, and its leaves continue to make the most commonly drunk beverage in the world today. The United States is the second-largest importer of tea, and more than half the U.S. population drinks it daily.

For thousands of years, people have loved tea because it tastes good and has stimulating properties similar to those of coffee. Today, more and more people are choosing to drink tea because of its highly popularized health benefits. But tea also offers us a benefit that doesn't commonly make the headlines. Drinking tea can give us precious moments of relaxation and connection, which in our perpetually stressed-out culture can be the most important medicine of all.

Scientific name: *Camellia sinensis*

Family: Theaceae

Parts used: leaves

Energetics: cooling, drying

Taste: sour (astringent)

Plant properties: stimulant, antioxidant, cardioprotective

Plant uses: energy, heart health, oral health, insulin resistance, type 2 diabetes

Plant preparations: tea, culinary

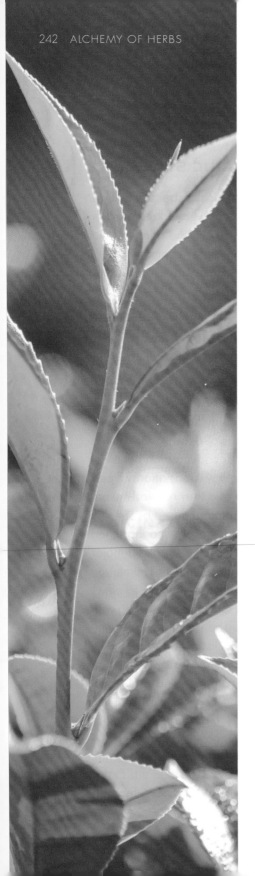

HOW TO USE TEA

In preparation for this section of the book, I made a visit to Floating Leaves Tea Shop in Seattle, where I took a class on oolong tea from the owner, Shiuwen Tai. Shiuwen is passionate about the art of tea as a way of contemplation and connection. For example, she states that not only is the tea in premade bags inferior to loose tea in terms of quality, but you also lose your connection with the leaves when you use bagged tea.

In fact, most of the tea consumed in the United States comes in tea bags or as a readymade tea drink. If you are drinking tea for your health, it is best to avoid these. Instead look for organic, fair trade, and loose-leaf tea from online distributors or tea specialty shops.

Shiuwen also told me that master tea connoisseurs can sip tea and taste the mountain it was grown on. While many people may never reach that level of discernment, regularly enjoying tea while being present in the moment can give us peace and contentment, something that many of us both lack and crave in our perpetually busy lives.

RECOMMENDED AMOUNTS

While tea offers lots of health benefits, it is also caffeinated. The healthy amount that can be enjoyed in a day will vary from person to person as well as by the type of tea. While I offer a recommended amount, you will ultimately have to determine what works best for you. Does a cup of tea leave you jittery? Does drinking tea throughout the day make it hard for you to sleep at night? All of these are signs that tea may not be working well for you.

The therapeutic amount of tea is the following:

As tea: 1 to 2 teaspoons brewed in 1 cup of water, 3 to 5 times per day

SPECIAL CONSIDERATIONS

All tea contains caffeine, and those sensitive to caffeine may be overly stimulated by tea. Black tea contains the most caffeine, green tea the least.

Most of the tea shipped to the United States, especially those in premade bags and drinks, is of the poorest quality. Low-quality tea has been found to have high concentrations of toxins like fluoride and heavy metals. Buy organic, loose-leaf tea to get the most benefits for your health.

A lot of tea is hand harvested, and much of it may be processed by hand too. Look for fair trade tea to ensure that the people involved in the harvesting and processing of your tea were paid a decent wage and treated with respect.

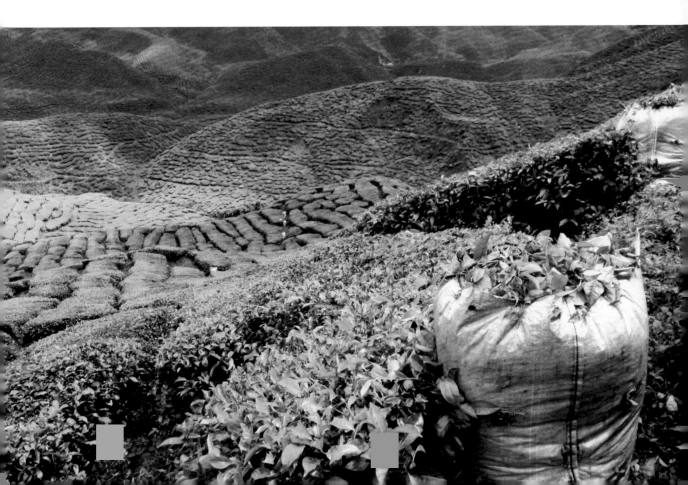

MAKE YOUR OWN
EARL GREY TEA

10 to 15 drops bergamot essential oil

1 cup loose-leaf black tea (I like Assam)

¼ cup dried orange peel* (20 grams)

2 tablespoons dried corn-flowers (optional)

1 vanilla bean, minced finely

cream, to taste (optional)

honey, to taste (optional)

Earl Grey tea is black tea that has been flavored with the citrus fruit bergamot (*Citrus bergamia*), which comes to us from Italy and other Mediterranean areas. Originally the tea may have been mixed with the actual bergamot peels, but these days it is usually made with essential oil.

You can easily make your own tea blend at home, so you can control the strength of flavor. Use less essential oil for a subtler effect, more oil for a stronger effect. The cornflower (*Centaurea cyanus*) doesn't add much flavor, but makes a beautiful blend; it can be omitted if you can't easily find it.

Yield: 1¼ cups loose-leaf tea, approximately 30 to 60 servings

1. Pour the bergamot essential oil into a 1-pint glass jar. Put a lid on the jar and shake well to distribute the essential oil all over the inside.

2. Add the tea leaves. Cover and shake well for about 30 seconds. Then add the rest of the ingredients and shake well.

3. This tea blend can be made into tea immediately, but I like to let mine cure for a couple of days to allow the flavors to combine. Store in a cool, dark place and use within 6 months.

4. To brew your Earl Grey: Bring 1¼ cups water to a boil. Place 1 to 2 teaspoons of the tea blend into a tea mug or large tea infuser. Avoid cramming the herbs into a small tea infuser; it's better for them to have room to expand and move around.

5. Cover your tea with just-boiled water. Let steep, covered, for 3 to 5 minutes. Strain.

6. Enjoy immediately with cream and honey to taste.

*Store-bought dried orange peel comes in small, uniform pieces. If you make your own, be sure to mince the orange peels finely before drying them, as they are difficult to cut once dried.

A TEA BREAK
WITH OOLONG

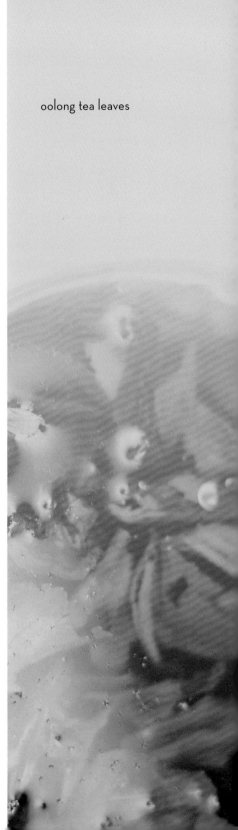

oolong tea leaves

You could take all the herbs and spices in the world for your health, but if you never take a moment to yourself, your efforts will be in vain. This recipe isn't just about the tea; it's also about taking time to rest and to be with yourself.

While drinking any tea can be a great way to relax and pause within your day, I chose a simple oolong tea here because I've been enamored with it ever since taking an oolong class with Shiuwen. One thing she mentioned in class was the difference between teaching how to make a tea in the United States versus Taiwan, China. She says in the States people are very concerned with the exact directions. They want to know: What exact temperature should the water be? Exactly how much tea do you use? How long do you steep? Instead of focusing on those details, this recipe is about relaxing into the process of making tea. Over time you'll find your own personal preferences.

I've been drinking a varietal blend of oolong called Oriental Beauty. While it is not the most sophisticated tea, I love its simplicity and mildly sweet taste. It is also very forgiving with steeping times and doesn't get overly astringent when steeped for a long time.

Yield: variable

1. Bring water to a boil. Let the water sit for a minute or two.

2. Place loose-leaf oolong tea into a small cup. Use enough tea to loosely cover the bottom of the cup.

3. Pour the hot water over the tea to fill the cup. Let steep. Eventually the leaves will sink to the bottom of the cup.

4. Put away your to-do lists and worries of the day. Find a quiet spot and enjoy your oolong tea.

GREEN TEA AND ROSE FACIAL CREAM

1 cup jojoba oil

30 grams green tea leaves

10 grams dried rose petals

1 gram alkanet root (optional; turns the oil red to make a pink cream)

20 grams beeswax

25 grams coconut oil

20 grams shea butter

⅓ cup rose hydrosol

⅓ cup aloe vera gel

1 teaspoon rosemary antioxidant extract

15 drops geranium essential oil (optional)

10 drops grapefruit essential oil (optional)

8 drops clary sage essential oil (optional)

One of my favorite recipes from herbalist Rosemary Gladstar is her recipe for the "Perfect Cream." I've made my own versions of this blend countless times over the years. I know it's a big hit because my friends are not shy about requesting another jar!

Admittedly, this may be the most complicated recipe in this entire book, but if you love decadent and nourishing facial creams, learning how to make them yourself will open a whole new world of luxury. Most facial creams you can buy at the store—even the "all natural" ones—have all sorts of weird ingredients. This cream is filled with the best and most nourishing ingredients for your skin.

Many of the ingredients in this recipe are oddly shaped, so you will need a scale to measure them by weight.

Because this cream doesn't have any harsh preservatives, make sure you use clean utensils, bowls, blenders, etc. Also, make sure all instruments are dry; you don't want to put any water in the mixture since this can increase the likelihood it will spoil. In many years of making this recipe, I've had only one batch ever go bad on me. You can tell a batch has spoiled if you see mold growing on the cream.

Jojoba oil is very luxurious. It is shelf stable, and it readily soaks into your skin. It's also expensive. Almond oil, grapeseed oil, and apricot kernel oil will also work. Rosemary antioxidant can be bought from herbal apothecaries like Mountain Rose Herbs. Besides helping to preserve the oils in the cream, rosemary antioxidant also has protective qualities for the skin.

Here's a tip for an easy cleanup: Wipe down all oily surfaces with a paper towel before using hot, soapy water to wash them.

Yield: 1½ cups

1. Your first step is to infuse the herbs into the oil. Put 1 to 2 inches of water in the bottom of a double boiler. Place the oil into the top. Add the green tea, rose petals, and alkanet root (if using), and stir well. Turn on the heat and heat the oil until it is fairly warm to the touch, about 100°F. Remove from the heat. Heat the oil 3 to 5 times per day for 1 to 2 days. You can also put this in a modified slow cooker or yogurt incubator as long as the temperature of the oil doesn't exceed 110°F.

2. Once the herbs and oil have infused, strain off the herbs, reserving the oil. When straining the oil I recommend using cheesecloth so you can squeeze all the oil out of the herbs. After you strain the herbs you should have ¾ cup jojoba oil. If you fall short of that, add enough pure jojoba oil to reach that amount.

3. In a double boiler, heat the beeswax, coconut oil, and shea butter until melted. Add the oil and stir until everything is liquid and combined. (I like to use a small wooden stick for stirring to avoid a messy cleanup.)

4. Pour the warm oil mixture into a food processor or blender. Let cool just until solid.

5. Mix together the rose hydrosol, aloe vera, rosemary antioxidant, and essential oils, if using. The next step is to emulsify these waters with the oils. For best results, the two mixtures should be roughly the same temperature.

6. Turn on the food processor or blender with the oils in it, and slowly drizzle in the water mixture. Continue to blend until the ingredients have combined to form a thick cream. Do not overblend. If necessary, use a spatula to scrape down the sides and around the blade as you blend.

7. Spoon the cream into containers. Store in a cool, dark place or the fridge.

8. *To use:* Massage a tiny amount of cream into your face and neck just after washing your face with warm water. It may feel oily for a few minutes but will soon soak in, leaving your skin feeling silky and smooth. Use within 3 months.

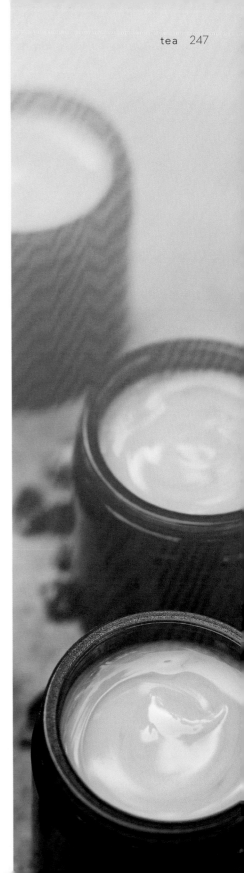

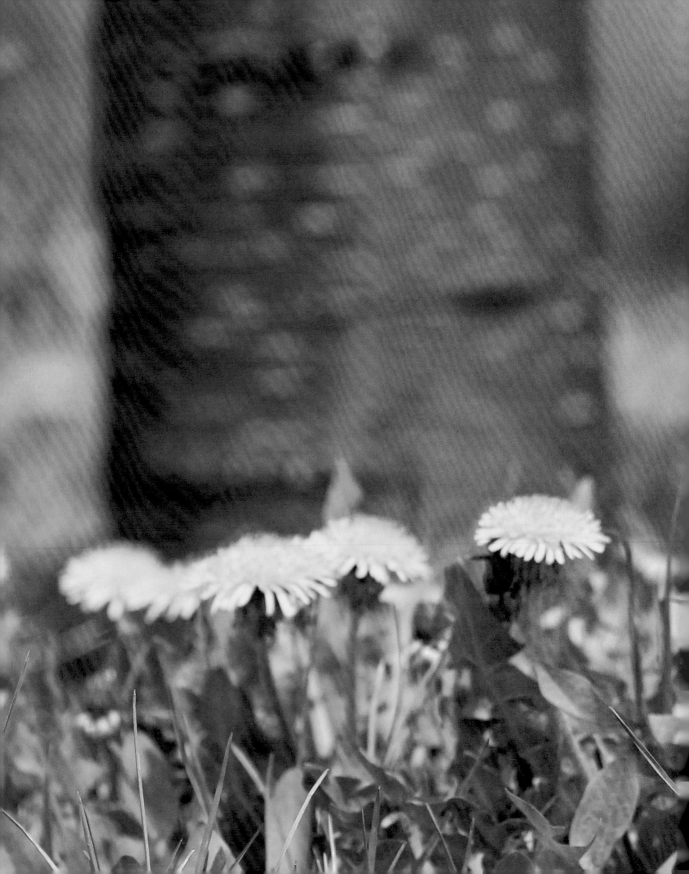

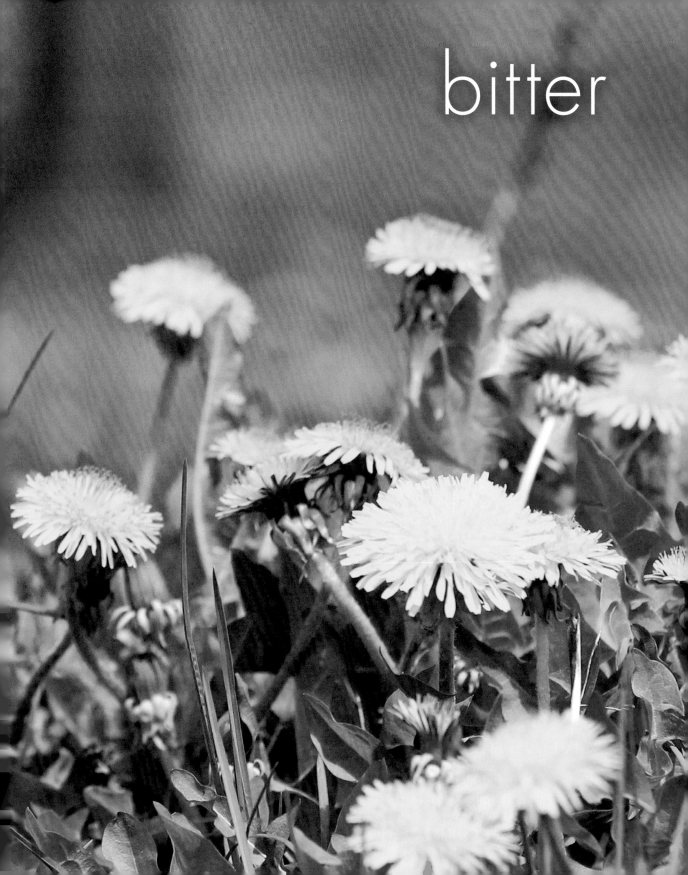

bitter

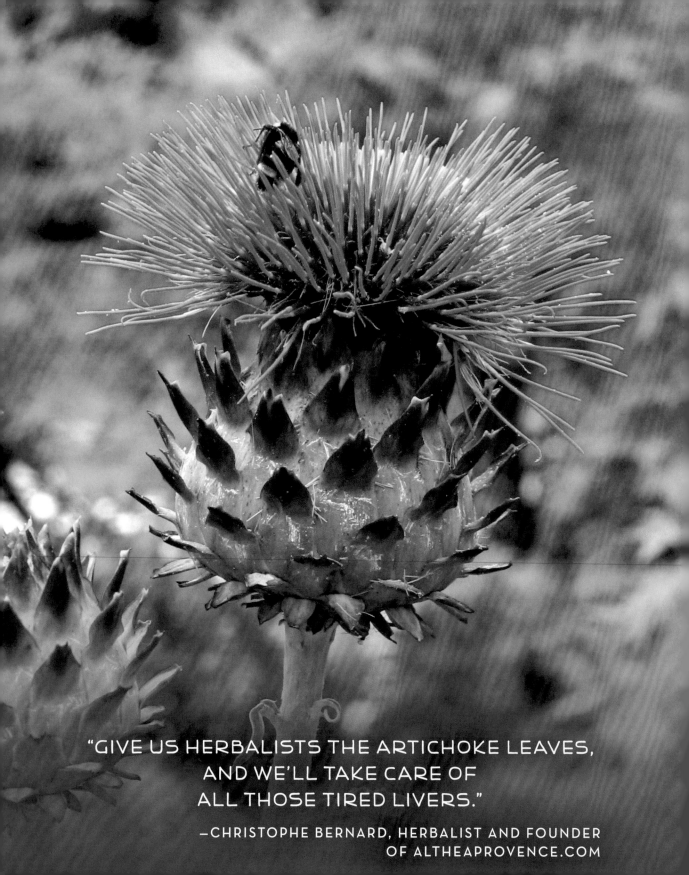

"GIVE US HERBALISTS THE ARTICHOKE LEAVES,
AND WE'LL TAKE CARE OF
ALL THOSE TIRED LIVERS."

—CHRISTOPHE BERNARD, HERBALIST AND FOUNDER
OF ALTHEAPROVENCE.COM

Artichoke

At first glance, artichoke might seem like a strange thing to include in an herb and spice book, but artichokes have long been used as food and medicine. They are among the most antioxidant-dense vegetables available. Their high levels of fiber and inulin (a prebiotic) make them a wonderful vegetable for digestive health. Historically they have long been used for liver health and were infamously used as an aphrodisiac.

As lovely as the artichoke vegetable is, this section is specifically about the leaves. What we typically eat (and see at the grocery store) is the flower bud. Artichoke leaves are lower down on the plant. Herbalists have long used bitter artichoke leaves for liver health and to aid digestion. New research has been validating these uses and also highlighting artichoke leaves' ability to reduce high cholesterol.

Botanical name: *Cynara scolymus*

Family: Asteraceae

Parts used: leaves, flower bud (vegetable)

Energetics: cooling, drying

Taste: bitter

Plant properties: bitter tonic, liver protective, heart protective, choleretic, cholagogue

Plant uses: high cholesterol, improving liver and heart health, troubled digestion

Plant preparations: tincture, tea, bitter digestive blends

Our modern-day artichokes are a type of thistle, probably derived from its older cousin, the cardoon. It is believed this plant originated in northern Africa or perhaps Sicily. The ancient Greeks and Romans were known to eat artichokes as well as use the leaves for medicine, but it seems they fell out of favor with the fall of Rome. By the Middle Ages, artichokes were being used by the elite in western Europe, and by the 18th century they were being cultivated in North America.

MEDICINAL PROPERTIES AND ENERGETICS OF ARTICHOKE LEAVES

Artichoke leaves strengthen our digestion, keep our liver healthy, and support heart health. When taken regularly, artichoke leaves also help support your body's natural detoxification strategies. When your detoxification pathways are working well, you will feel energized throughout the day. You'll have healthy-looking skin and hair, strong digestion, and optimally balanced hormones, resulting in a healthy and happy body.

FOR DIGESTION

One of the secrets to artichoke leaf's benefits lies in its bitter taste. While most people detest strong bitter tastes, herbalists are obsessed with bitterness and consider it one of the most important tastes for healthy digestion.

How can a taste be good for digestion? The bitter taste is challenging. It not only provokes our taste buds but also stimulates our entire digestive system. Our bodies recognize the bitter taste as being potentially poisonous. As a result, when bitterness is detected our systems go into full alert and digestive juices start flowing in order to mitigate any poisons entering our system. When you taste bitter foods and herbs regularly, your system is revved up and ready to go. Without these strong flavors, digestion can become sluggish and slow, resulting in gas, bloating, constipation, and other digestive maladies. In other words, we need bitterness daily in order to have good digestion.

Herbalists classify artichoke leaves as being both choleretic and cholagogue. Choleretics stimulate bile production in the liver, and cholagogues stimulate the release of bile from the gallbladder. Bile is what helps your body to break down and absorb fats and is also an important part of your body's natural detoxification system. Because of this, artichoke leaf is especially indicated when someone has a hard time digesting heavy foods and fats.

By challenging your entire digestive system, artichoke leaf can strengthen your digestion in a variety of ways. It stimulates your mouth to produce saliva, which helps to break down carbohydrates. That in turn stimulates digestive enzymes in the stomach. Artichoke leaves even stimulate pancreatic digestive enzymes. The flow of all these digestive juices signals the colon to perform its natural peristaltic rhythms, helping you to avoid constipation and keep your bowels moving regularly.

Researchers have been studying the positive effects of artichoke leaf in people with general digestive problems and those diagnosed with irritable bowel syndrome. One study split 244 people with functional dyspepsia (upper abdominal discomfort) into two groups. One group received artichoke leaf and the other a placebo. After six weeks, those taking the artichoke leaves tested significantly better in terms of their digestive symptoms.[1] Researchers also surveyed patients diagnosed with IBS who had been given artichoke leaf, and 96 percent responded that artichoke leaf was better than or equal to any previous therapies that they had tried.[2]

FOR LIVER HEALTH

Artichoke leaf helps stimulate bile production in the liver and is a powerful ally for this detoxification organ. Scientists have identified two constituents in artichoke leaf that are known to protect the liver. One, cynarin, is found only in artichoke. Another, silymarin, is also famously found in milk thistle, another wonderfully liver-protectant herb that has been used to protect people from liver poisoning after accidentally eating poisonous mushrooms.

Artichokes are also extremely high in antioxidants, which can further protect your liver. Regularly eating artichokes and using artichoke leaf can help protect your liver from harmful chemicals that may be found in your environment (such as pollutants, pesticides, etc.)

FOR HIGH CHOLESTEROL AND HIGH BLOOD PRESSURE

Christophe Bernard, herbalist and founder of Altheaprovence.com, writes: "Artichoke is a very dependable liver protecting

and lipid lowering plant. It is one of my go-to herbs for people suffering from metabolic syndrome with high cholesterol and triglycerides. And think about it—the world grows this bulky plant for the few flowers we put on our plates. And what happens to the huge mass of leaves? Discarded. Well, no more! Give us herbalists the leaves, and we'll take care of all those tired livers."[3]

While herbalists have long used artichokes and artichoke leaves to support the liver and improve digestion, researchers have been further validating artichoke leaves as a powerful herb for the heart. Extracts of artichoke leaf have been shown to reduce high levels of cholesterol and decrease mildly high blood pressure. While the exact mechanisms aren't known, it's probable that when liver health is supported, the body is better able to metabolize cholesterol. Since most imbalanced cholesterol levels are caused by systemic inflammation and complications of insulin resistance, another avenue of artichoke's beneficial action may be its high antioxidant levels that help to tame inflammation.

In one double-blind, placebo-controlled clinical trial, 46 people with high cholesterol were given artichoke leaf extract. After eight weeks, these patients had significant improvements in their lipid levels, including an increase in HDL ("good" cholesterol) and a decrease in LDL ("bad" cholesterol) and total serum cholesterol.[4]

Herbs rarely have just one benefit, and this is true for artichoke and heart health too. Researchers have shown that artichoke juice can improve endothelial function in adults with mildly high cholesterol.[5] Impaired endothelial function is one of the first stages of atherosclerotic heart disease.

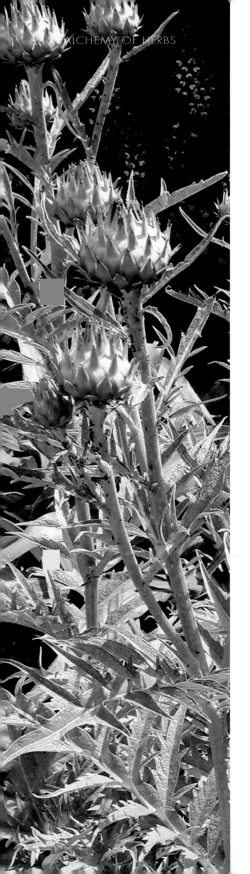

HOW TO USE ARTICHOKE

Artichoke leaf can be used as a tincture, tea, or capsule. My favorite way to use artichoke leaf is in digestive bitter blends (as in the following recipes), but to get the most benefits of artichoke leaves you may need to take them in larger amounts by using a tincture or tea. Since they are very bitter, it's difficult to take too much of them.

Remember, artichoke leaf is not what is found in the vegetable section of your grocery store. It can be special-ordered from herbal companies listed in the back of this book.

RECOMMENDED AMOUNTS

The therapeutic amount for artichoke is as follows:
As tea or capsule: 2 to 6 grams per day
As tincture: 1:5, 30% alcohol, 3 to 5 mL, 3 times per day[6]

SPECIAL CONSIDERATIONS

Avoid artichoke leaves if you have a known bile duct obstruction.

BITTER ARTICHOKE TEA

I am not going to lie to you. This tea is not going to be the best tea you've ever tasted. What it is going to be is *bitter*. And, as you've been learning, bitter is an incredibly important taste for stimulating digestion. I've tried to ease the bitterness a bit by combining the artichoke leaves with aromatic lemongrass and ginger. A small dollop of honey gives complexity to the tea but doesn't dampen the bitter benefits. Sip slowly before or after a meal to stimulate digestion.

Yield: 1¼ cup

small pinch dried
   artichoke leaves

1 tablespoon dried
   lemongrass

½ teaspoon ginger powder

honey, to taste (optional)

1. Bring 1¼ cups of water to a boil. Place the herbs in a mug or large tea infuser. Avoid cramming the herbs into a small tea infuser; it's better for them to have room to expand and move around.

2. Pour the just-boiled water over the herbs. Let steep, covered, for 5 minutes. Strain. Add honey for sweetness, if desired.

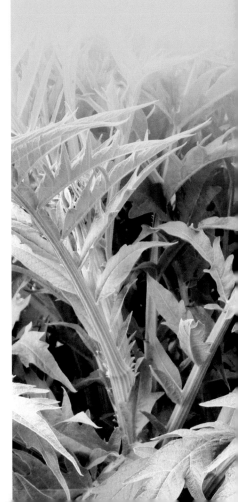

ARTICHOKE AND ORANGE BITTERS

¼ cup dried hawthorn
berries (20 grams)

¼ cup dried dandelion root
(30 grams)

1 tablespoon fennel seed
(5 grams)

1 teaspoon freshly ground
black pepper (3 grams)

¼ cup whole hibiscus
(7 grams)

1 tablespoon artichoke leaves
(1 gram)

2 tablespoons coriander
seeds (5 grams)

1 whole organic orange,
diced (including the peel
and seeds)

¼ to ½ cup honey, to taste

3 cups vodka (approximately)

This is a delicious bitter blend that can be taken 15 to 20 minutes before mealtime to help stimulate digestion. (I keep a tincture bottle of this on the dinner table and in my purse so it is readily available.) While the alcohol preserves the mixture and makes for a convenient way to take the herb, the amount of alcohol consumed each time is minimal. I like putting a teaspoon or two of this in a glass of sparkling water as a low-alcohol cocktail.

I've included both volume and weight measurements for this recipe because some ingredients are difficult to measure out. Use whichever measurement is convenient for you.

Yield: approximately 2 cups

1. Place all the herbs, spices, and orange into a 1-quart jar.

2. Add the desired amount of honey.

3. Fill the jar with the vodka. Stir well. Cover with a lid. Shake this 1 to 2 times per day.

4. Taste this after 1 week. If the flavors have infused to your liking, strain off the herbs, reserving the alcohol. Or leave it to infuse for an additional week.

5. Take ½ teaspoon or 5 to 10 drops in a small amount of water about 15 minutes before you eat, or whenever you remember. This will last indefinitely. Store in a dark bottle or dark location.

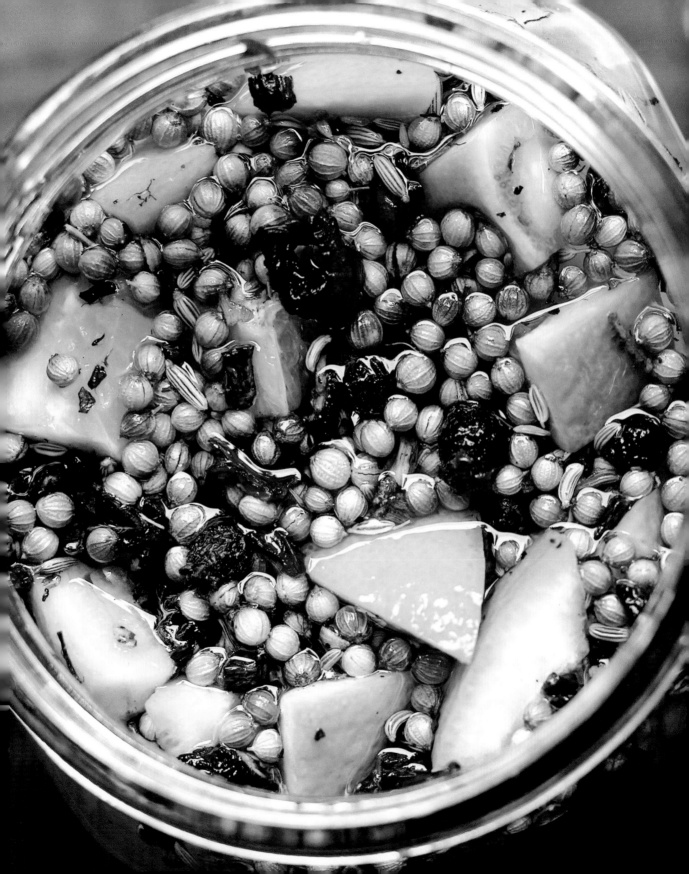

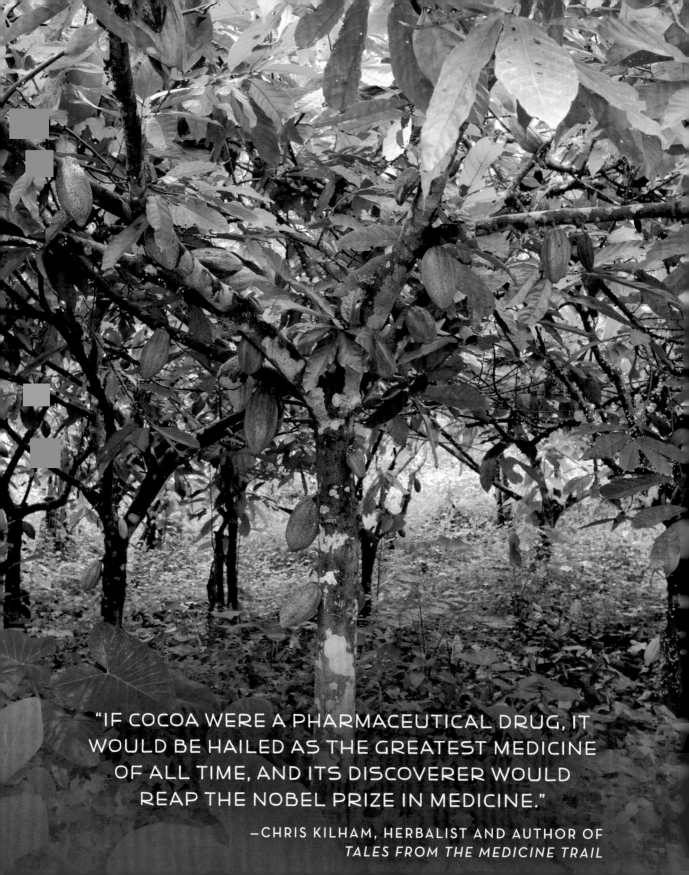

"IF COCOA WERE A PHARMACEUTICAL DRUG, IT WOULD BE HAILED AS THE GREATEST MEDICINE OF ALL TIME, AND ITS DISCOVERER WOULD REAP THE NOBEL PRIZE IN MEDICINE."

—CHRIS KILHAM, HERBALIST AND AUTHOR OF *TALES FROM THE MEDICINE TRAIL*

CARDAMOM CHOCOLATE MOUSSE CAKE

Chocolate lovers can celebrate this exceptionally dark chocolate mousse cake. Each bite slowly melts in your mouth while the cardamom spice enlivens the senses. This is my family's go-to dessert recipe for potlucks, and we've been asked for the recipe countless times. If you don't have a double boiler, fill a pot with 1 to 2 inches of water and place a tight-fitting bowl over the top.

Yield: 1 9-inch cake, approximately 16 small servings (or 8 large servings)

8 ounces bittersweet chocolate

⅓ cup coconut oil

½ cup honey

½ cup cocoa powder (plus extra, for garnish)

1 (13.5-oz.) can coconut milk

2 eggs

1 tablespoon cardamom powder

2 tablespoons vanilla extract

sliced almonds, for garnish (optional)

1. Preheat the oven to 350°F.
2. Put 1 to 2 inches of water in the bottom pan of a double boiler. Melt the bittersweet chocolate and coconut oil in the top.
3. When they are melted, remove from the heat. Add the honey and cocoa powder and mix well.
4. Add the coconut milk and mix well.
5. Whisk the eggs in a small bowl. Add the whisked eggs, cardamom, and vanilla extract to the chocolate mixture and combine well.
6. Pour the mixture into a slightly oiled 9-inch pie pan.
7. Bake in oven for 30 minutes.
8. When the cake is done, the top should be cracked but the middle should still be soft and wiggly.
9. Cool overnight to allow it to set. Sprinkle with sliced almonds, if desired.
10. Sprinkle some cocoa powder on top before serving.

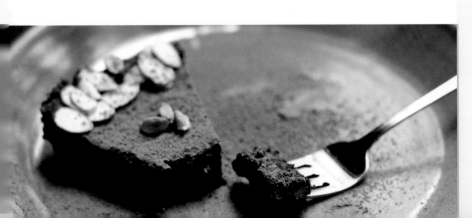

CHOCOLATE STRAWBERRY PUDDING

1 ounce 100% cacao unsweetened baking chocolate

¼ cup unsweetened cocoa powder

¼ cup honey

¾ cup coconut milk, full fat

1 teaspoon vanilla extract

⅛ teaspoon salt

½ teaspoon ground cinnamon

2 very ripe avocados, peeled and pitted

1 cup diced strawberries, stems removed

This light pudding is a perfect way to enjoy fresh spring and summer strawberries. The avocados give it a creamy consistency but otherwise don't distract from this delicious chocolate dessert.

Yield: approximately 3 cups

1. Put 1 to 2 inches of water in the bottom pan of a double boiler. Melt the baking chocolate in the top. Remove from heat when completely melted.

2. Into the same bowl, mix the cocoa powder, honey, coconut milk, vanilla extract, salt, and cinnamon.

3. Combine the chocolate mixture with the avocados and strawberries in a food processor. Puree until it has a smooth consistency.

4. Refrigerate for 2 to 3 hours, and enjoy within 24 hours.

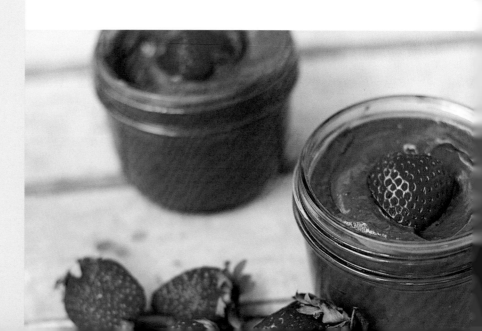

HOT CHOCOLATE

As I write this, it's a beautifully gloomy day, and I can hear raindrops pitter-pattering on our roof. It's exactly the kind of day that begs for the comfort of a rich hot chocolate.

This recipe isn't going to taste like the sugary, light chocolate of your youth. Instead this is a dark, frothy, and delicious blend for your grown-up taste. (If you are new to appreciating dark chocolate, you may want to start out using half cacao powder and half Dutch process cocoa.)

Yield: 2 cups, 2 servings

1. Put 2 cups of water in a medium saucepan and turn the heat to high. When the water is hot (not boiling), whisk in the cacao powder and cinnamon.

2. When fully mixed, remove from the heat, then add the butter, vanilla extract, and honey. Stir to combine until the butter and honey have melted.

3. Pour the liquid into a blender. Put the lid on loosely so steam can escape, and blend on high for 30 seconds.

4. Pour into cups and enjoy immediately.

¼ cup 100% cacao powder (16 grams)

1 teaspoon cinnamon powder

2 tablespoons butter (or coconut oil)

1 tablespoon vanilla extract

1 tablespoon honey, or to taste

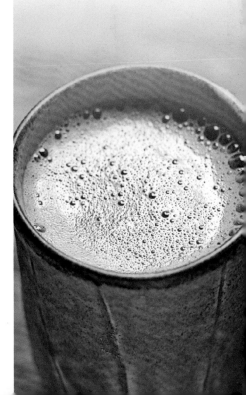

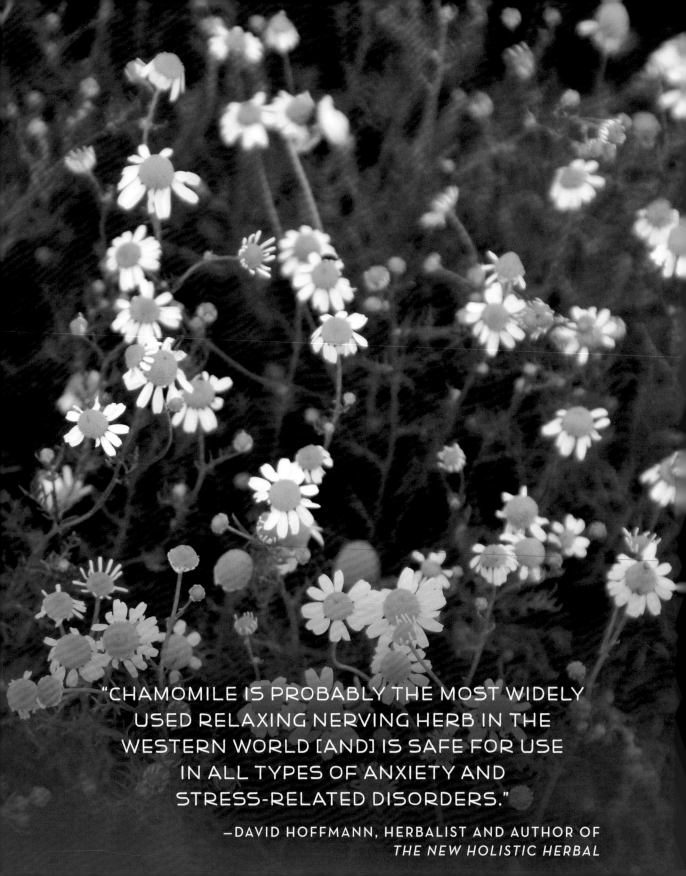

"CHAMOMILE IS PROBABLY THE MOST WIDELY
USED RELAXING NERVING HERB IN THE
WESTERN WORLD [AND] IS SAFE FOR USE
IN ALL TYPES OF ANXIETY AND
STRESS-RELATED DISORDERS."

—DAVID HOFFMANN, HERBALIST AND AUTHOR OF
THE NEW HOLISTIC HERBAL

CHAPTER 29

Chamomile

My introduction to herbal medicine may have been through *Peter Rabbit*, the classic story by Beatrix Potter. In the tale, Peter disobeys his mother, sneaks into Mr. McGregor's garden, and starts eating all the delicious vegetables he finds. The angry farmer spies Peter and chases him through the garden. Peter barely escapes, leaving his jacket and shoes behind. After such a tumultuous day, he doesn't feel well, so his mother puts him to bed and gives him chamomile tea. As a child, I had a plate depicting that scene and can still vividly see Peter's bunny ears sticking out of his bedcovers while his mother stands ready with the cup of tea.

Peter's mother was far smarter than I was. For years I was wrong about chamomile. I thought of it as gentle and, therefore, weak. I thought that because it was safe enough for little ones (like Peter Rabbit), it wasn't effective for the more serious problems of adults. But that is the beautiful secret of chamomile. As beloved herbalist Rosemary Gladstar so wisely says, "Chamomile demonstrates to us that gentle does not mean less effective."[1]

Other common names: German chamomile

Botanical name: *Matricaria chamomilla*

Family: Asteraceae

Parts used: flowering tops

Energetics: slightly cooling, drying

Taste: bitter

Plant properties: aromatic, relaxing nervine, carminative, relaxing diaphoretic, mild sedative, antispasmodic, vulnerary, anti-inflammatory

Plant uses: irritability, restlessness, insomnia, indigestion, dyspepsia, gas, fevers, colds, flu, teething, colic, externally for burns, rashes, conjunctivitis

Plant preparations: tea, tincture, essential oil, infused oil, hydrosol, steam inhalation

Chamomile is a member of the aster plant family and has an appearance similar to daisies. Each "flower" is actually a composite of smaller flowers, with a yellow center (made of disc flowers) and white petals (made up of ray flowers). It is native to southern and eastern Europe but has spread all over the world either in the garden or growing as a weed in disturbed soils.

Humans and Neanderthals have been interacting with chamomile for tens of thousands of years. Researchers analyzing the dental calculi of Neanderthals who lived around 50,000 years ago found evidence that they ate chamomile (and yarrow). They surmise that the only reason they would eat a bitter plant that doesn't contain a lot of nutrients would be for self-medication.[2]

TYPES OF CHAMOMILE

There are two plants that are commonly referred to as chamomile: German chamomile (*Matricaria chamomilla*) and Roman chamomile (*Chamaemelum nobile*). While there are some similarities between the two, there are also significant differences. This chapter is about German chamomile.

MEDICINAL PROPERTIES AND ENERGETICS OF CHAMOMILE

Drinking a cup of chamomile tea is like getting a warm hug from a loved one. It can help you relax and unwind after a stressful day, decrease pain caused by muscle tension or spasms, and strongly reduce inflammation. Chamomile's best gifts are that it is gentle while simultaneously offering profound relief. It can be enjoyed frequently as a tea, a massage oil, or a tincture. And because chamomile is gentle and effective, it works wonderfully for adults and children alike.

Parents often ask me what single herb they should have on hand for their children, and my answer is easily chamomile. It soothes the nervous system, promotes sleep, helps with digestive problems, and can be used for a variety of symptoms associated with a cold or flu. For example, chamomile gently relaxes muscle tension and can help soothe spasmodic or constricted coughs. Sometimes these types of coughs are caused by dryness or inflammation in the lungs. You can address this with chamomile, and it can also be combined with linden (*Tilia cordata*) and licorice (*Glycyrrhiza glabra*).

FOR ANXIETY AND INSOMNIA

Herbalists have long known of chamomile's ability to soothe someone who is distressed, anxious, or nervous. The genus name, *Matricaria*, is related to the Latin for "mother." Some say this is because it offers many benefits for mothers, while others say that sipping a cup of chamomile tea is like being soothed by a nurturing mother. A familiar saying in the herbal world is that chamomile works well for children who are whining or for adults who are acting like whining children. (Admittedly, I've had those kinds of days, and chamomile is a welcome gift.)

Sipping strongly brewed chamomile tea calms jangled nerves, which makes it a great companion after a stressful day or a good preventive measure before a difficult situation. I've often wondered if traveling would be a lot more enjoyable if everyone drank chamomile tea instead of coffee in airport terminals.

Herbalists have been relying on chamomile's relaxing properties for many centuries, and science is now catching up on validating its traditional use. In an exploratory study, researchers found that chamomile, even in a relatively small dose (220 mg), was more effective than a placebo in relieving both depression and anxiety in people.[3] Another clinical study found that chamomile relieved mild to moderate anxiety in people diagnosed with general anxiety disorder.[4]

Chamomile can also bring on a deep and restful sleep. I specifically think of chamomile if someone is having difficulty sleeping because of muscle tension or anxiety. For this use, it's best to drink a tea at least an hour before bed (to avoid nighttime bathroom trips) or use the tincture.

FOR PAIN RELIEF

Chamomile is an antispasmodic herb, which means that it relaxes muscle tension. As a result, it can decrease pain caused by tense muscles or cramping. I especially love chamomile for relieving menstrual cramps and pain associated with digestive cramping. A tincture or a strong cup of chamomile tea not only relieves pain quickly, but also lessens the worry or anxiety associated with those conditions.

While chamomile can effectively decrease pain, it goes beyond this simple use to address other common complaints of premenstrual syndrome (PMS). In one clinical study, nonsteroidal anti-inflammatory drugs (NSAIDs) were compared with chamomile in women with PMS. After two months, those using chamomile had a reduction in pain similar to that of the women using NSAIDs but also had significantly fewer emotional symptoms.[5]

Another common problem is shoulder tension, which leads to neck pain and headaches. A cup of chamomile tea along with a neck massage using chamomile-infused oil can do wonders for relaxing both the mind and the muscles, helping you unwind from the inside out.

FOR HEALING WOUNDS

Chamomile modulates inflammation and is slightly antimicrobial, making it a great choice for a variety of inflammatory conditions, such as wounds, burns, and rashes. For the best results, use chamomile both externally as an oil or wash and internally as a tea or tincture.

Science has shown chamomile's ability to modulate inflammation in a couple of powerful studies. In one, patients who had phlebitis (inflamed veins) due to intravenous chemotherapy were concurrently given chamomile. Those patients receiving a 2.5 percent and 5 percent concentration experienced a significantly shorter duration of phlebitis than those in the control group.[6] No one in this study had issues with toxicity, reminding us that chamomile is effective *and* gentle.

Another study compared the topical use of chamomile compresses with hydrocortisone cream for relieving itching and discomfort associated with skin lesions in people who have stomas (a surgically created opening in the abdomen that allows stool or urine to exit the body). Participants were either given a 1 percent hydrocortisone cream or instructed to use chamomile compresses twice a day. Those using the compresses had a significantly faster healing time as well as a considerable decrease in pain and itching compared with those using the steroid cream. The researchers pointed out that using chamomile in place of the steroid cream prevents serious side effects associated with topical steroid use, such as thinning of the skin.[7]

Another area where chamomile is effective is in the treatment of bleeding gums caused by gingivitis. Essentially, this condition is an infected wound in the mouth; however, the effects of gingivitis aren't just localized. They are often tied to inflammatory heart disease. In an interesting study, researchers compared the effectiveness of a chamomile mouthwash with the antiseptic chlorhexidine for bleeding gums associated with gingivitis. The results showed that the mouthwash had antimicrobial and anti-inflammatory properties similar to those of the chemical over-the-counter drug.[8]

FOR DIGESTION

Chamomile may be the perfect herb for many types of digestive complaints. As we've seen, it powerfully decreases inflammation, making it a great choice for inflammatory digestive problems such as Crohn's disease, diarrhea, ulcers, and irritations from food intolerances.

Not only can chamomile help relieve powerful inflammatory digestive problems in adults, but it can also bring gentle relief to children and has long been used for colic and children with diarrhea. In a study performed in 2006, children (aged six months to six years) with acute diarrhea were given a mixture of chamomile and apple pectin or a placebo. The symptoms of those receiving the chamomile/pectin mixture showed significant improvement as compared with those receiving the placebo.[9]

Chamomile really shines for digestive problems due to anxiety or worry, painful digestive spasms, or inflammatory digestive complaints. When consumed before a meal as a strong tea, it can, with its bitter taste, help stimulate a healthy appetite. Taken after a meal, it can help ease digestive problems such as bloating, gas, heartburn, and digestive spasms.

FOR FEVERS AND INFECTIONS

One of the most annoying symptoms of a cold or flu is sinus trouble. Being stuffed up and unable to breathe or having inflamed and irritated sinuses can affect your sense of smell and appetite and can just be altogether miserable. If left untreated, these symptoms can also make you more susceptible to developing a sinus infection. Chamomile inhaled as a steam can support the sinuses, help them to drain, and relieve inflammation.

Fever can be one of the most uncomfortable and scary symptoms of the flu. However, herbalists recognize that fevers are a beneficial immune system response and that, in most cases, a fever shouldn't be artificially lowered. Still, when someone is feeling hot, restless, and uncomfortable, chamomile can be used to release tension, promote healing sleep, and bring comfort.

Chamomile is also great at treating conjunctivitis or pinkeye. I've used this myself on several occasions. The most memorable happened years ago when I was teaching at my very first herb conference. I woke up the morning of my first class, and my eye was a gross, goopy mess. I could barely open it, and once I did, it was incredibly red and inflamed. Luckily, I had a few hours before class, and I had several bags of chamomile tea in my herbal first-aid kit. I wet a bag with warm water and put it over my eye for 30 minutes. I took a little break and then repeated it with a fresh tea bag. By the time I was in front of the class, my eye was almost back to normal. I repeated the process a couple more times that day, and by the next day, I was symptom-free.

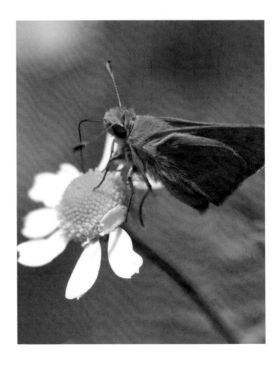

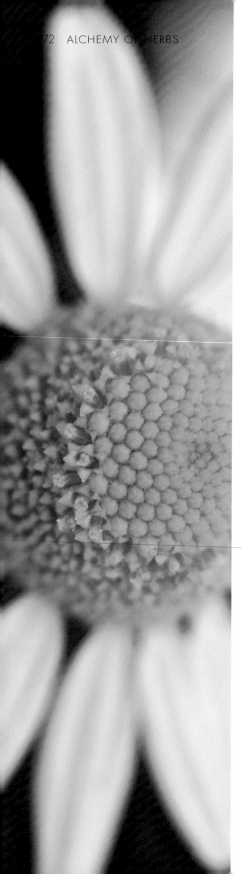

HOW TO USE CHAMOMILE

Probably most of us are familiar with dunking a chamomile tea bag in hot water for a couple of minutes and then drinking the slightly sweet, aromatic tea. While this does create a delicious beverage, stronger and more bitter brews of chamomile are what you need for profound relief of anxiety, insomnia, pain, inflammation, and cold and flu symptoms.

Instead of buying tea bags of chamomile, I recommend buying the loose herb in bulk. This makes it cheaper as well as easier to make a stronger brew. When buying chamomile in bulk, you'll know you have a quality product when it is strongly aromatic. Luckily, chamomile stores well and if kept in a cool, dark place may last a couple of years.

Chamomile works well as a steam inhalation for stuffy or inflamed sinuses. To make this, place a couple handfuls of chamomile into a medium bowl. Pour several cups of just-boiled water over the chamomile and stir well to soak the flowers. Place your face above the bowl and drape a towel over your head and the bowl so you trap the steam with the towel. Breathe deeply. Continue for as long as desired, filling the bowl with more hot water as needed.

RECOMMENDED AMOUNTS

Using small amounts of chamomile with a short steeping time makes a delicious tea. If using chamomile for more than a pleasing beverage, stronger and more bitter tea will give you more potent results.

The therapeutic amount for chamomile is as follows:

As tea: 9 to 15 grams per day

As tincture (dried flowers): 1:5, 40% alcohol, 3 to 6 mL, 3 times per day[10]

SPECIAL CONSIDERATIONS

Chamomile is generally considered safe for everyone; however, some people with sensitivities to the Asteraceae (aster) family may also be sensitive to chamomile.

CHAMOMILE EYEWASH

This is a simple saline wash. Saline solutions help to soothe irritated eyes and mucous membranes and are a lot gentler than using water alone.

You'll need an eyecup and cheesecloth or a coffee filter. Eyecups are made for treating for eye infections (like conjunctivitis) or eye irritations and can be purchased at most pharmacies.

Keep items as sterile as possible. Wash all instruments with hot, soapy water and consider boiling them before use. If you are addressing an eye infection, sterilize the eyecup after treating one eye and before treating the other, so you avoid spreading infection from the first to the second.

You can use this wash numerous times throughout the day. However, this solution needs to be made daily to avoid contamination.

Yield: 1 cup

1 cup distilled water*

½ teaspoon salt
(sea salt or real salt; avoid using table salt)

2 tablespoons dried chamomile

*Use distilled water only. Tap water can contain chlorine, fluoride, and other chemicals that are not eye friendly.

1. Combine water and salt in a saucepan. Bring to a boil and gently stir until salt is dissolved. Boil for 5 minutes, and then turn off the heat.

2. Add the chamomile and let steep, covered, for 10 minutes. Strain through several layers of cheesecloth or a coffee filter, but do not squeeze the cheesecloth at the end. It is important that there not be any little pieces of chamomile in your solution or it will irritate your eyes.

3. Let the solution cool in a glass measuring cup with a pouring spout.

4. When the solution is only slightly warm, pour it into a sterile eyecup. Fill the cup about halfway. Tilt your head forward and position the cup snugly against your eye. Hold the cup against your eye socket and tilt your head back. Blink your eye several times to get the solution in direct contact with your eye. Close your eye and continue to hold the cup in place for 1 to 2 minutes. (Repeat with other eye, if needed.)

1 tablespoon
    dried chamomile

1½ teaspoons oatstraw
    (*Avena sativa*)

1½ teaspoons rose petals

1 inch of vanilla bean, minced

honey to taste (optional)

CHAMOMILE TEA BLEND WITH ROSES AND VANILLA

This is a soothing chamomile tea blend that is a delicious after-meal beverage. One of my recipe testers, Cathy Izzi, described it as one might describe a fine wine. She said it was smooth, full bodied, and not overly floral while being very pleasant-tasting and comforting. She also noted that the vanilla bean gave it a nice, subtle finish.

Yield: 1½ cups

1. Bring 1½ cups of water to a boil. Steep the herbs, covered, in the just-boiled water for 15 minutes. Strain.

2. Add honey if desired.

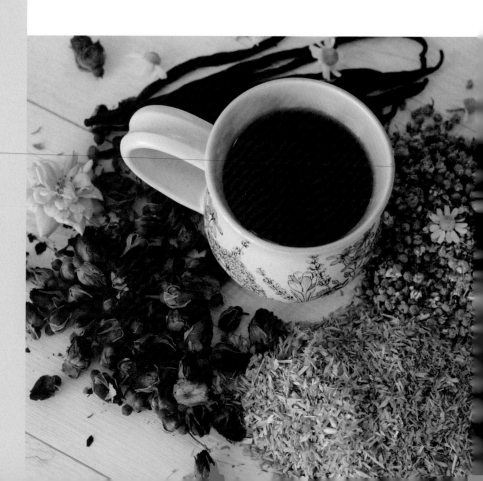

CHAMOMILE ICE POPS

These ice pops are a tasty treat for a hot summer day but are also a great herbal remedy for children of all ages. This recipe is formulated to replace electrolytes, helping to rehydrate kids who have been playing hard on a hot summer day as well as those recovering from a digestive illness such as diarrhea, upset tummy, or even vomiting. For this recipe, you will need small wooden sticks and some kind of ice cream mold—paper cups will do.

Yield: six 3-ounce desserts

2 tablespoons dried chamomile

1 tablespoon dried hibiscus

3 to 4 tablespoons honey, or to taste*

pinch of salt

1 tablespoon lemon juice

1 cup Greek yogurt

*If you are making this for children under the age of two, use sugar instead of honey due to botulism concerns.

1. Bring 1¼ cups of water to a boil. Put the chamomile and hibiscus in a cup, pour the boiling water over the herbs, and let steep for 10 minutes.

2. Strain the tea into a small bowl. While the mixture is still hot, add honey to taste. Stir well so the honey combines with the tea. (Since you will be mixing this with yogurt, you may want to make it more on the sweet side.)

3. Add the salt and lemon juice. Stir well. Let the mixture cool a little, approximately 5 minutes.

4. Add the yogurt and mix well.

5. Pour the mixture into molds or paper cups, and insert wooden sticks in the center. Place these in the freezer until frozen solid. (This will take several hours.)

6. These will be best if eaten within 1 week, before freezer burn sets in.

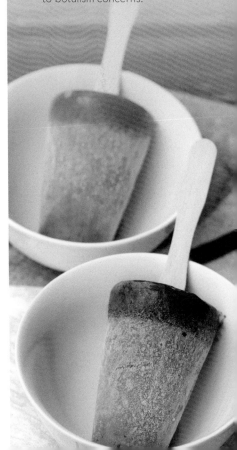

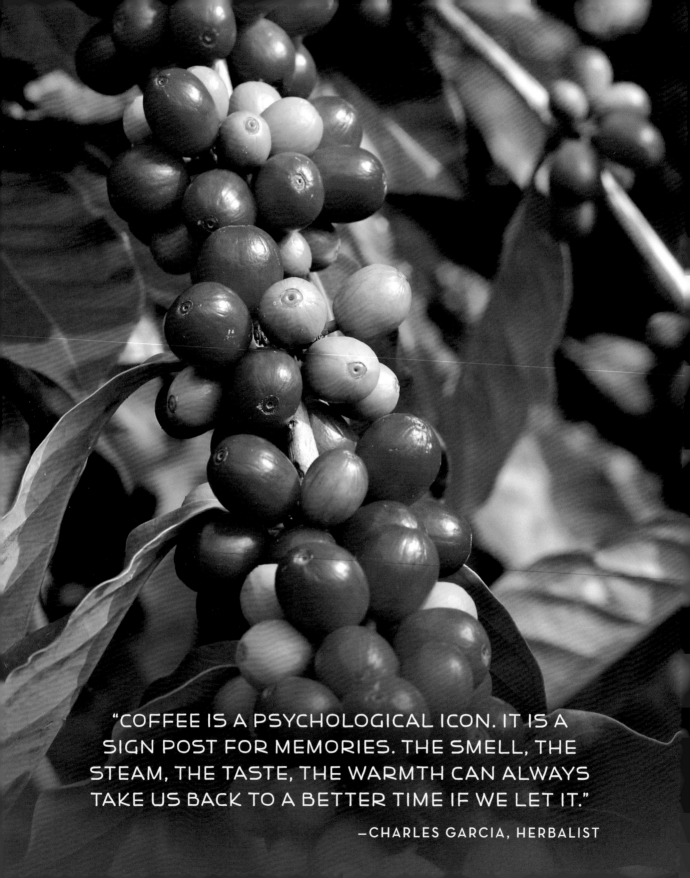

"COFFEE IS A PSYCHOLOGICAL ICON. IT IS A SIGN POST FOR MEMORIES. THE SMELL, THE STEAM, THE TASTE, THE WARMTH CAN ALWAYS TAKE US BACK TO A BETTER TIME IF WE LET IT."

—CHARLES GARCIA, HERBALIST

CHAPTER 30

Coffee

Most people don't think of coffee as an herb. However, if we define an herb as a medicinal plant, then coffee is not only an herb but also one of the most popular in the world. More than 500 billion cups of coffee are drunk annually, and more than 75 million people make their livelihood from it.

Perhaps the reason that coffee is commonly dismissed by the herbal world is because of our culture's overuse of this medicinal substance. It's rare to hear of an herbalist recommending coffee for someone's health, probably because 50 percent of the U.S. population is already self-dosing. Instead, herbalists are more likely to recommend against drinking coffee due to its side effects in susceptible people.

But there's more to coffee than a jolt of energy. Coffee can improve cognitive function, protect against neurodegenerative disease, prevent type 2 diabetes, support heart health, and more.

Though we often hear talk of "coffee beans," what we use is actually the seed of the plant. (However, for clarity, I'll use the word *beans* in this chapter.)

Botanical name: *Coffea arabica, Coffea robusta, Coffea liberica*

Family: Rubiaceae

Parts used: roasted seeds (commonly called "beans")

Energetics: cooling, drying

Taste: bitter

Plant properties: stimulating, diuretic, blood mover, laxative, blood sugar regulator, bronchial dilator, vasoconstrictor, antioxidant, cardioprotective, inflammatory modulator

Plant uses: fatigue, constipation, insulin resistance, stimulating digestion, improving cognition, symptomatic asthma, headaches, heart health, inflammation

Plant preparations: roasted coffee beverages, caffeine extracts, culinary

About 1,000 years ago, legend has it, a goat herder in Ethiopia noticed his animals were more rambunctious and frisky after eating the berries and leaves of a small shrub. Testing it out for himself, the goat herder felt more energized—and thus the fascination with coffee began.

The Arabs are credited with figuring out how to roast coffee beans and then brew them into a delicious beverage. For centuries the Arabs controlled the flow of coffee beans to other parts of the world, until coffee plants slowly but surely were smuggled out of controlled plantations and cultivated throughout equatorial regions of the world.

There is also a dark side to coffee's history. As the demand for coffee grew, profit-driven governments and entrepreneurs slashed down native forests and destroyed numerous indigenous cultures to make room for coffee plantations. Millions of people who were once independent subsistence farmers were forced into coffee cultivation, leaving families and entire countries vulnerable to the rise and fall of coffee prices.

Starting in the 1990s, awareness about the negative economic and environmental impacts of coffee began to rise. Organizations and cooperatives were created to ensure a fair price for farmers. Today coffee is the largest fair trade product in the world. Fair trade is the only ethical choice when buying coffee. "Shade grown" and "organic" coffees are further sustainable choices, adding layers of environmental protection by plantations maintaining biodiverse forests and growing coffee without pesticides.

TYPES OF COFFEE

Okay, I'll admit it . . . I adore coffee. That's why I am very grateful that in my small rural valley we have an exceptional coffee roaster, Blue Star Coffee Roasters. Blue Star buys green coffee beans from fair trade, organic, and shade-grown coffee farms around the world. (*Green* denotes beans that are raw and unroasted.) Dan Donohue, one of the owners, explained to me that the taste of coffee beans varies widely depending on the growing conditions and the climate. From year to year, coffee beans produced from a single coffee shrub can vary dramatically. As an herbalist, I found this especially interesting and further proof that nature can't be standardized.

Decaffeinated coffee is often wrongly thought to be completely caffeine free. In fact, while it has had the majority of the caffeine taken out of it, it may still have up to 3 percent of the original caffeine content, which can adversely affect people who are sensitive to caffeine.

Historically, caffeine was extracted from coffee by soaking the beans in chemical solvents like benzene, a known carcinogen. These days, dichloromethane and ethyl acetate are used to decaffeinate coffee. Proponents of this method claim that very little solvent remains on the coffee beans. However, concerns about these chemicals aren't just about the end product, but also about what we introduce into the environment in the process. If you want to avoid known carcinogens and the creation of chemical waste, then look for coffee that has been decaffeinated using water or carbon dioxide instead of harsh chemical solvents.

MEDICINAL PROPERTIES AND ENERGETICS OF COFFEE

The simplest way to describe the medicinal benefit of coffee is to say it's a stimulant. It stimulates energy, circulation, digestion, and even urination. Coffee acts by affecting the central nervous system, suppressing the parasympathetic "rest and relax" nervous system and bolstering the sympathetic "fight or flight" nervous system. The most obvious effect we feel after drinking coffee is more energy—it's no wonder we especially love this beverage upon waking in the morning.

In essence, coffee wakes things up and gets them moving. Physiologically, heart rate increases, as does circulation, diuresis, gastric enzymes, and peristalsis. The stimulation of gastric enzymes, which are an important factor in the digestive process, and peristalsis, the natural movement of the colon, are one reason that many habitual coffee drinkers rely on their morning cup to get their bowels moving.

Coffee is high in antioxidants. In fact, it may be the number one source of antioxidants for many people in the United States.

FOR FATIGUE AND DEPRESSION

People love coffee for its taste and for the comfort of a warm morning ritual. Some people say it's the best part of waking up. If you've ever enjoyed a morning cup of coffee, then you know exactly how this feels.

Many people depend on coffee to help them fight fatigue and increase their energy. Many studies have shown the positive effects of coffee for people who work the night shift, work exceptionally long hours, or do monotonous work throughout the day. In the short term, coffee can provide a relatively safe way to stay awake and increase alertness.[1,2]

That morning cup of coffee makes many people happy, and research says it may have a long-term effect on happiness as well. Epidemiological studies have shown an inverse relationship between coffee, tea, and caffeine consumption and levels of depression.[3]

FOR YOUR BRAIN

Numerous studies have shown that drinking coffee benefits cognitive performance. One interesting study on the effects of caffeine and extroversion showed that while caffeine improved reaction time and the speed of encoding of new information in everyone, people who identify as being more extroverted showed more improvement in terms of serial recall and running memory tasks.[4] This study validates what many herbalists already know: everyone is different, and therefore each person needs personalized recommendations rather than a silver bullet "cure."

Studies also show that drinking coffee decreases the risk for Alzheimer's and Parkinson's, two of the most prevalent neurodegenerative diseases.[5] One study found that drinking "3–5 cups per day at midlife was associated with a decreased risk of dementia/ AD [Alzheimer's disease] by about 65% at late-life."[6] While researchers don't know the exact mechanism of action, they hypothesize these results could be due to coffee's antioxidant content or its positive effects on insulin resistance.

FOR DETOXIFICATION

Studies have also shown regular coffee consumption supports the health of your liver, which is a powerful organ for detoxification. One study showed that its beneficial effects on the liver were especially helpful for people who drink alcohol.[7] Another study showed that even decaffeinated coffee consumption is correlated with a decrease in abnormal liver enzymes, leading researchers to theorize that caffeine is not the only medicinal substance in coffee.[8] There have even been studies showing coffee to be beneficial for people with chronic hepatitis C infections.[9, 10]

Coffee mildly increases the kidneys' rate of filtration, thus increasing urination. However, people quickly create a tolerance to this effect. It was once widely believed that coffee caused dehydration, but this is no longer thought to be the case.[11]

FOR INSULIN RESISTANCE, INFLAMMATION, AND HEART DISEASE

Clinical trials have shown that both light- and medium-roast coffee reduce oxidative stress and inflammation in humans.[12] Researchers hypothesize that the antioxidants in coffee may be the reason it has positive effects on many chronic diseases that are linked to oxidative damage (e.g., diabetes, heart disease, neurodegenerative diseases, and liver cirrhosis).[13]

Coffee has numerous benefits for preventing insulin resistance or mitigating the negative effects of this inflammatory metabolic disease. People who drink three to five cups of coffee a day have a significantly decreased risk for developing type 2 diabetes.[14] Some studies show as many as seven cups of coffee a day to be beneficial, although many people would experience adverse effects, such as anxiety or jitters, when drinking that much coffee daily.[15]

Several studies have shown that inflammatory heart disease, often strongly tied to type 2 diabetes, is decreased in people who regularly drink coffee. Coffee has been shown to improve endothelial function, reduce the risk of sudden cardiac death in women, and reduce coronary heart disease in women.[16,17] It's long been thought that coffee can increase blood pressure. Clinical trials have had conflicting results on this effect, which may point to an individual susceptibility.

HOW TO USE COFFEE

Raw (green) coffee beans stay fresh for about a year. Properly stored whole roasted coffee beans are best consumed within six months. For the best flavor, use your beans as soon as possible after grinding. Roasted, preground coffee is not ideal; it is preferable to grind your coffee fresh at home or at the store.

Grinding beans is another critical part of brewing that perfect cup of coffee. Finely ground beans lend themselves to a quick, pressurized-water extraction like espresso. A medium grind lends itself better to drip or pour-over coffee.

To get that incredible cup of coffee, look for a small coffee roasting company near you that offers fair trade, organic, and shade-grown coffee. If that's not available, many small roasters, like Blue Star Coffee Roasters, can ship you freshly roasted coffee.

In recent years, single-serving coffee-brewing machines have risen in popularity. While some may argue that these beans-plus-filter devices are convenient, they are also considered to be of low quality and produce an embarrassing amount of plastic and aluminum waste. The coffee in these single-cup preparations is rarely fair trade, organic, or shade-grown, which means it has already wreaked human and environmental damage before it even reaches the coffeepot.

SPECIAL CONSIDERATIONS

There are some potentially serious adverse effects to drinking too much coffee. Whether or not it is a health choice for you depends on who you are and your current health.

Those who experience negative effects from a cup of coffee, such as hyperactivity or jitteriness, should heed the wisdom of their bodies and entirely avoid caffeinated coffee. Also avoid coffee if you are continually stressed, have a lot of anxiety, aren't sleeping well, and/or have significant ups and downs in energy level during the day, as coffee could exacerbate these symptoms.

In choosing decaffeinated coffee, look for coffee that has been decaffeinated using water or carbon dioxide instead of harsh chemical solvents such as benzene, dichloromethane, and ethyl acetate.

Some people may abuse coffee, which can lead to both short- and long-term negative effects on overall health. For example, coffee can disrupt someone's sleep patterns. Then, when a person doesn't sleep well, they tend to feel tired the next day, thus fueling the desire for more coffee. This again disrupts sleep, leading to a self-perpetuating negative cycle.

Coffee can be addictive. As coffee consumption is increased, the body becomes tolerant to it, resulting in the perception that more coffee is needed. Suddenly stopping coffee can lead to withdrawal symptoms including headaches, fatigue, and foggy mental capabilities. It's generally better to slowly reduce coffee intake rather than stop all at once ("cold turkey").

Coffee can create or exacerbate heartburn.

Coffee is not recommended during pregnancy.

SPICED COLD-BREW COFFEE

1 cup coarsely ground
coffee beans

½ teaspoon
cinnamon powder

¼ teaspoon
cardamom powder

cream (optional)

honey or sugar,
to taste (optional)

Cold-brewed coffee makes a delicious drink that has less bitterness than traditional coffee that has been brewed with hot water. This recipe spices it up with the addition of cinnamon and cardamom. I like to keep a jar of this in the fridge for a cold coffee drink during the hot summer months.

Yield: approximately 2¾ cups

1. Place the coarsely ground beans and spices in a 1-quart jar. Fill the jar with water and stir well. Place a lid on this and let it sit in the fridge for 12 hours.

2. Strain off the coffee and spices through a coffee filter or several layers of cheesecloth. This creates a cold brew concentrate that will last for up to a week in the fridge.

3. *To use:* When ready to drink, mix 1 part of the coffee brew with 2 parts of liquid (for example, ¼ cup of cold-brew coffee with ½ cup of water). I like to add 1 part water and 1 part cream: ¼ cup of cold-brew coffee, ¼ cup of water, and ¼ cup of cream. If desired, add sweetener and ice before serving.

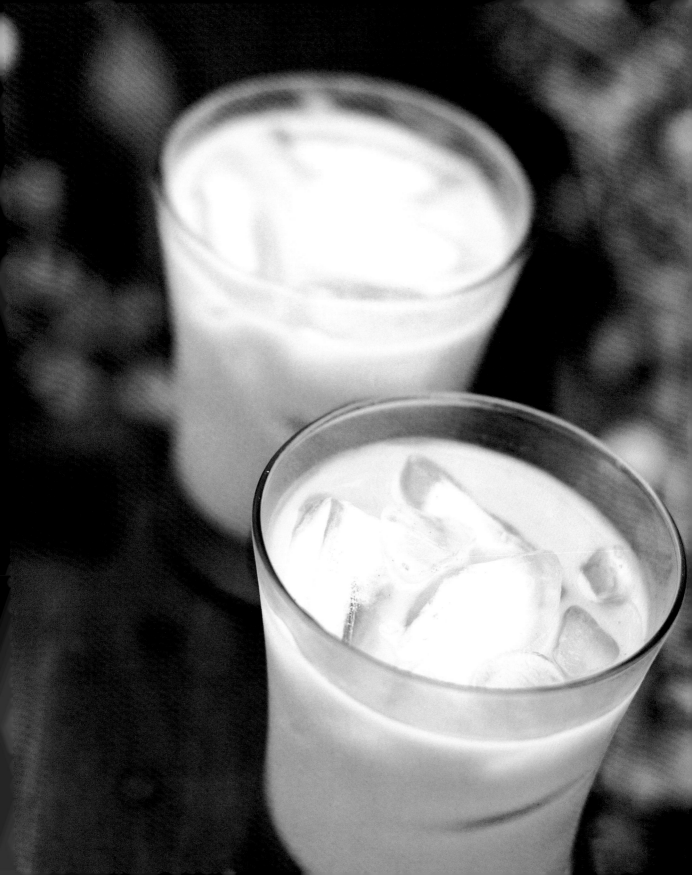

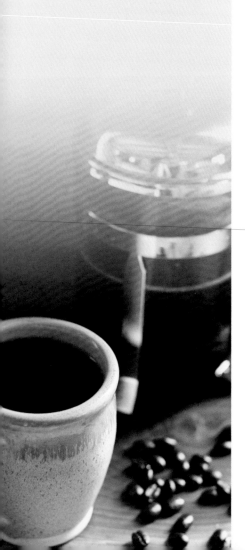

2 tablespoons coarsely
ground coffee

¾ cup to 1 cup of
spring water
(or water fresh from
the tap)

THE PERFECT CUP OF
FRENCH PRESS COFFEE

You might be wondering how French press coffee is different from other methods. During a tour of Blue Star Coffee Roasters, co-owner Dan Donohue explained to me, "The French press method has no paper filter that traps the finest particles and also some of the oils from the roasted bean. It produces a fuller cup, with accentuated body than other filtering methods."

He also reminds us that it's important to grind the coffee correctly: "The ground coffee is steeping in very hot water, and particle size will have an effect on how much extraction happens. If too fine, overextraction will draw out the woody flavor of the beans. Too coarse will underextract the flavor and lessen the depth of flavor and body in the cup." He suggests using a good burr grinder to grind your coffee, because it will "achieve relatively uniform pieces that are large enough to brew with this method." He advises that you set the grinder to a coarse setting relative to drip. When finished grinding, the coffee will be of similar size to very coarse sand.

This man knows his coffee, and his expert directions will give you the perfect brew of French press coffee. Before you start, keep the following notes in mind:

Measure the coffee carefully, as the amount of coffee relative to water volume will affect the strength of the brew. A good starting point is 2 tablespoons of coffee for every 6 to 8 fluid ounces (¾ to 1 cup) of water; then you can adjust to your personal preference. The ratio is important for good flavor extraction; if the resulting strength is too much for your taste, you can add hot water or milk to your cup to adjust.

You'll need to be ready to remove the water from the heat source as soon as it's brought to a boil, then pour it into your French press. The boiling point of water is 212°F, and by using water just off the boil, you are able to get the water to the perfect brewing temperature of 200 to 204°F.

Yield: 1 cup

1. Bring your fresh water to a boil. As it's heating, measure your ground coffee and add it to your French press.

2. As soon as the water comes to a boil, remove it from the heat source, then add some of this water to the French press, just enough to wet the grounds. Use a spoon or gently swirl the ground coffee to be sure all of it is moistened. Don't agitate the mix much.

3. Give the coffee a moment to bloom if the beans are very fresh, then add the rest of the measure of hot water.

4. Fit the plunger to the pot and press it just enough to keep all of your ground beans immersed. Coffee floats, so be sure to push the plunger gently because the floating coffee might try to rise above it.

5. For best results, time how long the coffee is in contact with the water. Four minutes is generally accepted. (Donohue says he usually prefers an extra 10 seconds.) Then carefully press the plunger all the way down to separate the grounds from the beverage.

6. Pour your perfect cup of French press coffee. Add cream and sweetener as desired, and enjoy immediately.

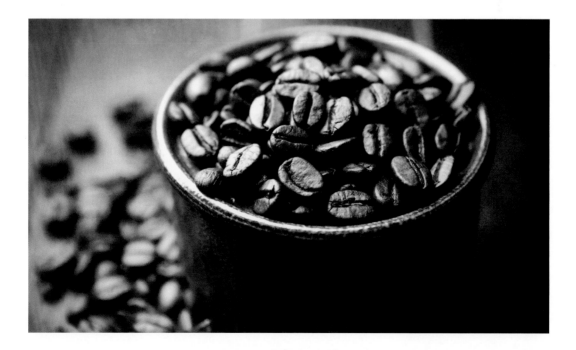

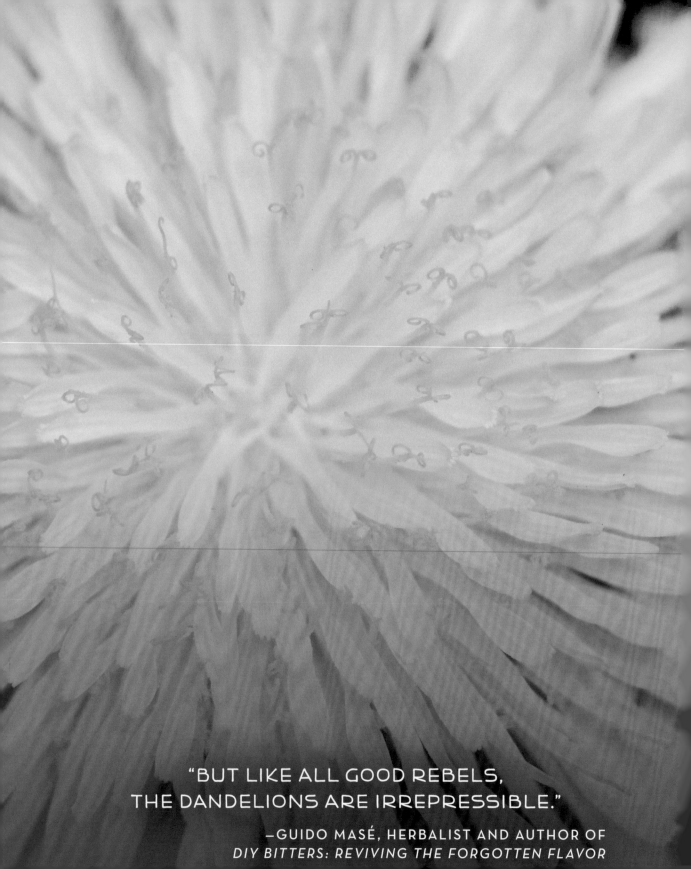

"BUT LIKE ALL GOOD REBELS,
THE DANDELIONS ARE IRREPRESSIBLE."

—GUIDO MASÉ, HERBALIST AND AUTHOR OF
DIY BITTERS: REVIVING THE FORGOTTEN FLAVOR

CHAPTER 31

Dandelion

Spring is one of my favorite times in the Methow Valley, the place where I live. The yellow blooms of our native sunflowers transforms our hillsides into gold while my favorite weed covers our lawns in little sunny buttons.

It might sound strange to have a favorite weed, but dandelion has so many virtues that it's an easy choice. Dandelion is a generous plant in that every part of it can be used as food or medicine. Blowing on a dandelion seed puff offers both children and adults cheap entertainment—and, some say, a free wish.

Because this is such a delicious and medicinal plant it completely confounds me that so many people despise it. Instead of rushing out with their harvesting tools to enjoy this free food and medicine, they spray harmful chemicals to kill them. Many of those herbicides are known to promote cancer, poison our soils and waters, and kill countless birds and bees.

Why is there all this hatred against dandelions? Because lawns should be "pure"? Because dandelions make an area look unkempt? Are those good enough reasons to poison our beautiful earth? I say it's time to end our war on dandelions and embrace them for the many benefits they so freely offer.

Botanical name: *Taraxacum officinale*

Family: Asteraceae

Parts used: root, leaves, flowers

Energetics: cooling, drying

Taste: bitter (leaf); bitter, sweet (root)

Properties (leaf): diuretic, alterative, nutritive, digestive stimulant, choleretic

Properties (root): alterative, nutritive, cholagogue

Plant uses: poor digestion, water retention, nourishment, skin eruptions, supporting healthy liver function

Plant preparations: decoction, tincture, food

Because dandelions are so adept at spreading, it's hard to pinpoint where they originated beyond the vast area of Europe and Asia. In modern times dandelion grows all over the world, usually in sunny disturbed soils.

It's believed that the humble dandelion was intentionally brought to North America by European settlers who couldn't bear the thought of leaving this important food and medicine behind. In fact, dandelions are still admired in many European countries. The flowers are routinely made into jams and wine, and my French husband fondly remembers harvesting the leaves with his mother in the spring in order to make a delicious salad. In this chapter, we focus on the therapeutic use of the dandelion roots and leaves.

MEDICINAL PROPERTIES AND ENERGETICS OF DANDELION LEAVES

Dandelion leaves are among our most nutrient-dense greens. The tender spring leaves are full of nutrients, including vitamin C, vitamin K1, potassium, magnesium, and beta-carotene. It's a time-honored tradition in many countries in Europe to pick those spring greens and eat them, not only for their valuable nutrition, but also for their ability to stimulate healthy digestion.

FOR DIGESTION

Dandelion leaves have a pleasantly bitter taste. As I've said, eating something bitter, even just a bite, stimulates a cascade of digestive secretions. It increases saliva, which helps to break down carbohydrates. It stimulates gastric secretions like HCL, which breaks down proteins, and it helps to release bile, which breaks down fats. So dandelion is not only high in nutrients itself but also helps you digest and assimilate the nutrients from your food.

AS A DIURETIC

Dandelions have another important use: as a diuretic. The French refer to this in their common name for dandelion, pissenlit (which literally translates to "pee the bed"). If you've ever drunk dandelion tea before bed, you'll know exactly what the French are referring to, as you make your fifth trip to the bathroom that night!

Herbalists have long used dandelion leaves to remove excess fluids or dampness from the body, treating conditions such as edema and hypertension. If you eat the leaves or make a tea from them, you can directly experience the diuretic properties yourself.

One clinical trial has shown the efficacy of dandelion leaf as a diuretic.[1] The leaves are considered to be a potassium-sparing diuretic. That is, unlike many pharmaceutical diuretic drugs, dandelions are naturally high in potassium and do not promote potassium excretion or deficiency.

MEDICINAL PROPERTIES AND ENERGETICS OF DANDELION ROOT

Dandelion root offers powerful support to the liver by increasing function and decreasing inflammation. Herbalists mainly use dandelion root for supporting liver health by helping to move a stagnant or sluggish liver. In herbal theory, a sluggish liver can be related to poor digestion, skin rashes like eczema or acne, and hormonal imbalances like tension due to premenstrual syndrome (PMS).

FOR DIGESTIVE ISSUES AND HEALTHY GUT FLORA

Dandelion root supports healthy digestion by its action on the liver. Poor digestion due to a sluggish liver may be seen in an inability to digest fats, clay-colored stools, nausea, gas, bloating, and headaches. Dandelion root gently nudges the liver into action to relieve these common digestive complaints.

Dandelion root is also really high in inulin, a type of carbohydrate that supports healthy gut flora. Because humans are unable to digest inulin, it passes to the colon where it ferments and feeds the healthy bacteria in your intestines. (Dandelion leaves also contain a healthy amount of inulin.)

After decades of overusing antibiotics, we are beginning to realize the importance of a healthy and complex microbiome. Researchers have shown correlations with gut flora and inflammatory digestive problems, obesity, poor immune system function, and even allergies. Some of the best ways to ensure we have healthy digestive flora include: eating fermented foods, living in a nonsanitary environment (playing in the dirt is good for you!), avoiding frequent and unnecessary antibiotics, and eating a nutritious diet that includes prebiotics like the inulin found in dandelion roots.

FOR HEALTHY HORMONE LEVELS

There is a lot of discussion about "balancing hormones" in the natural health field, with many practitioners recommending using exogenous (external) synthetic hormones to create an internal hormonal balance. While this may sometimes be necessary, I believe it is essential to first address our internal environment, especially in regard to our liver health.

The liver plays an important role in metabolizing hormones. Keeping the liver healthy with gentle herbs like dandelion root can help us maintain a healthy hormonal balance. Herbalists regularly use dandelion root for women with signs of hormonal imbalance including menstrual cramps, mood swings, and irregular periods.

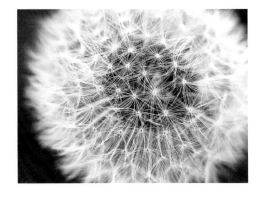

FOR ARTHRITIS

Herbalists have long used dandelion root for people with painful arthritis. It may work by relieving fluid buildup in the joints, modulating inflammation, or increasing nutrient absorption. So far scientists have isolated one constituent, taraxasterol, that may be responsible for relieving the inflammation and pain of arthritis.[2]

FOR CANCER

Traditionally, herbalists have recommended dandelion root to support the health of people with cancer. In recent years scientists have started to take note, and there are a handful of in vitro and constituent-based studies showing dandelion's promising results in supporting the immune system and even fighting against cancer cells. I look forward to seeing human clinical trials validating this traditional use of dandelion.

HOW TO USE DANDELION

If you are lucky enough to have dandelions growing near you, then you can easily harvest this plant yourself. However, be sure to consult a field guide or have someone knowledgeable point out the correct plant to you, as there are a couple of dandelion look-alikes. When harvesting plants in the wild, or even in your own backyard, be sure the area is free of herbicides and other pollutants.

When harvesting the leaves, you'll find the young, tender leaves of the spring to be the most palatable. If you sample mature leaves, you'll find they are very bitter and perhaps not even edible.

Dandelion leaves (and their close cousins, chicory leaves) can be found more and more readily in grocery stores. If you don't see them in your local store, ask if they can be ordered. Dried leaves can be used as a tea.

Dried dandelion root can easily be found in herb stores.

The flowers are also edible. They can can be made into a lovely jam and even wine.

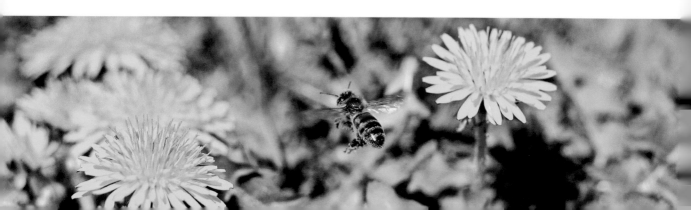

RECOMMENDED AMOUNTS

Dandelions are considered to be both food and medicine and can be eaten in fairly high amounts.

The therapeutic amount for dandelion leaves and root is as follows:

Leaves, as tea: 5 to 9 grams total, taken in small doses throughout the day

Leaves (dried), as tincture: 1:5, 30% alcohol, 3 to 4 mL, 3 times per day.[3]

Root, as decoction: 9 to 15 grams per day

Root (fresh), as tincture: 1:2, 30% alcohol, 4 to 5 mL, 3 times per day.[4]

SPECIAL CONSIDERATIONS

More than 80 million pounds of herbicides are used on lawns, most specifically against dandelions, each year. Many of these chemicals either have not been tested for safety or have been shown to have a strong correlation with cancer. Children and fetuses are the most susceptible. If harvesting your own dandelions, be sure to harvest in an area free from harmful chemicals.

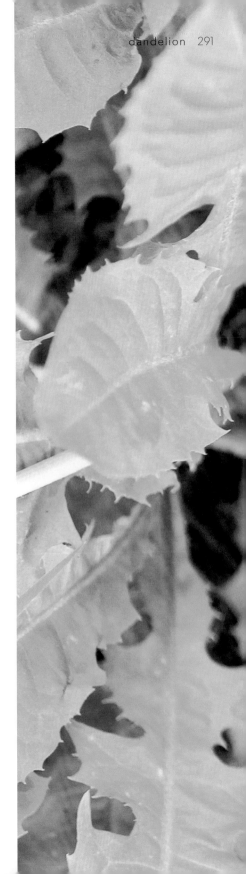

ROASTED DANDELION
AND REISHI TEA

6 grams dried sliced reishi

**10 grams roasted
dandelion root**

This is one of my favorite tea blends. The roasted, nutty flavor of the dandelion root hides the somewhat bitter flavor of the reishi, which is a mushroom known for its many health benefits. Both are outstanding for supporting liver health. If you don't have reishi, you can simply omit the reishi and use dandelion root.

You can buy dandelion root already roasted. To roast your own, heat dried minced roots on medium heat, preferably in a cast iron pan (use a stainless steel pan otherwise). The roots are done when they turn a deeper brown and become aromatic. Because dandelion root and reishi come in various sizes and shapes, it's best to measure the amounts by weight.

Yield: approximately 1¼ cup to 1½ cup

1. Simmer the reishi and dandelion in 2 cups of water for 30 minutes to 1 hour. You can also put this in a slow cooker on a low setting overnight, but you may need to add more water.

2. Strain when done. Drink within 1 day.

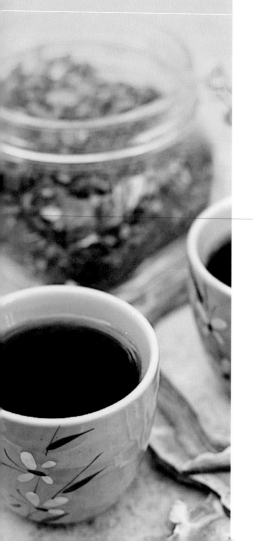

DANDELION ROOT VINEGAR

Dandelion root is high in minerals, and apple cider vinegar helps extract the mineral content. It is a convenient way for you to incorporate dandelion into your life. You can use this herbal vinegar to make your own salad dressing, as part of a marinade, or even as a digestive (try a tablespoon diluted in water) prior to eating a meal.

Instead of giving specific amounts of each ingredient, I've written this recipe exactly as I make it at home. This allows you to choose the amount you want to make and shows you how easy it is to prepare. For example, if you choose to make a pint (2 cups), you would need roughly 2 cups of fresh root or ⅔ cup of dried root, and approximately 1½ cups of vinegar.

Yield: variable

fresh or dried dandelion root

apple cider vinegar

jar with glass or plastic lid

1. If using fresh dandelion root, fill the jar with the finely chopped root. If using dried, fill the jar ⅓ full (to leave room for the root to expand).

2. Fill the jar with apple cider vinegar. Cover with a glass or plastic lid, or if using a metal lid, place parchment or wax paper between the lid and the jar (vinegar will corrode metal).

3. Infuse this for 2 weeks, shaking once daily. Strain when ready. This does not need to be refrigerated (although it can be). Use within 1 year.

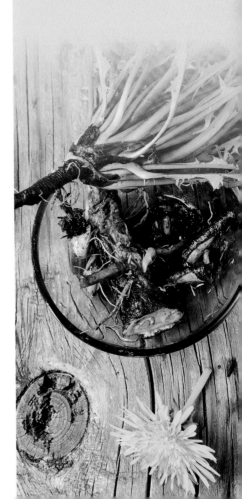

DANDELION PESTO

½ cup shelled pine nuts

3 garlic cloves, minced

2 cups chopped fresh dandelion leaves, loosely packed

1 tablespoon lemon juice, plus
   1 tablespoon lemon zest

½ cup extra-virgin olive oil

½ teaspoon sea salt

1 teaspoon turmeric powder

½ teaspoon freshly ground
   black pepper

¼ cup freshly grated
   Parmesan

This bitter pesto is tempered by the nutty, sweet flavor of pine nuts and the zing of lemon. If you aren't up for foraging your own dandelion greens, look for them at your grocery store in the produce section. Enjoy this as a dip with crackers, bread, or carrots. It's also great as a topping on meats, veggies, and eggs.

Yield: 2 cups

1.   Place all the ingredients except the Parmesan into a blender or food processor. Process until smooth. If it's too thick, slowly add a bit more olive oil.

2.   Add the Parmesan and continue to blend until the mixture has a smooth consistency.

3.   Refrigerate, and eat within 3 days.

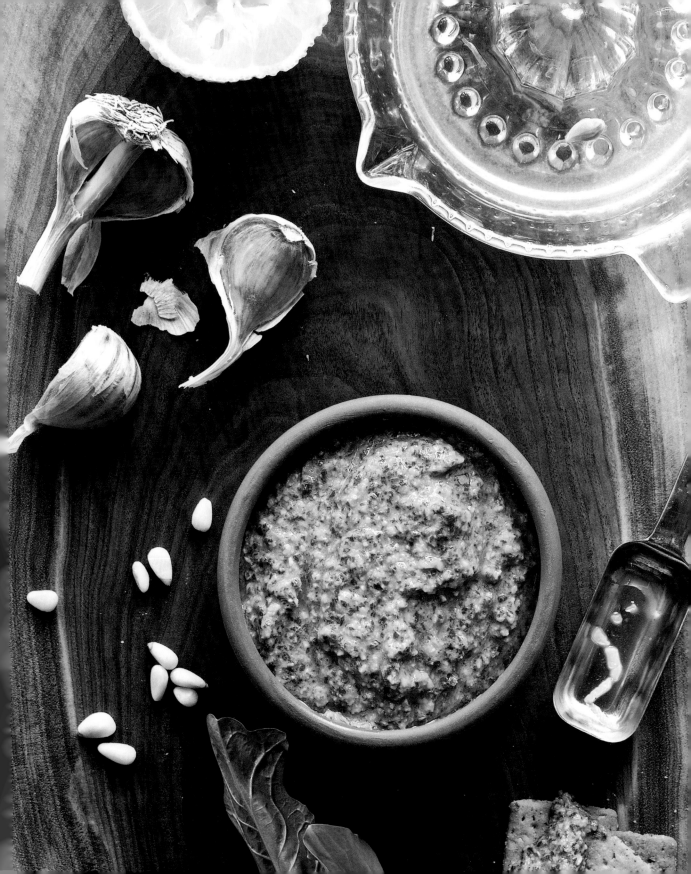

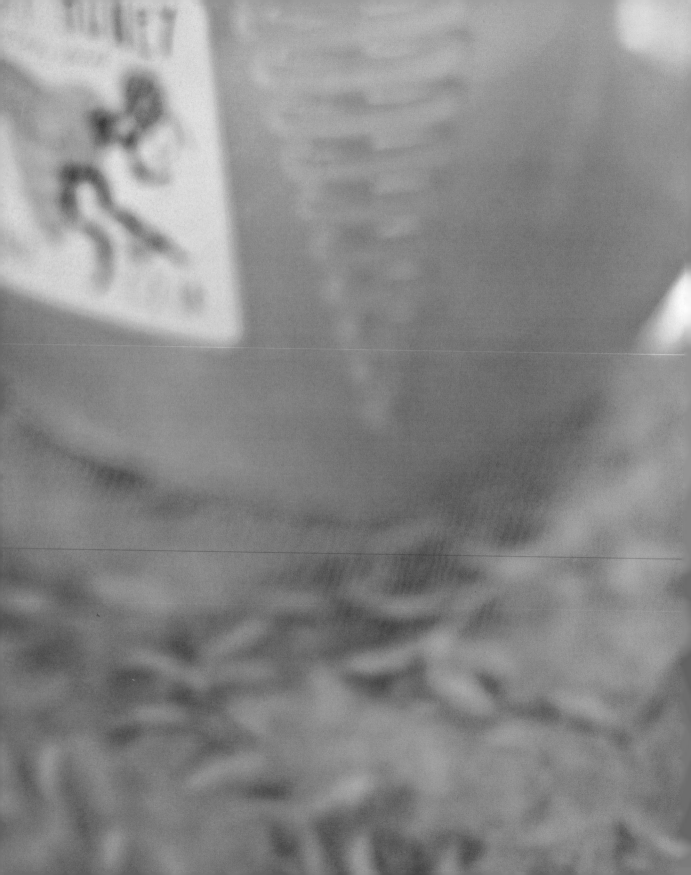

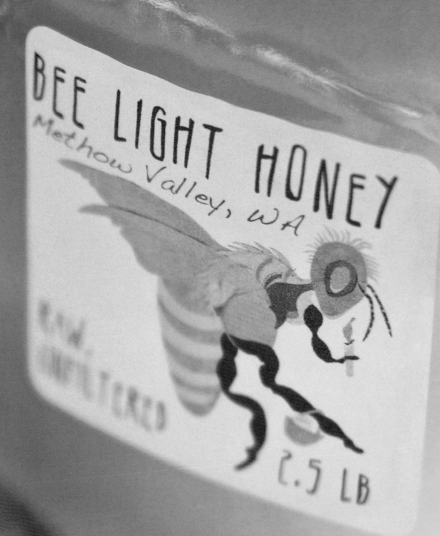

sweet

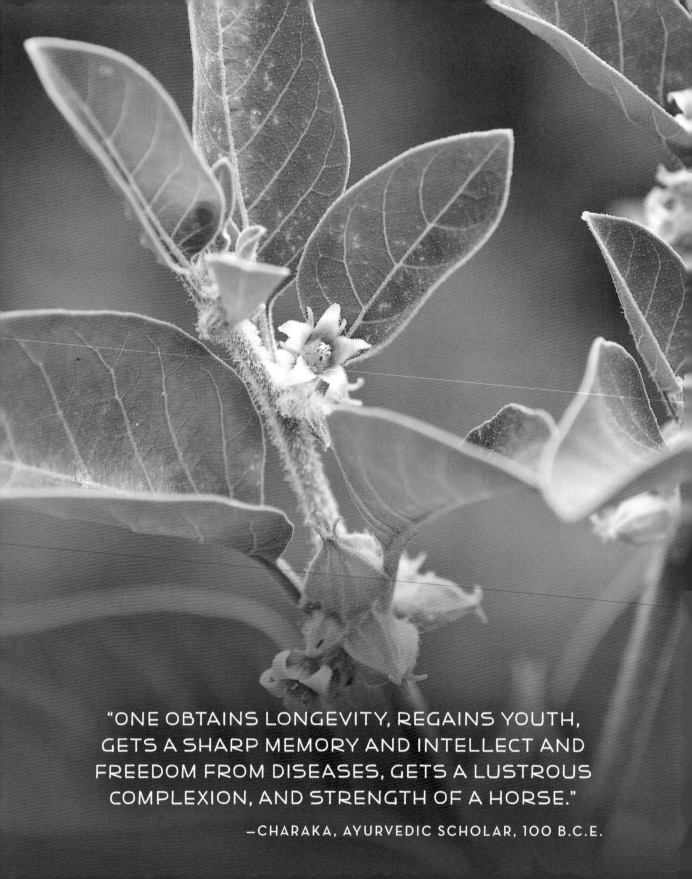

"ONE OBTAINS LONGEVITY, REGAINS YOUTH, GETS A SHARP MEMORY AND INTELLECT AND FREEDOM FROM DISEASES, GETS A LUSTROUS COMPLEXION, AND STRENGTH OF A HORSE."

—CHARAKA, AYURVEDIC SCHOLAR, 100 B.C.E.

CHAPTER 32

Ashwagandha

Ashwagandha has long been a revered medicinal plant in India and Africa, and in recent years it has enamored Western herbalists with its ability to both strengthen those who are tired and calm those who are stressed and anxious.

The word *ashwaganda* can be translated to mean "smell of a horse's urine or sweat." Don't let this description stop you from trying this incredible herb! While it may not smell like roses, there is a common saying for ashwaganda: it gives you the strength of a stallion. This is a safe and powerfully rejuvenating herb that could benefit many people faced with the chronic health problems of modern society.

Other common names: Winter cherry, Indian ginseng

Botanical name: *Withania somnifera*

Family: Solanaceae

Parts used: root (mainly), leaf, berries

Energetics: warming, moistening

Taste: sweet, bitter

Plant properties: adaptogen, anti-inflammatory, antioxidant, anxiolytic, aphrodisiac, immunomodulator, cardioprotective

Plant uses: fatigue, emaciation, reproductive health, hypothyroid, insomnia, longevity, low libido, degenerative disease, anxiety, asthma, arthritis, fibromyalgia, insulin resistance

Plant preparations: powder, tincture, decoction

Ashwagandha is in the same plant family as potatoes and tomatoes, and it grows in a fashion similar to that of tomatoes (including growing conditions and growing structure). The first writings about ashwagandha are in Ayurveda texts from roughly 3,000 to 4,000 years ago. Ayurveda classifies ashwagandha as a *rasayana*, an herb that deeply rejuvenates and promotes longevity. Rasayana herbs are especially revered for sustaining good health into the elder years.

MEDICINAL PROPERTIES AND ENERGETICS OF ASHWAGANDHA

In Western herbalism we classify ashwagandha as an adaptogen herb. Adaptogens are herbs used to build and nourish a person as a whole. They are commonly used when someone is depleted, fatigued, and just plain worn out.

FOR IMPROVING SLEEP AND DECREASING ANXIETY

Are you tired, anxious, or run-down? Do you struggle to get a good night's sleep? Ashwagandha strengthens and calms the nervous system. Taken over time, it can restore healthy sleep cycles and relieve anxiety. While there are numerous causes for anxiety, I commonly see people who have symptoms of anxiety along with an inability to get restful sleep. This creates a vicious cycle that ashwagandha can often reset.

Ashwagandha has been nicknamed the "ginseng of India" for its ability to strengthen vitality. But while *Panax ginseng* can be overstimulating to people with anxiety, ashwagandha excels at decreasing anxiety and soothing the nervous system.

In a study on anxiety, two groups of people received either a small dose of ashwagandha, a multivitamin, deep breathing exercises, and dietary counseling; or psychotherapy, the same breathing exercises, and a placebo to replace the ashwagandha. After eight weeks, those taking ashwagandha showed more improvement in their anxiety levels than the placebo group.[1] (I love how this study incorporated holistic health, not only a dose of an herb, to address a complex health challenge!)

FOR ENERGY

Ashwagandha helps with day-to-day fatigue and can also support the energy levels of patients undergoing chemotherapy for breast cancer. In one particular study, patients taking the ashwagandha for cancer-related fatigue had a higher survival rate. The researchers said that this increase wasn't statistically significant, but called for more studies to validate their findings.[2]

Ashwagandha may also support energy levels due to its ability to improve thyroid function, although more human clinical trials are warranted.[3]

FOR REPRODUCTIVE HEALTH

Ashwagandha has long been used to support sexual desire and fertility. Science is now validating that use. In one study, 75 men taking ashwagandha were shown to have improved semen quality, which researchers credited to decreased levels of oxidative stress and regulated hormone levels.[4] Another study looked at 180 men taking 5 grams of ashwagandha for three months. The researchers reported that: "*Withania somnifera* not only reboots enzymatic activity of metabolic pathways and energy metabolism but also invigorates the harmonic balance of seminal plasma metabolites and reproductive hormones in infertile men."[5]

Ashwagandha has also been shown to improve the sexual function of healthy women. In one pilot study, 25 women were given a concentrated root extract of ashwagandha and 25 were given a starch-based placebo. After eight weeks, those taking the ashwagandha root showed numerous significant improvements in sexual function including lubrication and orgasm.[6]

FOR YOUR BRAIN

Ashwagandha is well known to have memory-enhancement properties. In one double-blind, placebo-controlled clinical trial, 20 men who took an extract of dried ashwagandha leaves and roots twice daily showed significant improvements in cognitive ability. The authors of this study hypothesize that ashwagandha may help in the treatment of disorders that affect cognitive performance.[7]

In another double-blind, placebo-controlled, randomized trial, ashwagandha was shown to improve working memory, reaction time, and social function in people diagnosed with bipolar disorder.[8]

FOR IMMUNE SYSTEM SUPPORT

Ashwagandha's benefits include support for the immune system. In one trial, ashwagandha was shown to increase four different immune system cells, indicating a major change in immune cell activation.[9]

Cancer specialist and herbalist Donald Yance reports: "I use ashwagandha in adaptogenic formulas for all my patients with cancer during and after chemotherapy, radiation, and surgery. The immune-modulating activities of ashwagandha have been well researched and are significant."[10]

FOR SUPPORT WITH DEGENERATIVE DISEASES

Herbalists use ashwagandha for a variety of degenerative, wasting, and chronic diseases, including arthritis, fibromyalgia, and chronic fatigue. Because it builds tissue and supports overall health, it can help people regain their strength. In *The Way of Ayurvedic Herbs*, authors Khalsa and Tierra write, "Ayurveda considers it a 'grounding' herb—one that nourishes and regulates metabolic processes and stabilizes mood."[11]

Studies have shown that ashwagandha has a beneficial hypoglycemic effect and can regulate cholesterol levels, indicating it could be an important herb to use with people who have insulin resistance and type 2 diabetes.[12]

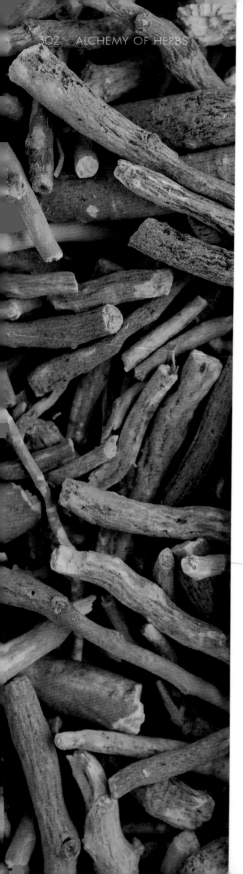

HOW TO USE ASHWAGANDHA

Ashwagandha is traditionally used as a powder, and this is my preferred way to use it as well. While ashwagandha can be taken alone, Ayurveda often uses it in formulations. There are some complex formulations with ashwagandha, but it is often simply mixed with pungent herbs like pipali (*Piper longum*) or the classic Ayurvedic herbal blend known as trikatu (see the recipe for Trikatu Pastilles on page 43).

RECOMMENDED AMOUNTS

Unlike many of our aromatic herbs, ashwagandha is not considered tasty. Rather than using it to flavor a meal, we more often put it in recipes to hide the flavor.

The therapeutic amount of ashwagandha is:

As powder: 3 to 6 grams per day[13]

As decoction: 20 to 30 grams per day, added to heated milk[14]

As tincture: 1:4, 60% alcohol, 2 to 8 mL per day[15]

SPECIAL CONSIDERATIONS

Use ashwagandha during pregnancy only under the advice of a qualified herbalist or health professional.

Do not take with barbiturates, as ashwagandha may potentiate their sedative effects.

Some people with nightshade sensitivities may not tolerate ashwagandha, although this seems to be a small percentage. (Ashwagandha is a member of the nightshade family.)

In Ayurvedic theory, ashwagandha shouldn't be used if there is a current upper respiratory infection or lots of mucus congestion.

ASHWAGANDHA GHEE

Combining ashwagandha with pungent spices and ghee (clarified butter) is a traditional Ayurvedic practice. You can make your ghee, or buy it at health food stores or online. You can also substitute coconut oil for the ghee.

Trikatu powder is an Ayurvedic herbal formula that is a simple combination of three pungent herbs. You can make your own (see the recipe for Trikatu Pastilles on page 43), or simply substitute an equal amount of black pepper.

The spices in this recipe increase the absorption of the ashwagandha, while the ghee is a good source of healthy fats. The sweet taste of honey is commonly added for people who have a cold and dry constitution. I often recommend a spoonful a day for people who have anxiety or insomnia.

Yield: ⅓ cup

3 tablespoons ghee

1 tablespoon honey

½ cup ashwagandha powder (25 grams)

1 teaspoon trikatu powder (1 gram)

1. Gently heat the ghee and honey in a small pot over very low heat. Do not overheat. You simply want it to be melted and have a thin consistency.

2. Add the ashwagandha and trikatu powders to the honey mixture, and stir well. Pour into a glass jar to let cool.

3. This can be stored at room temperature and is best consumed within 1 week.

1½ cups pitted and chopped dates (approximately 250 grams)

2 tablespoons cocoa powder

⅓ cup ashwagandha powder (40 grams)

⅔ cup coconut flakes (plus extra for rolling)

¼ cup tahini

2 teaspoons vanilla extract

½ teaspoon organic orange extract

1 teaspoon cinnamon powder

1 teaspoon ginger powder

pinch of salt

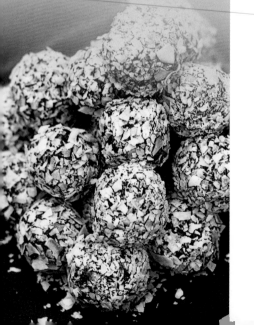

ASHWAGANDHA DATE TREATS

Powdering herbs and using them in a dried-fruit, nut, or seed butter is a great way to enjoy herbs without having to use capsules. These delicious snacks are a variation of a recipe my friend Emily is fond of making. Emily recommends making these on a full stomach. "Otherwise, you may end up eating half the mix before you form the balls. True story."

I recommend eating 2 or 3 of these per day.

Yield: roughly 40 teaspoon-size balls

1. Soak pitted dates in 2 cups hot water for 30 minutes.

2. Strain dates well. (The water can be reserved for cooking sweet rice or oatmeal; see the recipe for Astragalus and Cardamom Rice, page 312.)

3. Place the dates and the rest of the ingredients into a food processor. Blend until it forms a consistent paste.

4. Chill the mixture in the refrigerator for 30 minutes.

5. Roll the paste into teaspoon-size balls and roll in coconut. Store these in the refrigerator and eat within 1 week.

ASHWAGANDHA BANANA SMOOTHIE

This yummy treat is a great way to share the nourishing and supportive qualities of ashwagandha. If you have a sensitivity to dairy, use any nondairy yogurt of your choice. For the nut or seed butter, peanut, almond, cashew, and sunflower seed butters are all good options.

Yield: 5 cups, 3 to 5 servings

1. Place all the ingredients into a blender. Blend until smooth.

2. Pour the mixture into glasses. Use a spatula to get all the liquid from the sides of the blender—there are lots of good herbs in there.

3. Drink immediately.

2 bananas

2 cups almond milk

1 cup plain yogurt

½ cup nut or seed butter

¼ cup coconut oil

2 tablespoons ashwagandha powder

2 teaspoons cinnamon powder

maple syrup or honey, to taste

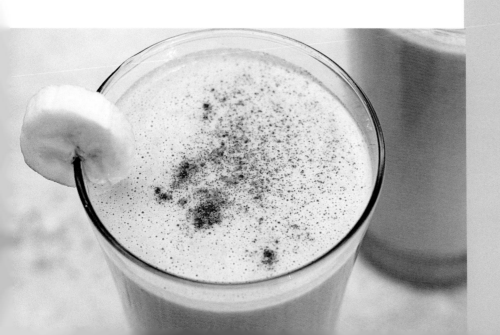

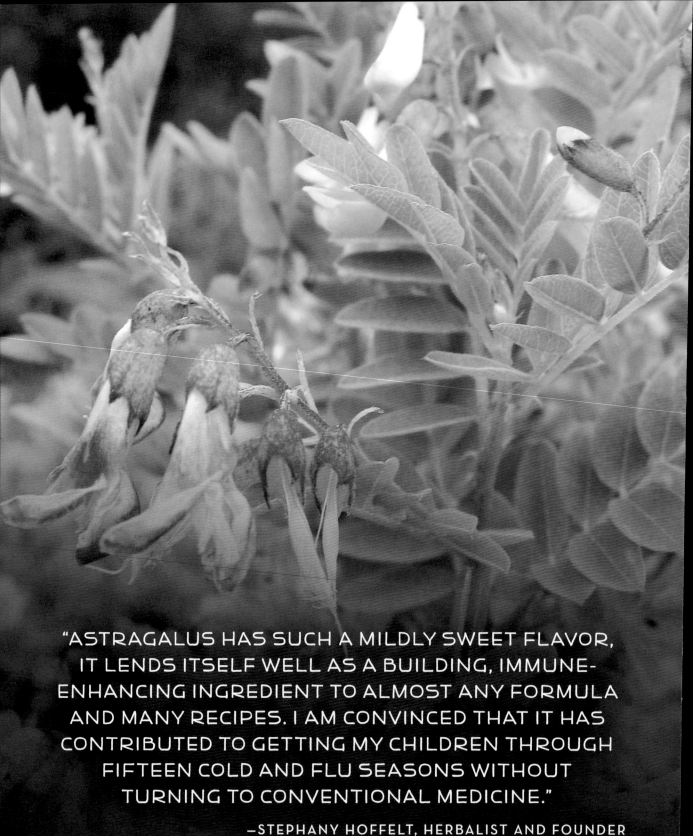

"ASTRAGALUS HAS SUCH A MILDLY SWEET FLAVOR, IT LENDS ITSELF WELL AS A BUILDING, IMMUNE-ENHANCING INGREDIENT TO ALMOST ANY FORMULA AND MANY RECIPES. I AM CONVINCED THAT IT HAS CONTRIBUTED TO GETTING MY CHILDREN THROUGH FIFTEEN COLD AND FLU SEASONS WITHOUT TURNING TO CONVENTIONAL MEDICINE."

—STEPHANY HOFFELT, HERBALIST AND FOUNDER

CHAPTER 33

Astragalus

Do you frequently get colds every winter? Do you often come down with the flu? While avoiding sick people and washing your hands can help you to avoid sickness, strengthening your immune system is your best defense. Consistently restful sleep, daily exercise, a whole foods diet, and keeping your vitamin D3 at an optimal level are powerful ways to strengthen the immune system. Herbs, including astragalus, can also be an important part of your immune system support.

Other common names: milk vetch, huang qi, radix astragali

Botanical name: *Astragalus propinquus* (syn. *Astragalus membranaceus*)

Family: Fabaceae (pea)

Parts used: root

Energetics: slightly warming, slightly drying

Taste: sweet

Plant properties: immunomodulator, antioxidant, hepatoprotective, cardioprotective, adaptogen, diuretic

Plant uses: immune system dysfunction (from frequent colds and flu, seasonal allergies, HIV, cancer), angina, hypertension, hepatitis, fatigue, asthma, prolapsed organs, weak limbs, anemia

Plant preparations: decoctions, cooked with food, powdered, capsules, tincture

Astragalus comes to us from China, where it has been used for thousands of years to strengthen the immune system. However, it has quickly integrated itself into Western herbalism. In a poll of practicing herbalists, it placed 16th among the top 50 herbs commonly used by Western practitioners. There have been no high-quality clinical trials using astragalus, so most of our knowledge comes from its extensive use in Traditional Chinese Medicine and, more recently, its use by Western herbalists.

TYPES OF ASTRAGALUS

There are more than 2,000 different species in the *Astragalus* genus. Some of these plants are toxic, and no other species are known to have the same qualities as *Astragalus propinquus* (syn. *Astragalus membranaceus*), although a few are used medicinally. Make sure you buy or grow *Astragalus propinquus* and not one of the many other plants in the same genus.

MEDICINAL PROPERTIES AND ENERGETICS OF ASTRAGALUS

Astragalus root is a supreme herb for the immune system and an adaptogen, an herb that helps build and restore overall health to the body. Numerous studies have shown it to be a valuable ally for illnesses as serious as cancer, and it also powerfully protects people from getting frequent upper respiratory ailments such as colds and the flu. Astragalus root also contains many protective properties for the heart, liver, and kidneys, making it a wonderful herb to consider for preventive care.

Astragalus is a key herb in the classical Chinese formula Yu Ping Feng Pian, also known as Jade Screen Formula. This formula is used to form a protective shield and keep pathogens from entering the body. Herbalist Paul Bergner explains, "In Chinese medical terms, astragalus builds up the protective chi. Imagine that there is a protective shield around your body, just below the surface of the skin, that keep out cold and other external influences. It vitalizes the non-specific immune defenses and wards off infections. This is the protective chi, and astragalus is the premier herb in Chinese herbalism to strengthen it."[1]

FOR IMMUNE SYSTEM SUPPORT

Herbalists refer to astragalus as an immunomodulator, a broad term that basically means that it positively influences the immune system, making it stronger. From limited human clinical trials and from in vitro studies, we know that astragalus increases the white blood cell count, decreases viral replication, and stimulates the production of T killer cells.[2,3,4,5]

I used to get colds throughout the winter and suffer through the flu nearly every year. My immune system was clearly defeated and falling prey to everything that came my way. Now I rarely catch an upper-respiratory infection, and I attribute that to regularly drinking astragalus chai and keeping my vitamin D3 level in the optimum range. I've seen many people reduce the frequency of their own colds and flu by doing these two things. (I've included a recipe for Astragalus Chai in this chapter.)

Herbalists recommend astragalus to alleviate the side effects of chemotherapy treatments. One study used astragalus injections alongside chemotherapy in patients with malignant tumors. As compared to the patients receiving chemotherapy alone, the patients receiving the astragalus injections had inhibited tumor development, less functional impairment, elevated immune function, and improved quality of life.[6]

FOR IMPROVED ENERGY

Herbalists regularly recommend astragalus for people with adrenal fatigue, fibromyalgia, and chronic fatigue syndrome. But you don't have to be ill to get benefits from astragalus. In one study two groups of athletes received either a Chinese herbal formula with astragalus as a main ingredient, or a placebo. After eight weeks those taking the astragalus formula had increased endurance and enhanced recovery from fatigue. The researchers concluded that it worked "by increasing the oxygen uptake and the systemic utility of oxygen."[7]

FOR YOUR HEART, KIDNEYS, AND LIVER

Astragalus has been studied extensively for its effects on improving heart function, even in patients with extreme cases of congestive heart failure.[8] In one study, patients with congestive heart failure were divided into two groups. One group was given an injection of astragalus (roughly 80 grams of the bulk herb), and the other group was given conventional treatment. After four weeks, both groups showed improvements, but cardiac function was significantly better in the group receiving the astragalus injections.[9]

This herb has also been shown to prevent and repair damage to the kidneys and liver due to medications or viral infections. In one study, a combination of astragalus and angelica was shown to improve renal function in chronic kidney disease patients.[10]

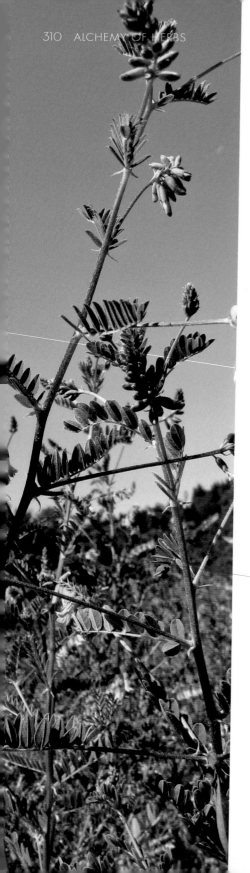

HOW TO USE ASTRAGALUS

Astragalus slowly nourishes the body deeply over time, so don't expect immediate results. Because it is food-like, herbalists recommend that it be taken daily, in large amounts and for an extended period. Astragalus has a mild, sweet taste and can be cooked into foods or enjoyed in teas.

You can often find astragalus root sold in bulk in three different ways: sliced, cut and sifted, and powdered. Avoid buying roots that look like long tongue depressors, as these often contain chemical yellow dyes.

I like to buy the sliced root for soups (since it is easy to remove) and the finely cut and sifted root for use in tea blends. When using the sliced whole root in food (soups, rice, quinoa, etc.), you will always have to remove the root since it is too fibrous to eat.

RECOMMENDED AMOUNTS

I recommend people use large amounts of astragalus, anywhere from 10 to 30 grams per day, as they do in Traditional Chinese Medicine. It is difficult to get this dose using a tincture or capsules.

SPECIAL CONSIDERATIONS

Make sure you buy or grow *Astragalus membranaceus*, not one of the many other plants in the same genus.

Take astragalus to prevent colds and the flu; however, avoid it during acute illness. (One exception is that if someone is sick and has a lot of deficiency symptoms, astragalus might be used to strengthen the person to boost them toward wellness.)

Do not use astragalus with immunosuppressive drugs. (It interacts with recombinant interleukin 2 and recombinant alpha interferon 1 and 2.)

ASTRAGALUS CHAI

Drinking this delicious chai is a wonderful way to support your immune system during the winter months. The spices warm you up from the inside out, making this a perfect tea for the colder times of the year. Because astragalus root comes in a variety of shapes and sizes and are hard to measure out by volume, I recommend using a scale to measure it by weight.

Yield: 1 serving

1. *Stove method:* Place all the ingredients in a pan with 2½ cups of water. Bring to a boil. Reduce heat and simmer for 20 minutes, covered. Strain, then add milk and honey as desired. Drink within 36 hours.

2. *Slow cooker method:* Place all ingredients in a slow cooker with 2½ cups water. Set it to low heat and let it cook overnight, covered. Inspect the amount; if it looks low, add more water. Strain, then add milk and honey as desired. Drink within 36 hours.

20 to 30 grams astragalus root (approximately 15 to 20 small slices)

1 tablespoon dried orange peel*

2 teaspoons minced fresh or dried ginger

½ tablespoon cinnamon chips

½ teaspoon whole peppercorns

1 or 2 cardamom pods

2 whole cloves

* Store-bought dried orange peel comes in small, uniform pieces. If you make your own, be sure to mince the orange peels finely before drying them, as they are difficult to cut once dried.

ASTRAGALUS AND CARDAMOM RICE

1 cup basmati rice

1 (13.5-oz.) can coconut milk

2 tablespoons astragalus
    root powder

2 tablespoons
    cardamom powder

2 tablespoons honey,
    or to taste

My husband and I love this simple dessert, which features one of my favorite spices, cardamom, as well as the nourishing qualities of astragalus. It's easy to make for a nice after-dinner sweet treat. This rice has a creamy or thick, souplike consistency.

Yield: 4 cups, 4 to 8 servings

1.   Add 1⅔ cups water to the rice, coconut milk, and astragalus in a saucepan.

2.   Heat on medium-high until mixture starts to simmer. Reduce the heat to low, stir the rice, then cover and cook for 20 minutes, or until the rice is cooked through.

3.   Remove the pan from the heat. Add the cardamom and honey. Mix well.

4.   Enjoy while warm and eat within 3 days.

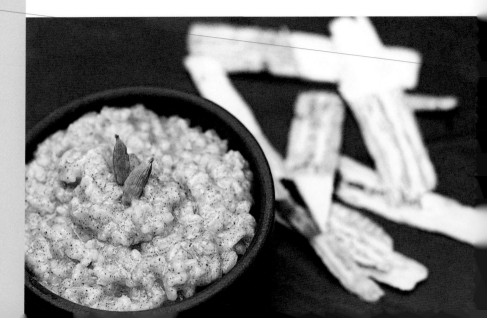

ASTRAGALUS BONE BROTH

Bone broth stock is both the secret of delicious soups and a wonderful way to get immunomodulating herbs like astragalus into your daily diet. It's high in calcium, magnesium, phosphorus, silicon, sulfur, trace minerals, chondroitin sulfates, and glucosamine. Apple cider vinegar helps draw out the minerals and calcium from the bones. Boiling the bones releases gelatin into the broth (which is why it gels slightly when cooled).

This recipe is more of a general guideline, because there are many different ways to make bone broth. It can be made in whatever quantity you like. I like to make big batches and freeze what I don't need immediately. This broth can then be the base for soups or can simply be enjoyed as is, perhaps with a bit of miso added to it. Yum!

Yield: variable

enough chicken or beef bones to fill ⅓ of a large soup pot

2 tablespoons apple cider vinegar

1 onion, coarsely chopped (including skin)

2 carrots, greens removed, coarsely chopped

3 large handfuls of sliced dried astragalus root (approximately 2½ ounces or 75 grams)

1. Preheat the oven to 375°F. Place the bones in an oven pan and roast them for 20 to 30 minutes.

2. Place the roasted bones, apple cider vinegar, onion, carrots, and astragalus in a large soup pot. Fill the pot with water and bring to a boil, then reduce the heat to a simmer.

3. After a while, you will see some foam forming at the top. Gently skim this off every couple of minutes.

4. Once the broth is clear, cover the pot with a lid. Continue to simmer on low heat for 12 to 24 hours. When ready, strain and discard the solids.

5. Store the broth in the fridge or freezer until ready to use. If storing for more than 2 days, keep in the freezer.

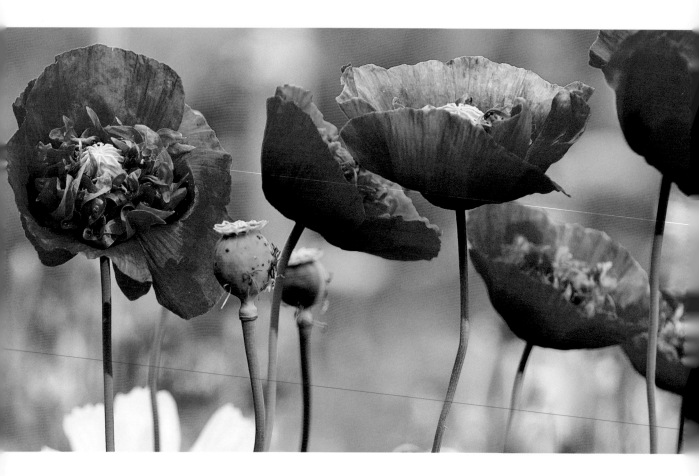

AFTERWORD

You have come to the end of this book, and yet it is still just the beginning of your exciting journey. As you continue to experiment with the different herbs, you will learn more about who you are and what herbs and spices really work for you because you will feel those beneficial changes within your body. The observation and awareness skills you've developed will empower you with the wisdom to effectively choose the remedies that work best for you. This is a type of wisdom that can't be bought, and it's not as readily forgotten as memorizing lists of herbal properties and "superfood" benefits. Instead, it's your own personal transformation. You own it. You are your own specialized expert!

As you begin to home in on what really works for you, you will also probably notice your preferences shifting. You'll find that what works for you could change with the time of day, the seasons of the year, or the seasons of your life, or in special situations like an illness. For example, you may find that elderberry works best for one cold but at another time you need to turn to ginger. There are no strict rules here. Instead of identifying your one mystical solution, you've gained the skills to make the best choices for yourself under continually changing circumstances. Through this transformative journey, you will deepen your connection to nature and further recognize your own ebb and flow within it.

One of the best ways to continue your learning is to create a community around sharing herbal inspiration. I have continually seen people learn more (and have lots of fun) by getting together with friends to harvest herbs, garden, and make herbal remedies. For free ongoing herbal inspiration, please visit LearningHerbs.com. If you want to connect with others online, I suggest joining the supportive community on HerbMentor.com.

It is my hope that the tools and recipes you've learned in this book will serve you for the rest of your life; that your meals can now be seen as opportunities to add delicious and healing herbs and spices to your diet; and that should you reach for herbs for minor ailments like a sore throat or achy muscles, you'll know that you have safe and natural solutions just waiting to be whipped up in your kitchen.

METRIC CONVERSION CHART

The recipes in this book use the standard United States method for measuring liquid and dry or solid ingredients (teaspoons, tablespoons, and cups). The following charts are provided to help cooks outside the U.S. successfully use these recipes. All equivalents are approximate.

Standard Cup	Fine Powder (e.g., flour)	Grain (e.g., rice)	Granular (e.g., sugar)	Liquid Solids (e.g., butter)	Liquid (e.g., milk)
1	140 g	150 g	190 g	200 g	240 ml
¾	105 g	113 g	143 g	150 g	180 ml
⅔	93 g	100 g	125 g	133 g	160 ml
½	70 g	75 g	95 g	100 g	120 ml
⅓	47 g	50 g	63 g	67 g	80 ml
¼	35 g	38 g	48 g	50 g	60 ml
⅛	18 g	19 g	24 g	25 g	30 ml

Useful Equivalents for Liquid Ingredients by Volume				
¼ tsp				1 ml
½ tsp				2 ml
1 tsp				5 ml
3 tsp	1 tbsp		½ fl oz	15 ml
	2 tbsp	⅛ cup	1 fl oz	30 ml
	4 tbsp	¼ cup	2 fl oz	60 ml
	5⅓ tbsp	⅓ cup	3 fl oz	80 ml
	8 tbsp	½ cup	4 fl oz	120 ml
	10⅔ tbsp	⅔ cup	5 fl oz	160 ml
	12 tbsp	¾ cup	6 fl oz	180 ml
	16 tbsp	1 cup	8 fl oz	240 ml
	1 pt	2 cups	16 fl oz	480 ml
	1 qt	4 cups	32 fl oz	960 ml
			33 fl oz	1000 ml 1 L

Useful Equivalents for Dry Ingredients by Weight		
(To convert ounces to grams, multiply the number of ounces by 30.)		
1 oz	1/16 lb	30 g
4 oz	¼ lb	120 g
8 oz	½ lb	240 g
12 oz	¾ lb	360 g
16 oz	1 lb	480 g

Useful Equivalents for Cooking/Oven Temperatures			
Process	Fahrenheit	Celsius	Gas Mark
Freeze Water	32° F	0° C	
Room Temperature	68° F	20° C	
Boil Water	212° F	100° C	
Bake	325° F	160° C	3
	350° F	180° C	4
	375° F	190° C	5
	400° F	200° C	6
	425° F	220° C	7
	450° F	230° C	8
Broil			Grill

Useful Equivalents for Length				
(To convert inches to centimeters, multiply the number of inches by 2.5.)				
1 in			2.5 cm	
6 in	½ ft		15 cm	
12 in	1 ft		30 cm	
36 in	3 ft	1 yd	90 cm	
40 in			100 cm	1 m

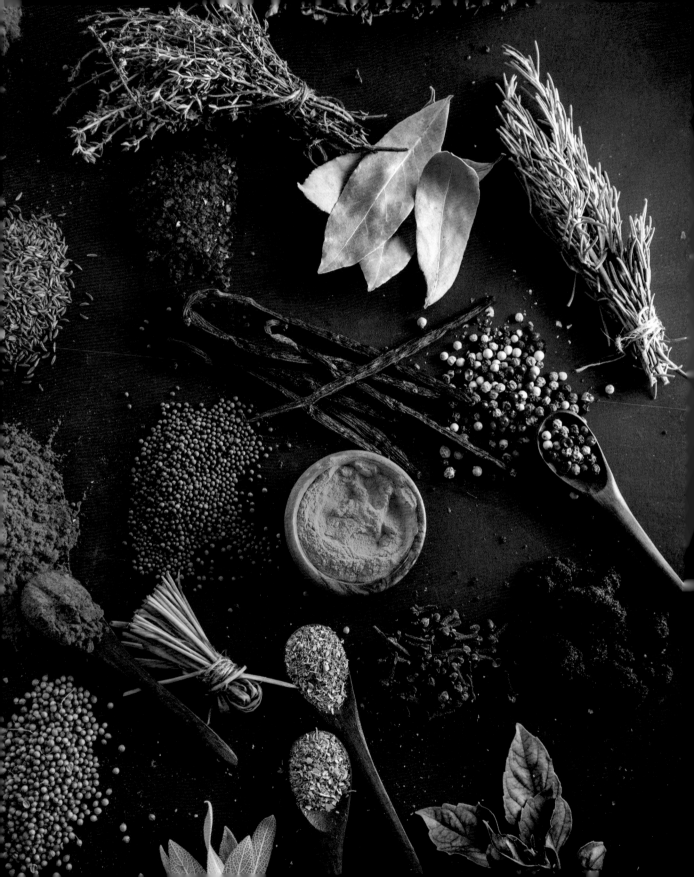

GLOSSARY

This glossary is a quick guide to some of the terms in this book that may be unfamiliar to you. While I've included the basics—what you need to know to get the most out of this book—many of these terms have more complex or nuanced meanings that come into play when you study herbalism further. For an in-depth explanation of many of these terms, check out my Herbal Glossary video series on HerbMentor.com.

A

adaptogen: Broadly defined, this is essentially something that helps the body adapt well to stress. Adaptogens are considered to be building herbs that are often used for people with signs of weakness or deficiency such as chronic fatigue. The herbs in this category have a wide range of energetics and are most effective when the herb is chosen to match the person. Astragalus, ashwagandha, holy basil, and ginseng are examples of adaptogen herbs.

aerial portions: This refers to all of the parts of the plant that grows aboveground (as opposed to roots).

alterative: Alterative herbs generally support detoxification by aiding specific elimination pathways of the body. Various herbs support different organs or systems including the liver, urinary system, skin, lymph, lungs, colon, etc. Many alterative herbs are bitter; they include artichoke, dandelion, and echinacea.

amenorrhea: This condition is characterized by the absence of a menstrual period in a woman of reproductive age.

analgesic: An analgesic is any substance that relieves pain. Analgesic herbs dull pain in a variety of ways. Some relieve muscle tension, some resolve blood stagnation (bruises or contusions), and some relieve pain by affecting the nervous system.

antiemetic: Antiemetic herbs relieve nausea and the urge to vomit. Ginger is an example.

antispasmodic: Muscular tension or cramping can be relieved with antispasmodic herbs. Chamomile is an example.

antitussive: An antitussive stops coughing. Herbs do this in a variety of ways. Some moisten a dry cough, some are antispasmodics that inhibit spasmodic coughing, and others are expectorants that relieve the congestion that is causing a cough. Thyme is one example of an antitussive.

anxiolytic: These herbs help relieve anxiety by affecting the nervous system. Lavender is an example.

astringent: Astringency is an important herbal action related to the tightening and toning of muco-sal tissues. This is useful for healing wounds or reducing excessive discharges (e.g., runny nose or diarrhea). Sage, rose, and oak bark are astringent herbs.

B

bioavailability: This term refers to how well a substance (nutrients, drugs, etc.) can be absorbed by the body. Certain herbs, such as black pepper, are known to increase bioavailability of other herbs or nutrients.

C

carminative: Carminatives are herbs that help with symptoms of stagnant digestion. Have you ever eaten a meal that felt like it was stuck in your stomach? Or had aches in your belly due to gas? That's when carminatives come in handy. These herbs are often aromatic (meaning they have a strong scent) and contain volatile oils. Fennel, ginger, parsley, and chamomile are examples of carminative herbs.

cholagogue: Cholagogue herbs stimulate the gallbladder to release bile. These herbs are useful when someone has trouble digesting fats. They should not be used if there is a known gallbladder obstruction. Turmeric, dandelion, and artichoke are examples.

choleretic: Choleretic herbs support liver health by increasing bile production. Many bitter herbs are choleretics.

constitution: Your personal constitution is your unique blend of energetic qualities as they relate to hot and cold and dry and damp.

D

decoction: This is an herbal preparation that involves simmering herbs (or sometimes boiling them) for an extended period of time.

demulcent: Demulcent herbs are moistening and often slimy in nature. These herbs coat and pro-tect mucous membranes. Cinnamon, oatmeal, and aloe gel are examples of demulcents.

diaphoretic: Diaphoretics induce perspiration and are often used to support the fever process. In herbalism we break these into two categories: relaxing diaphoretics and stimulating diaphoretics. (*See also:* relaxing diaphoretic, stimulating diaphoretic.)

diffusive: Diffusive herbs break up stagnant energy and move it throughout the body. Have you ever eaten a hot pepper and felt the heat in your toes and fingers? That's diffusion. Diffusive herbs are often used for stagnant digestion and are often added in small quantities to herbal formulas. Ginger is an example of a diffusive herb.

diuretic: Diuretic herbs stimulate urination. Dandelion leaf is an example.

dysbiosis: Dysbiosis is an imbalance of the beneficial bacteria (gut flora) in the digestive tract that is causing general digestive problems.

E

edema: This condition is characterized by excess fluid trapped in your body's tissues, causing swelling.

emmenagogue: This is a substance that stimulates blood flow in the uterus; some herbs in the category can induce menstruation.

endothelial function: Your endothelium is a single layer of cells that lines various organs and blood and lymph vessels. Endothelium dysfunction occurs when the endothelium has an impaired ability to vasodilate when stimulated; this is associated with cardiovascular disease.

essential oil: Essential oils are concentrated and naturally occurring volatile liquids that are usually obtained by distilling aromatic plants.

expectorant: Expectorant herbs help to expel excess mucus from the body. Herbalists break these into two categories: relaxing expectorants and stimulating expectorants. (See also: relaxing expectorant, stimulating expectorant.)

F

fomentation: An herbal preparation that involves soaking a cloth in an herbal tea and then applying it to a specific area. These are used for pain, rashes, and headaches. See the Peppermint Fomentation on page 146.

G

galactagogue: Galactagogue herbs stimulate the production of breast milk. Fennel is an example.

ghee: This is a type of clarified butter.

gut flora: This refers to the variety of bacteria living within each person's intestines. The human body has an important relationship with its gut flora. Having a disrupted gut flora has been linked to many health problems, so it's important to be cautious with antibiotics that indiscriminately kill all bacteria, even the beneficial bacteria. Eating fermented foods, living in a non-overly sanitized environment (playing in the dirt is good for us!), avoiding frequent and unnecessary antibiotics, and eating a nutritious diet that includes prebiotics help support healthy gut flora.

H

hemostatic: Hemostatic herbs stop bleeding. Turmeric and yarrow are examples of hemostatic herbs.

hepatoprotective: Hepatoprotective herbs protect the liver. Dandelion, astragalus, and milk thistle are examples of hepatoprotective herbs.

homocysteine: Homocysteine is an amino acid. Elevated levels of homocysteine have been associated with cardiovascular disease.

hydrosol: A hydrosol is an aqueous solution that comes from steam-distilling aromatic plants, often a by-product of essential oils. These are also called floral waters. Rose, lavender, and neroli are commonly used as hydrosols.

I

immunomodulator: Herbs in this category broadly support the immune system. These herbs are generally used for people who frequently get sick or who have seasonal allergies or autoimmunity concerns. Astragalus, ashwagandha, and holy basil are examples.

insulin resistance: This is a state of metabolic dysfunction in the body in which cells do not respond properly to the hormone insulin. It can be a precursor to diabetes.

in vitro studies: These are studies done in a controlled environment outside the living organism, such as the testing of cells in a petri dish.

in vivo studies: These are studies done on a living organism, whether animal, human, or plant.

L

liniment: This herbal preparation is a topical, alcohol-based product.

M

metabolic syndrome: This is a state of metabolic dysfunction in which a person has three or more symptoms out of a group of certain risk factors that raises the risk for heart disease and other health problems, such as type 2 diabetes.

N

nervine: A "nervine" can refer to a medicine that calms the nerves but in herbalism, this broad term refers to any herbs that affect the nervous system. Herbalists break them down into two categories: relaxing and stimulating. (*See also:* relaxing nervine, stimulating nervine.)

NSAID: NSAID stands for nonsteroidal anti-inflammatory drug. Examples include aspirin, ibuprofen (Advil, Motrin), and naproxen sodium (Aleve).

O

oxymel: An oxymel is an herbal preparation made with honey and vinegar. See page 173 for an example.

P

parasympathetic nervous system: This is the rest-and-relax branch of the nervous system. (*See also:* sympathetic nervous system.)

pastille: This from the French word for "pill" and is often used to describe handmade pills made with powdered herbs and honey.

peristalsis: Peristalsis is the normal contracting action of the digestive tract, which moves food from the mouth to the anus.

poultice: This is a soft moist mass of herbs applied externally to the body for a therapeutic effect. It helps you get herbs directly to the area that needs it most.

prebiotic: Prebiotics are substances high in carbohydrates that feed the beneficial bacteria of your digestive tract (gut flora). Dandelion is an herb that is high in prebiotics.

R

rasayana: This is an Ayurvedic term for herbs that support overall health and increase longevity.

relaxing diaphoretic: Relaxing diaphoretics are often used during a fever when a person feels hot and tense but is not sweating. They open up the periphery of the body and allow heat to escape. Elderflower is an example of a relaxing diaphoretic. (*See also:* diaphoretic, stimulating diaphoretic.)

relaxing expectorant: Relaxing or moistening expectorants are herbs that increase healthy mucosal flow to address congestion that has become dried and stuck in the lungs. Marshmallow root and plantain are examples of relaxing expectorants. (*See also:* expectorant, stimulating expectorant.)

relaxing nervine: Relaxing nervines are herbs that calm the nervous system and are commonly used for people with high stress, anxiety, or difficulties with sleep. Chamomile, lavender, and hawthorn are examples of relaxing nervines. (*See also:* nervine, stimulating nervine.)

rubefacient: Rubefacient herbs are applied topically to increase blood circulation to an area. They cause the capillaries to dilate and increase blood circulation. Cayenne, ginger, mustard, and arnica are examples of rubefacient herbs.

S

stagnant digestion: People with cold and stagnant digestion have a difficult time transforming food into the nutrients needed for good health. Symptoms of this condition include a sensation of food sitting heavy in your stomach (like you have an immobile rock in your belly), bloating, nausea, decreased appetite, belching, flatulence, painful stuck gas, and constipation.

stimulating diaphoretic: Stimulating diaphoretics are often used during a fever when a person feels cold and is shivering. These herbs spread heat from the core of the body to the periphery, helping the body to warm up. Ginger, cayenne, and garlic are stimulating diaphoretics. (*See also:* diaphoretic, relaxing diaphoretic.)

stimulating expectorant: Stimulating expectorants are herbs that are often spicy in nature; they thin mucus to help expel it from the body. Ginger, mustard, and thyme are examples of stimulating expectorants. (*See also:* expectorant, relaxing expectorant.)

stimulating nervine: Stimulating nervines are herbs that rev up the nervous system. Some do this through constituents like caffeine (coffee, tea), and others, like rosemary, have specific aromatic qualities that are stimulating in nature. (*See also:* nervine, relaxing nervine.)

styptic: A styptic is a substance that stops bleeding.

sympathetic nervous system: This is the fight-or-flight branch of the nervous system. (*See also:* parasympathetic nervous system.)

synergist: This is something that increases the potency of herbs and pharmaceuticals.

T

tea: A tea is a simple water extraction of an herb or spice. Generally it is made with a small amount of herbs (1 teaspoon) and a short steeping time (5 to 10 minutes).

tincture: A tincture is an alcohol extract of a plant..

trophorestorative: Trophorestorative herbs support the health of a particular organ by restoring normal function, often because of nutritive qualities. For example, hawthorn is a cardiac trophorestorative herb because it supports the heart in a myriad of ways.

V

vasoconstriction: This is a narrowing of the blood vessels.

vermifuge: Vermifuge herbs help to expel worms and other parasites from the body. Garlic, ginger, and thyme are examples.

vulnerary: Vulnerary herbs help to heal wounds. Turmeric, chamomile, and rose are examples.

W

wildcrafting: This is the identifying and harvesting of medicinal herbs in nature.

RECOMMENDED RESOURCES

The best places to find herbs and spices are your local grassroots herbalist, apothecary, food co-op, or even small organic farm. Buying local ensures that the herbs are at their freshest, and you get to support people doing important work in the herbal community.

If you aren't able to find something locally, then the following online resources may be helpful to you.

Mountain Rose Herbs: This is my favorite place to go for bulk organic herbs and spices. Not only do I appreciate their high-quality herbs, but I also love their commitment to the environment. This is also a great place to go for supplies for everything from oils, cheesecloth, and beeswax to bottles, tins, and tea accessories. www.mountainroseherbs.com

Pacific Botanicals: Pacific Botanicals offers high-quality fresh and dried herbs. You'll need to order fresh herbs in advance; check the website for details. www.pacificbotanicals.com

Dandelion Botanical Company: Dandelion Botanical is my favorite apothecary to visit in person; whenever I am in Seattle I make sure to drop by to browse the shelves and say hi to the friendly folks who work there. They also offer online ordering. www.dandelionbotanical.com

Zack Woods Herb Farm: The people running this small farm offer many dried and fresh herbs that they carefully grow and harvest themselves. They offer exceptional-quality herbs while demonstrating how to be good stewards of the land. www.zackwoodsherbs.com

Banyan Botanicals: Banyan Botanicals offers organic Ayurvedic herbs and spices. Look here for ashwagandha, trikatu, long pepper, turmeric, cardamom, and many more. www.banyanbotanicals.com

Frontier Co-op: Frontier Co-op is another great place to find bulk organic herbs and spices as well as supplies. www.frontiercoop.com

Blue Star Coffee Roasters: If you don't have an excellent coffee roaster near you, or if you just want to taste some amazing coffee, check out Blue Star Coffee Roasters. My favorite is the Highway 20 House Blend. www.bluestarcoffeeroasters.com

Floating Leaves Tea: Floating Leaves Tea is a Seattle-based tea importer and retailer that offers online ordering. The owner, Shiuwen Tai, has a passion for Japanese and Chinese tea, teaware, and tea culture. Her teas are seasonal, unblended, and for the most part single-estate. If you are in Seattle, I recommend taking one of her tasting classes. www.floatingleaves.com

The following online resources will help you learn more about herbs.

Apothecary: The Alchemy of Herbs Video Companion: This inspiring video collection will show you how to build your first herbal medicine chest using recipes from this book. Learn the 15 most important herbal remedy preparations that everyone should have on hand. www.alchemyofherbs.com/apothecary

LearningHerbs.com: LearningHerbs makes learning about herbs simple and fun. There are tons of free articles and recipes written by yours truly. The Herbal Remedy Kit is a great place to start. You can learn right alongside your kids or grandkids with the board game Wildcraft! and the Herb Fairies book series.

HerbsWithRosalee.com: My website has lots of free articles about herbs, health, and herbal recipes. Sign up for my newsletter and get instant access to my free mini course on Herbal Energetics.

HerbMentor.com: HerbMentor has exceptional online courses and a supportive community and curates amazing herbal resources. It provides inspiration for ongoing learning and features videos, articles, and recipes from herbalists around the world.

Taste of Herbs Online Course: A keen sense of taste is one of the most important tools an herbalist can develop. This course gives you the confidence you need to choose the best herbs for each person. www.tasteofherbs.com

Herbal Cold Care Online Course: Break the cycle of sickness and explore how to use herbs to prevent a cold or flu and to address many of the symptoms. This course gives you the whole picture for working with an individual and not simply using herbs to suppress symptoms. www.herbalcoldcare.com

Herb Rally: There are many herbalist gatherings, classes, and even podcasts popping up all over the country. Check out this free resource to find classes and events near you. www.herbrally.com

United Plant Savers: This nonprofit organization is dedicated to protecting at-risk herbal species. It does incredibly important work for the plants and offers some great learning experiences. I am proud to be a member of this organization. www.unitedplantsavers.org

American Herbalists Guild: Would you like to work with an herbalist for your health challenges? Check out the American Herbalists Guild directory to find an herbalist near you. I am proud to be a Registered Professional Herbalist with this organization. www.americanherbalistsguild.com

American Botanical Council: The American Botanical Council is an independent, nonprofit research and education organization dedicated to providing accurate and reliable information for consumers, health care practitioners, researchers, educators, industry, and the media. http://abc.herbalgram.org

ENDNOTES

Introduction

1. "Number of U.S. Farmers' Markets Continues to Rise." U.S. Department of Agriculture Economic Research Service. August 4, 2014. Accessed October 18, 2015.

2. "Chronic Disease Overview." Centers for Disease Control and Prevention. August 26, 2015. Accessed October 18, 2015.

3. "Health Expenditure, Total (% of GDP)." World Bank, Accessed October 18, 2015. http://data.worldbank.org/indicator /SH.XPD.TOTL.ZS.

4. Edelson, Mat. "Take Two Carrots and Call Me in the Morning." *Hopkins Medicine*, Winter 2010. Accessed October 18, 2015.

Chapter 1: The Benefits of Herbs and Spices

1. Salleh, Mohd Razali. "Life Event, Stress and Illness." *Malaysian Journal of Medical Sciences* 15, no. 4 (2008): 9–18.

2. "Antibiotic Resistance Threats in the United States, 2013." Centers for Disease Control and Prevention. July 17, 2014. Accessed October 18, 2015.

3. Stermitz, F. R., et al. "Synergy in a Medicinal Plant: Antimicrobial Action of Berberine Potentiated by 5′-methoxyhydnocarpin, a Multidrug Pump Inhibitor." *Proceedings of the National Academy of Sciences of the United States of America* 97, no. 4 (2000). doi:10.1073/pnas.030540597.

Chapter 2: How Do We Know Herbs Can Do That?

1. Snitz, Beth E., et al. "Ginkgo Biloba for Preventing Cognitive Decline in Older Adults: A Randomized Trial." *JAMA* 302, no. 24 (2009). doi:10.1001/jama.2009.1913.

2. Rabin, Roni. "Ginkgo Biloba Ineffective Against Dementia, Researchers Find." *New York Times*, November 18, 2008. Accessed October 18, 2015.

3. "Herbal Science Organization Clarifies New Ginkgo Study." American Botanical Council. December 29, 2009. Accessed October 18, 2015.

Chapter 4: How to Get the Most Out of This Book

1. Robinson, Jo. *Eating on the Wild Side: The Missing Link to Optimum Health* (New York: Little, Brown, 2014).

2. Aubrey, Allison. "The Average American Ate (Literally) a Ton This Year." National Public Radio. December 2011. Accessed October 18, 2015.

3. "By Any Other Name It's Still Sweetener." American Heart Association. Accessed February 22, 2016. http://www.heart .org/HEARTORG/HealthyLiving/HealthyEating/Nutrition /By-Any-Other-Name-Its-Still-Sweetener_UCM_437368 _Article.jsp#.

Chapter 5: Black Pepper

1. Jaffee, Steven. "Delivering and Taking the Heat: Indian Spices and Evolving Product and Process Standards." The World Bank. 2005. Accessed October 12, 2015.

2. Kasibhatta, Ravisekhar, and M. U. R. Naidu. "Influence of Piperine on the Pharmacokinetics of Nevirapine under Fasting Conditions: A Randomised, Crossover, Placebo-Controlled Study." *Drugs in R&D* 8, no. 6 (2007): 383–91.

3. Shoba, G., et al. "Influence of Piperine on the Pharmacokinetics of Curcumin in Animals and Human Volunteers." *Planta Medica* 64, no. 4 (May 1998): 353–56. doi:10.1055/s-2006-957450.

4. Buhner, Stephen Harrod. *Herbal Antibiotics: Natural Alternatives for Treating Drug-Resistant Bacteria* (North Adams, MA: Storey Publishing, 2012).

5. Ibid., 161.

6. Badmaev, V., M. Majeed, and L. Prakash. "Piperine Derived from Black Pepper Increases the Plasma Levels of Coenzyme Q10 Following Oral Supplementation." *Journal of Nutritional Biochemistry* 11, no. 2 (February 2000): 109–13.

7. Badmaev, Vladimir, Muhammed Majeed, and Edward P. Norkus. "Piperine, an Alkaloid Derived from Black Pepper Increases Serum Response of Beta-Carotene during 14 Days of Oral Beta-Carotene Supplementation." *Nutrition Research* 19, no. 3 (1999): 381–88. doi:10.1016/S0271-5317(99)00007-X.

8. Umesh, Patil, Amrit Singh, and Anup Chakraborty. "Role of Piperine as a Bioavailability Enhancer." *International Journal of Recent Advances in Pharm. Research* 1, no. 4 (October 2011): 16–23.

9. Ibid.

10. Jin, Cheng-Qiang, et al. "Stir-Fried White Pepper Can Treat Diarrhea in Infants and Children Efficiently: A Randomized Controlled Trial." *American Journal of Chinese Medicine* 41, no. 4 (2013): 765–72. doi:10.1142/S0192415X13500511.

Chapter 6: Cayenne

1. Bortolotti, M., and S. Porta. "Effect of Red Pepper on Symptoms of Irritable Bowel Syndrome: Preliminary Study." *Digestive Diseases and Sciences* 56, no. 11 (2011): 3288–95. doi:10.1007/ s10620-011-1740-9.

2. Bortolotti, M., et al. "The Treatment of Functional Dyspepsia with Red Pepper." *Alimentary Pharmacology & Therapeutics* 16, no. 6 (2002): 1075–82. doi:10.1046/j.1365-2036.2002.01280.x.

3. Yeoh, K. G., et al. "Chili Protects against Aspirin-Induced Gastroduodenal Mucosal Injury in Humans." *Digestive Diseases and Sciences* 40, no. 3 (1995): 580–83. doi:10.1007/BF02064374.

4. Kang, J. Y., et al. "Chili—Protective Factor against Peptic Ulcer?" *Digestive Diseases and Sciences* 40, no. 3 (1995): 576–79. doi:10.1007/BF02064373.

5. Snitker, Soren, et al. "Effects of Novel Capsinoid Treatment on Fatness and Energy Metabolism in Humans: Possible Pharmacogenetic Implications." *American Journal of Clinical Nutrition* 89, no. 1 (2009): 45–50. doi:10.3945/ajcn.2008.26561.

6. Ludy, Mary-Jon, and Richard D. Mattes. "The Effects of Hedonically Acceptable Red Pepper Doses on Thermogenesis and Appetite." *Physiology & Behavior* 102, no. 3–4 (2011): 251–58. doi:10.1016/j.physbeh.2010.11.018.

7. Ahuja, K. D. K., et al. "The Effect of 4-Week Chilli Supplementation on Metabolic and Arterial Function in Humans." *European Journal of Clinical Nutrition* 61, no. 3 (2007): 326–33.

8. Ahuja, Kiran D. K., and Madeleine J. Ball. "Effects of Daily Ingestion of Chili on Serum Lipoprotein Oxidation in Adult Men and Women." *British Journal of Nutrition* 96, no. 02 (2006): 239–42. doi:10.1079/BJN20061788.

9. Raghavendra, R. H., and K. Akhilender Naidu. "Spice Active Principles as the Inhibitors of Human Platelet Aggregation and Thromboxane Biosynthesis." *Prostaglandins, Leukotrienes and Essential Fatty Acids* 81, no. 1 (2009): 73–78. doi:10.1016/j.plefa.2009.04.009.

10. Ahuja, Kiran D.K., et al. "Effects of Chili Consumption on Postprandial Glucose, Insulin, and Energy Metabolism." *American Journal of Clinical Nutrition* 84, no. 1 (2006): 63–69.

11. Weerapan Khovidhunkit, M. D. "Pharmacokinetic and the Effect of Capsaicin in Capsicum frutescens on Decreasing Plasma Glucose Level." *J Med Assoc Thai* 92, no. 1 (2009): 108–13.

12. Landis, Robyn, and Karta Purkh Singh Khalsa. *Herbal Defense: Positioning Yourself to Triumph over Illness and Aging* (New York: Hachette, 1997).

13. Frerick, Helmut, et al. "Topical Treatment of Chronic Low Back Pain with a Capsicum Plaster." *Pain* 106, no. 1–2 (2003): 59–64. doi:10.1016/S0304-3959(03)00278-1.

14. Chrubasik, S., T. Weiser, and B. Beime. "Effectiveness and Safety of Topical Capsaicin Cream in the Treatment of Chronic Soft Tissue Pain." *Phytotherapy Research* 24, no. 12 (2010): 1877–85. doi:10.1002/ptr.3335.

15. Forst, T., et al. "The Influence of Local Capsaicin Treatment on Small Nerve Fibre Function and Neurovascular Control in Symptomatic Diabetic Neuropathy." *Acta Diabetologica* 39, no. 1 (2002): 1–6. doi:10.1007/s005920200005.

16. Tandan, Rup, et al. "Topical Capsaicin in Painful Diabetic Neuropathy: Controlled Study with Long-Term Follow-Up." *Diabetes Care* 15, no. 1 (1992): 8–14. doi:10.2337/diacare.15.1.8.

17. Henson, Shari. "Re: Use of Herbs to Treat Shingles—A Review." American Botanical Council. December 2005. http://cms.herbalgram.org/herbclip/295/review44338.html.

Chapter 7: Cinnamon

1. Wood, Matthew. *The Earthwise Herbal: A Complete Guide to Old World Medicinal Plants.* (Berkeley, CA: North Atlantic Books, 2008).

2. Tierra, Lesley. *Healing with the Herbs of Life* (New York: Crossing Press/Random House, 2003).

3. mcdonald, jim. "Herbs, Vitalism & Holistic Immunity," seminar, White Lake, Michigan, 2011.

4. McIntyre, Anne. "Preparing for the Cold Season." *Positive Health* 69, October 2001. http://www.positivehealth.com/article/herbal-medicine/preparing-for-the-cold-season.

5. "National Diabetes Statistics Report: Estimates of Diabetes and Its Burden in the United States, 2014." Centers for Disease Control and Prevention, June 10, 2014. http://www.cdc.gov/diabetes/pubs/statsreport14/national-diabetes-report-web.pdf.

6. Akilen, R., et al. "Glycated Haemoglobin and Blood Pressure-Lowering Effect of Cinnamon in Multi-Ethnic Type 2 Diabetic Patients in the UK: A Randomized, Placebo-Controlled, Double-Blind Clinical Trial." *Diabetic Medicine* 27, no. 10 (October 1, 2010): 1159–67. doi:10.1111/j.1464-5491.2010.03079.x.

7. Khan, Alam, et al. "Cinnamon Improves Glucose and Lipids of People with Type 2 Diabetes." *Diabetes Care* 26, no. 12 (2003): 3215–18. doi:10.2337/diacare.26.12.3215.

8. Solomon, Thomas P. J., and Andrew K. Blannin. "Changes in Glucose Tolerance and Insulin Sensitivity Following 2 Weeks of Daily Cinnamon Ingestion in Healthy Humans." *European Journal of Applied Physiology* 105, no. 6 (2009): 969–76. doi:10.1007/s00421-009-0986-9.

Chapter 8: Fennel

1. Von Bingen, Hildegard. *Hildegard Von Bingen's Physica: The Complete English Translation of Her Classic Work on Health and Healing,* translated by Priscilla Throop (Rochester, VT: Healing Arts Press, 1998).

2. Hoffmann, David. *Medical Herbalism: The Science and Practice of Herbal Medicine* (Rochester, VT: Healing Arts Press, 2003).

3. Modaress, Nejad V., and M. Asadipour. "Comparison of the Effectiveness of Fennel and Mefenamic Acid on Pain Intensity in Dysmenorrhoea," 2006.

4. Nordqvist, Christian. "What Is Colic? What Causes Colic?" *Medical News Today,* September 8, 2014. http://www.medicalnewstoday.com/articles/162806.php.

5. Alexandrovich, Irina, et al. "The Effect of Fennel (Foeniculum vulgare) Seed Oil Emulsion in Infantile Colic: A Randomized, Placebo-Controlled Study." *Alternative Therapies in Health and Medicine* 9, no. 4 (2003): 58–61.

6. Savino, Francesco, et al. "A Randomized Double-blind, placebo-controlled Trial of a Standardized Extract of Matricariae recutita, Foeniculum vulgare and Melissa officinalis (ColiMil®) in the Treatment of Breastfed Colicky Infants." *Phytotherapy Research* 19, no. 4 (2005): 335–40.

7. "Fennel." In *The World's Healthiest Foods,* George Mateljan Foundation. Accessed June 26, 2015. http://www.whfoods.com/genpage.php?tname=foodspice&dbid=23.

Chapter 9: Garlic

1. Bergner, Paul. *The Healing Power of Garlic* (Roseville, CA: Prima Lifestyles, 1996).

2. Ishikawa, Hideki, et al. "Aged Garlic Extract Prevents a Decline of NK Cell Number and Activity in Patients with Advanced Cancer." *Journal of Nutrition* 136, no. 3 (2006): 816S–820S.

3. Mozaffari-Khosravi, Hassan, et al. "The Effect of Garlic Tablet on Pro-Inflammatory Cytokines in Postmenopausal Osteoporotic Women: A Randomized Controlled Clinical Trial." *Journal of Dietary Supplements* 9, no. 4 (2012): 262–71. doi:10.3109/19390211.2012.726703.

4. Bakhshi, Mahin, et al. "Comparison of Therapeutic Effect of Aqueous Extract of Garlic and Nystatin Mouthwash in Denture Stomatitis." *Gerodontology* 29, no. 2 (2012): e680–84. doi:10.1111/j.1741-2358.2011.00544.x.

5. Chavan, S. D., N. L. Shetty, and M. Kanuri. "Comparative Evaluation of Garlic Extract Mouthwash and Chlorhexidine Mouthwash on Salivary Streptococcus Mutans Count—An in Vitro Study." *Oral Health & Preventive Dentistry* 8, no. 4 (2009): 369–74.

6. Ishikawa, Hideki, et al. "Aged Garlic Extract Prevents a Decline of NK Cell Number and Activity in Patients with Advanced Cancer." *Journal of Nutrition* 136, no. 3 (2006): 816S–820S.

7. Andrianova, I. V., et al. "[Effect of Long-Acting Garlic Tablets 'Allicor' on the Incidence of Acute Respiratory Viral Infections in Children]." *Terapevticheskii Arkhiv* 75, no. 3 (2002): 53–56.

8. Nantz, Meri P., et al. "Supplementation with Aged Garlic Extract Improves Both NK and γδ-T Cell Function and Reduces the Severity of Cold and Flu Symptoms: A Randomized, Double-Blind, Placebo-Controlled Nutrition Intervention." *Clinical Nutrition* 31, no. 3 (2012): 337–44. doi:10.1016/j.clnu.2011.11.019.

9. Ried, K., O. R. Frank, and N. P. Stocks. "Aged Garlic Extract Reduces Blood Pressure in Hypertensives: A Dose–Response Trial." *European Journal of Clinical Nutrition* 67, no. 1 (2013): 64–70. doi:10.1038/ejcn.2012.178.

10. Ried, Karin, Oliver R. Frank, and Nigel P. Stocks. "Aged Garlic Extract Lowers Blood Pressure in Patients with Treated but Uncontrolled Hypertension: A Randomised Controlled Trial." *Maturitas* 67, no. 2 (2010): 144–50. doi:10.1016/j.maturitas.2010.06.001.

11. Ashraf, Rizwan, Rafeeq Alam Khan, and Imran Ashraf. "Garlic (Allium sativum) Supplementation with Standard Antidiabetic Agent Provides Better Diabetic Control in Type 2 Diabetes Patients." *Pakistan Journal of Pharmaceutical Sciences* 24 (2011): 565–70.

12. Hoffmann, David. *Medical Herbalism: The Science and Practice of Herbal Medicine* (Rochester, VT: Healing Arts Press, 2003).

13. Mohammed, Abdul M. I., et al. "Pharmacodynamic Interaction of Warfarin with Cranberry but Not with Garlic in Healthy Subjects." *British Journal of Pharmacology* 154, no. 8 (August 1, 2008): 1691–1700. doi:10.1038/bjp.2008.210.

14. Scharbert, Gisela, et al. "Garlic at Dietary Doses Does Not Impair Platelet Function." *Anesthesia & Analgesia* 105, no. 5 (2007): 1214–18. doi:10.1213/01.ane.0000287253.92211.06.

15. Wojcikowski, Ken, Stephen Myers, and Lyndon Brooks. "Effects of Garlic Oil on Platelet Aggregation: A Double-blind, placebo-controlled Crossover Study." *Platelets* 18, no. 1 (2007): 29–34. doi:10.1080/09537100600800636.

Chapter 10: Ginger

1. Bode, Ann M., and Zigang Dong. "The Amazing and Mighty Ginger." In *Herbal Medicine: Biomolecular and Clinical Aspects*. Edited by Iris F. F. Benzie and Sissi Wachtel-Galor (Boca Raton, FL: CRC Press/Taylor & Francis, 2011).

2. Buhner, Stephen Harrod. *Herbal Antibiotics: Natural Alternatives for Treating Drug-Resistant Bacteria* (North Adams, MA: Storey Publishing, 2012).

3. Jenabi, Ensiyeh. "The Effect of Ginger for Relieving of Primary Dysmenorrhoea." *J Pak Med Assoc* 63, no. 1 (2013): 8–10.

4. Paramdeep, G. I. L. L. "Efficacy and Tolerability of Ginger (Zingiber officinale) in Patients of Osteoarthritis of Knee." *Indian J Physiol Pharmacol* 57, no. 2 (2013): 177–83.

5. Al-Nahain, Abdullah, Rownak Jahan, and Mohammed Rahmatullah. "Zingiber Officinale: A Plant against Rheumatoid Arthritis." *Arthritis* 2014 (2014): e159089. doi:10.1155/2014/159089.

6. Therkleson, Tessa. "Topical Ginger Treatment with a Compress or Patch for Osteoarthritis Symptoms." *Journal of Holistic Nursing* 32, no. 3 (2014): 173–82. doi:10.1177/0898010113512182.

7. Black, Christopher D., et al. "Ginger (Zingiber Officinale) Reduces Muscle Pain Caused by Eccentric Exercise." *Journal of Pain* 11, no. 9 (2010): 894–903. doi:10.1016/j.jpain.2009.12.013.

8. Sritoomma, Netchanok, et al. "The Effectiveness of Swedish Massage with Aromatic Ginger Oil in Treating Chronic Low Back Pain in Older Adults: A Randomized Controlled Trial." *Complementary Therapies in Medicine* 22, no. 1 (2014): 26–33. doi:10.1016/j.ctim.2013.11.002.

9. Maghbooli, Mehdi, et al. "Comparison between the Efficacy of Ginger and Sumatriptan in the Ablative Treatment of the Common Migraine." *Phytotherapy Research* 28, no. 3 (2014): 412–15. doi:10.1002/ptr.4996.

10. Khalsa, Karta Purkh Singh. "Culinary Herbalism Course" on LearningHerbs.com. Accessed August 31, 2016. http://courses.learningherbs.com/culinary-herbalism.

11. Wu, Keng-Liang, et al. "Effects of Ginger on Gastric Emptying and Motility in Healthy Humans" *European Journal of Gastroenterology & Hepatology* 20, no. 5 (May 2008): 436–40. doi:10.1097/MEG.0b013e3282f4b224.

12. Hu, Ming-Luen, et al. "Effect of Ginger on Gastric Motility and Symptoms of Functional Dyspepsia." *World Journal of Gastroenterology* 17, no. 1 (2011): 105–10. doi:10.3748/wjg.v17.i1.105.

13. Ozgoli, Giti, Marjan Goli, and Masoumeh Simbar. "Effects of Ginger Capsules on Pregnancy, Nausea, and Vomiting." *Journal of Alternative and Complementary Medicine* 15, no. 3 (February 28, 2009): 243–46. doi:10.1089/acm.2008.0406.

14. Dabaghzadeh, Fatemeh, et al. "Ginger for Prevention of Antiretroviral-Induced Nausea and Vomiting: A Randomized Clinical Trial." *Expert Opinion on Drug Safety* 13, no. 7 (July 1, 2014): 859–66. doi:10.1517/14740338.2014.914170.

15. Ryan, Julie L., et al. "Ginger (Zingiber officinale) Reduces Acute Chemotherapy-Induced Nausea: A URCC CCOP Study of 576 Patients." *Supportive Care in Cancer* 20, no. 7 (2011): 1479–89. doi:10.1007/s00520-011-1236-3.

16. Pillai, Anu Kochanujan, et al. "Anti-Emetic Effect of Ginger Powder versus Placebo as an Add-on Therapy in Children and Young Adults Receiving High Emetogenic Chemotherapy." *Pediatric Blood & Cancer* 56, no. 2 (February 1, 2011): 234–38. doi:10.1002/pbc.22778.

17. Mozaffari-Khosravi, Hassan, et al. "The Effect of Ginger Powder Supplementation on Insulin Resistance and Glycemic Indices in Patients with Type 2 Diabetes: A Randomized, Double-Blind, Placebo-Controlled Trial." *Complementary Therapies in Medicine* 22, no. 1 (February 2014): 9–16. doi:10.1016/j.ctim.2013.12.017.

18. Arablou, Tahereh, et al. "The Effect of Ginger Consumption on Glycemic Status, Lipid Profile and Some Inflammatory Markers in Patients with Type 2 Diabetes Mellitus." *International Journal of Food Sciences and Nutrition* 65, no. 4 (June 1, 2014): 515–20. doi:10.3109/09637486.2014.880671.

19. Alizadeh-Navaei, Reza, et al. "Investigation of the Effect of Ginger on the Lipid Levels. A Double-blind Controlled Clinical Trial." *Saudi Medical Journal* 29, no. 9 (2008): 1280–84.

20. Giriraju, Anjan, and G. Y. Yunus. "Assessment of Antimicrobial Potential of 10% Ginger Extract against Streptococcus mutans, Candida albicans, and Enterococcus faecalis : An in Vitro Study." *Indian Journal of Dental Research* 24, no. 4 (2013): 397. doi:10.4103/0970-9290.118356.

21. Karuppiah, Ponmurugan, and Shyamkumar Rajaram. "Antibacterial Effect of Allium Sativum Cloves and Zingiber officinale Rhizomes against Multiple-Drug Resistant Clinical Pathogens." *Asian Pacific Journal of Tropical Biomedicine* 2, no. 8 (2012): 597–601. doi:10.1016/S2221-1691(12)60104-X.

22. Chang, Jung San, et al. "Fresh Ginger (Zingiber officinale) Has Anti-Viral Activity against Human Respiratory Syncytial Virus in Human Respiratory Tract Cell Lines." *Journal of Ethnopharmacology* 145, no. 1 (2013): 146–51. doi:10.1016/j.jep.2012.10.043.

23. Kuhn, Merrily A., and David Winston. *Winston & Kuhn's Herbal Therapy & Supplements: A Scientific & Traditional Approach.* 2nd ed. (Philadelphia: Lippincott Williams & Wilkins, 2008), 217.

24. Shalansky, Stephen, et al. "Risk of Warfarin-Related Bleeding Events and Supratherapeutic International Normalized Ratios Associated with Complementary and Alternative Medicine: A Longitudinal Analysis." *Pharmacotherapy: The Journal of Human Pharmacology and Drug Therapy* 27, no. 9 (2007): 1237–47. doi:10.1592/phco.27.9.1237.

Chapter 11: Holy Basil

1. Winston, David, and Steven Maimes. *Adaptogens: Herbs for Strength, Stamina, and Stress Relief* (Rochester, VT: Healing Arts Press, 2007).

2. Bhattacharyya, D., et al. "Controlled Programmed Trial of Ocimum Sanctum Leaf on Generalized Anxiety Disorders." *Nepal Medical College Journal* 10, no. 3 (2008): 176–79.

3. Winston, David, and Steven Maimes. *Adaptogens: Herbs for Strength, Stamina, and Stress Relief* (Rochester, VT: Healing Arts Press, 2007), 170.

4. Khalsa, Karta Purkh Singh, and Michael Tierra. *The Way of Ayurvedic Herbs: The Most Complete Guide to Natural Healing and Health With Traditional Ayurvedic Herbalism* (Twin Lakes, WI: Lotus, 2008), 98.

5. Agrawal, P., V. Rai, and R. B. Singh. "Randomized Placebo-Controlled, Single Blind Trial of Holy Basil Leaves in Patients with Noninsulin-Dependent Diabetes Mellitus." *International Journal of Clinical Pharmacology and Therapeutics* 34, no. 9 (1996): 406-9.

6. Rai, V., U. V. Mani, and U.M. Iyer. "Effect of Ocimum Sanctum Leaf Powder on Blood Lipoproteins, Glycated Proteins and Total Amino Acids in Patients with Non-Insulin-Dependent Diabetes Mellitus." *Journal of Nutritional & Environmental Medicine* 7, no. 2 (1997): 113-18. doi:10.1080/13590849762709.

7. Kelm, M. A., et al. "Antioxidant and Cyclooxygenase Inhibitory Phenolic Compounds from Ocimum Sanctum Linn." *Phytomedicine* 7, no. 1 (2000): 7-13. doi:10.1016/S0944-7113(00)80015-X.

8. Mondal, Shankar, et al. "Double-Blinded Randomized Controlled Trial for Immunomodulatory Effects of Tulsi (Ocimum Sanctum Linn.) Leaf Extract on Healthy Volunteers." *Journal of Ethnopharmacology* 136, no. 3 (2011): 452-56. doi:10.1016/j.jep.2011.05.012.

9. Bhat, Jyoti, et al. "In Vivo Enhancement of Natural Killer Cell Activity through Tea Fortified with Ayurvedic Herbs." *Phytotherapy Research* 24, no. 1 (January 1, 2010): 129-35. doi:10.1002/ptr.2889.

10. Jadhav, Priyanka, et al. "Antiviral Potential of Selected Indian Medicinal (Ayurvedic) Plants Against Herpes Simplex Virus 1 and 2." *North American Journal of Medical Sciences* 4, no. 12 (2012): 641-47. doi:10.4103/1947-2714.104316.

11. Shimizu, Tomohiro, et al. "Holy Basil Leaf Extract Decreases Tumorigenicity and Metastasis of Aggressive Human Pancreatic Cancer Cells in Vitro and in Vivo: Potential Role in Therapy." *Cancer Letters* 336, no. 2 (August 2013): 270-80. doi:10.1016/j.canlet.2013.03.017.

Chapter 12: Lavender

1. Hardin, Kiva Rose. "The Soothing Magic of Lavender." *The Medicine Womans Roots.* Accessed August 31, 2016. http://bearmedicineherbals.com/tag/lavender.

2. Lehrner, J., et al. "Ambient Odors of Orange and Lavender Reduce Anxiety and Improve Mood in a Dental Office." *Physiology & Behavior* 86, no. 1-2 (September 15, 2005): 92-95. doi:10.1016/j.physbeh.2005.06.031.

3. Lytle, Jamie, Catherine Mwatha, and Karen K. Davis. "Effect of Lavender Aromatherapy on Vital Signs and Perceived Quality of Sleep in the Intermediate Care Unit: A Pilot Study." *American Journal of Critical Care* 23, no. 1 (2014): 24-29. doi:10.4037/ajcc2014958.

4. Woelk, H., and S. Schläfke. "A Multi-Center, Double-Blind, Randomised Study of the Lavender Oil Preparation Silexan in Comparison to Lorazepam for Generalized Anxiety Disorder." *Phytomedicine* 17, no. 2 (2010): 94-99. doi:10.1016/j.phymed.2009.10.006.

5. Pham, M., Winai Sayorwan, and Vorasith Siripornpanich. "The Effects of Lavender Oil Inhalation on Emotional States, Autonomic Nervous System, and Brain Electrical Activity." *J Med Assoc Thai* 95, no. 4 (2012): 598-606.

6. Lagopoulos, Jim, et al. "Increased Theta and Alpha EEG Activity during Nondirective Meditation." *Journal of Alternative and Complementary Medicine* 15, no. 11 (2009): 1187-92. doi:10.1089/acm.2009.0113.

7. Atsumi, Toshiko, and Keiichi Tonosaki. "Smelling Lavender and Rosemary Increases Free Radical Scavenging Activity and Decreases Cortisol Level in Saliva." *Psychiatry Research* 150, no. 1 (2007): 89-96. doi:10.1016/j.psychres.2005.12.012.

8. Winston, David. "Differential Treatment of Depression and Anxiety with Botanical and Nutritional Medicines." In *17th Annual AHG Symposium Proceedings Book.* Millennium Hotel, Boulder, Colorado, 2006.

9. Conrad, Pam, and Cindy Adams. "The Effects of Clinical Aromatherapy for Anxiety and Depression in the High Risk Postpartum Woman—A Pilot Study." *Complementary Therapies in Clinical Practice* 18, no. 3 (2012): 164-68. doi:10.1016/j.ctcp.2012.05.002.

10. Salmon, William. *Botanologia. The English Herbal or History of Plants* (London: Dawks, Rhodes and Taylor, 1710).

11. Grieve, Maud. *A Modern Herbal: The Medicinal, Culinary, Cosmetic and Economic Properties, Cultivation and Folk-Lore of Herbs, Grasses, Fungi, Shrubs, & Trees with All Their Modern Scientific Uses.* Vol. 2. (New York: Dover, 1971).

12. Sheikhan, Fatemeh, et al. "Episiotomy Pain Relief: Use of Lavender Oil Essence in Primiparous Iranian Women." *Complementary Therapies in Clinical Practice* 18, no. 1 (2012): 66-70. doi:10.1016/j.ctcp.2011.02.003.

13. Vakilian, Katayon, et al. "Healing Advantages of Lavender Essential Oil during Episiotomy Recovery: A Clinical Trial." *Complementary Therapies in Clinical Practice* 17, no. 1 (2011): 50-53. doi:10.1016/j.ctcp.2010.05.006.

14. Altaei, D. T. "Topical Lavender Oil for the Treatment of Recurrent Aphthous Ulceration." *American Journal of Dentistry* 25, no. 1 (2012): 39-43.

15. Tisserand, Robert. "Gattefossé's Burn." roberttisserand.com. April 22, 2011. http://roberttisserand.com/2011/04/gattefosses-burn.

16. Culpeper, Nicholas. *The English Physician: OR An Astrologo-Physical Discourse of the Vulgar Herbs of This Nation* (London: Commonwealth of England, 1652).

17. Sasannejad, Payam, et al. "Lavender Essential Oil in the Treatment of Migraine Headache: A Placebo-Controlled Clinical Trial." *European Neurology* 67, no. 5 (2012): 288-91. doi:10.1159/000335249.

18. Hadi, Niaz, and Ali Akbar Hanid. "Lavender Essence for Post-Cesarean Pain." *Pakistan Journal of Biological Sciences* 14, no. 11 (2011): 664.

19. Soltani, Rasool, et al. "Evaluation of the Effect of Aromatherapy with Lavender Essential Oil on Post-Tonsillectomy Pain in Pediatric Patients: A Randomized Controlled Trial." *International Journal of Pediatric Otorhinolaryngology* 77, no. 9 (2013): 1579-81. doi:10.1016/j.ijporl.2013.07.014.

20. Apay, Serap Ejder, et al. "Effect of Aromatherapy Massage on Dysmenorrhea in Turkish Students." *Pain Management Nursing* 13, no. 4 (2012): 236-40. doi:10.1016/j.pmn.2010.04.002.

21. Kuhn, Merrily A., and David Winston. *Winston & Kuhn's Herbal Therapy & Supplements: A Scientific & Traditional Approach.* 2nd ed. (Philadelphia: Lippincott Williams & Wilkins, 2008), 286.

22. Gardner, Zoë, and Michael McGuffin, editors. *American Herbal Products Association's Botanical Safety Handbook.* 2nd ed. (Boca Raton, FL: CRC Press, 2013).

Chapter 13: Mustard

1. Saul, Hayley, et al. "Phytoliths in Pottery Reveal the Use of Spice in European Prehistoric Cuisine." *PloS One* 8, no. 8 (2013). doi:10.1371/journal.pone.0070583.

2. Jordan, Michele Anna. *The Good Cook's Book of Mustard: One of the World's Most Beloved Condiments, with More than 100 Recipes* (New York: Skyhorse Publishing, 2015).

3. Robinson, Jo. *Eating on the Wild Side: The Missing Link to Optimum Health* (Boston: Little, Brown, 2013).

4. Lamy, Evelyn, et al. "Antigenotoxic Action of Isothiocyanate-Containing Mustard as Determined by Two Cancer Biomarkers in a Human Intervention Trial." *European Journal of Cancer Prevention* 21, no. 4 (2012): 400-406. doi:10.1097/CEJ.0b013e32834ef140.

5. Singh, Ram B., et al. "Randomized, Double-Blind, Placebo-Controlled Trial of Fish Oil and Mustard Oil in Patients with Suspected Acute Myocardial Infarction: The Indian Experiment of Infarct Survival—4." *Cardiovascular Drugs and Therapy* 11, no. 3 (1997): 485-91. doi:10.1023/A:1007757724505.

6. Huo, G. R., L. Q. Ma, and C. H. Huang. "[Clinical Study on Treatment of Chronic Bronchitis by Tracheitis Plaster.]" *Zhongguo Zhong Xi Yi Jie He Za Zhi* [Chinese Journal of Integrated Traditional and Western Medicine] 21, no. 11 (November 2001): 816-18.

Chapter 14: Nutmeg

1. Lad, Vasant, and David Frawley. *The Yoga of Herbs: An Ayurvedic Guide to Herbal Medicine* (Santa Fe, NM: Lotus Press), 1986.

2. Von Bingen, Hildegard. *Hildegard Von Bingen's Physica: The Complete English Translation of Her Classic Work on Health and Healing*. Translated by Priscilla Throop (Rochester, VT: Healing Arts Press, 1998).

3. Gardner, Zoë, and Michael McGuffin, editors. *American Herbal Products Association's Botanical Safety Handbook*. 2nd ed. (Boca Raton, FL: CRC Press, 2013), 587.

Chapter 15: Parsley

1. George Mateljan Foundation. "Parsley." *The World's Healthiest Foods*. Accessed August 15, 2015. http://www.whfoods.com/genpage.php?tname=foodspice&dbid=100.

2. Shea, M. Kyla, Christopher J. O'Donnell, Udo Hoffmann, Gerard E. Dallal, Bess Dawson-Hughes, José M. Ordovas, Paul A. Price, Matthew K. Williamson, and Sarah L. Booth. "Vitamin K Supplementation and Progression of Coronary Artery Calcium in Older Men and Women." *The American Journal of Clinical Nutrition* 89, no. 6 (2009): 1799–1807. doi:10.3945/ajcn.2008.27338.

3. Nielsen, S. E., et al. "Effect of Parsley (Petroselinum Crispum) Intake on Urinary Apigenin Excretion, Blood Antioxidant Enzymes and Biomarkers for Oxidative Stress in Human Subjects." *British Journal of Nutrition* 81, no. 06 (1999): 447–55. doi:10.1017/S000711459900080X.

4. Aggarwal, Bharat B., and Debora Yost. *Healing Spices: How to Use 50 Everyday and Exotic Spices to Boost Health and Beat Disease* (New York: Sterling Pub., 2011).

5. Gadi, Dounia, et al. "Flavonoids Purified from Parsley Inhibit Human Blood Platelet Aggregation and Adhesion to Collagen under Flow." *Journal of Complementary and Integrative Medicine* 9, no. 1 (2012).

Chapter 16: Peppermint

1. Merat, Shahin, et al. "The Effect of Enteric-Coated, Delayed-Release Peppermint Oil on Irritable Bowel Syndrome." *Digestive Diseases and Sciences* 55, no. 5 (2009): 1385–90. doi:10.1007/s10620-009-0854-9.

2. Alam, M. S., et al. "Efficacy of Peppermint Oil in Diarrhea Predominant IBS —A Double-blind Randomized Placebo-Controlled Study." *Mymensingh Medical Journal* 22, no. 1 (2013): 27–30.

3. Papathanasopoulos, A., et al. "Effect of Acute Peppermint Oil Administration on Gastric Sensorimotor Function and Nutrient Tolerance in Health." *Neurogastroenterology & Motility* 25, no. 4 (2013): e263–71. doi:10.1111/nmo.12102.

4. Kline, Robert M., et al. "Enteric-Coated, pH-Dependent Peppermint Oil Capsules for the Treatment of Irritable Bowel Syndrome in Children." *Journal of Pediatrics* 138, no. 1 (2001): 125–28. doi:10.1067/mpd.2001.109606.

5. Moss, Mark, et al. "Modulation of Cognitive Performance and Mood by Aromas of Peppermint and Ylang-Ylang." *International Journal of Neuroscience* 118, no. 1 (2008): 59–77. doi:10.1080/00207450601042094.

6. Varney, Elizabeth, and Jane Buckle. "Effect of Inhaled Essential Oils on Mental Exhaustion and Moderate Burnout: A Small Pilot Study." *Journal of Alternative and Complementary Medicine* 19, no. 1 (2012): 69–71. doi:10.1089/acm.2012.0089.

7. Gladstar, Rosemary. *Rosemary Gladstar's Medicinal Herbs: A Beginner's Guide* (North Adams, MA: Storey Pub., 2012).

8. Göbel, H., G. Schmidt, and D. Soyka. "Effect of Peppermint and Eucalyptus Oil Preparations on Neurophysiological and Experimental Algesimetric Headache Parameters." *Cephalalgia* 14, no. 3 (1994): 228–34. doi:10.1046/j.1468-2982.1994.014003228.x.

9. Davies, Simon J., Louise M. Harding, and Andrew P. Baranowski. "A Novel Treatment of Postherpetic Neuralgia Using Peppermint Oil." *Clinical Journal of Pain* 18, no. 3 (2002): 200–202.

10. Kuhn, Merrily A., and David Winston. *Winston & Kuhn's Herbal Therapy & Supplements: A Scientific & Traditional Approach*. 2nd ed. (Philadelphia: Lippincott Williams & Wilkins, 2008), 342.

Chapter 17: Rosemary

1. Karpińska-Tymoszczyk, M. "Effect of the Addition of Ground Rosemary on the Quality and Shelf-Life of Turkey Meatballs during Refrigerated Storage." *British Poultry Science* 49, no. 6 (2008): 742–50. doi:10.1080/00071660802454665.

2. Puangsombat, Kanithaporn, and J. Scott Smith. "Inhibition of Heterocyclic Amine Formation in Beef Patties by Ethanolic Extracts of Rosemary." *Journal of Food Science* 75, no. 2 (2010): T40–47. doi:10.1111/j.1750-3841.2009.01491.x.

3. Pérez-Sánchez, A., et al. "Protective Effects of Citrus and Rosemary Extracts on UV-Induced Damage in Skin Cell Model and Human Volunteers." *Journal of Photochemistry and Photobiology B: Biology* 136 (July 5, 2014): 12–18. doi:10.1016/j.jphotobiol.2014.04.007.

4. Ross, Jeremy. *Combining Western Herbs and Chinese Medicine* (Bristol, UK: Greenfields Press, 2010), 640.

5. Lukaczer, Daniel, et al. "A Pilot Trial Evaluating meta050, a Proprietary Combination of Reduced Iso-Alpha Acids, Rosemary Extract and Oleanolic Acid in Patients with Arthritis and Fibromyalgia." *Phytotherapy Research* 19, no. 10 (2005): 864–69. doi:10.1002/ptr.1709.

6. Gedney, Jeffrey J., Toni L. Glover, and Roger B. Fillingim. "Sensory and Affective Pain Discrimination after Inhalation of Essential Oils." *Psychosomatic Medicine* 66, no. 4 (2004): 599–606.

7. Park, M. K., and E. S. Lee. "[The Effect of Aroma Inhalation Method on Stress Responses of Nursing Students]." *Taehan Kanho Hakhoe Chi* 34, no. 2 (2004): 344–51.

8. McCaffrey, Ruth, Debra J. Thomas, and Ann Orth Kinzelman. "The Effects of Lavender and Rosemary Essential Oils on Test-Taking Anxiety among Graduate Nursing Students." *Holistic Nursing Practice* 23, no. 2 (2009): 88–93. doi:10.1097/HNP.0b013e3181a110aa.

9. Moss, Mark, et al. "Aromas of Rosemary and Lavender Essential Oils Differentially Affect Cognition and Mood in Healthy Adults." *International Journal of Neuroscience* 113, no. 1 (2003): 15–38. doi:10.1080/00207450390161903.

10. "Alzheimer's Statistics." Alzheimers.net. Accessed September 27, 2015. http://www.alzheimers.net/resources/alzheimers-statistics.

11. Pengelly, Andrew, et al. "Short-Term Study on the Effects of Rosemary on Cognitive Function in an Elderly Population." *Journal of Medicinal Food* 15, no. 1 (2011): 10–17. doi:10.1089/jmf.2011.0005.

12. Jimbo, Daiki, et al. "Effect of Aromatherapy on Patients with Alzheimer's Disease." *Psychogeriatrics* 9, no. 4 (2009): 173–79. doi:10.1111/j.1479-8301.2009.00299.x.

13. Hay, I. C., M. Jamieson, and A. D. Ormerod. "Randomized Trial of Aromatherapy: Successful Treatment for Alopecia Areata." *Archives of Dermatology* 134, no. 11 (1998): 1349–52. doi:10.1001/archderm.134.11.1349.

14. Tierra, Lesley. *Healing with the Herbs of Life* (New York: Crossing Press/Random House, 2003).

15. Kuhn, Merrily A., and David Winston. *Winston & Kuhn's Herbal Therapy & Supplements: A Scientific & Traditional Approach*. 2nd ed. (Philadelphia: Lippincott Williams & Wilkins, 2008).

16. Gardner, Zoë, and Michael McGuffin, editors. *American Herbal Products Association's Botanical Safety Handbook*. 2nd ed. (Boca Raton, FL: CRC Press, 2013).

17. Ibid.

18. Ibid.

Chapter 18: Sage

1. Grieve, M. *A Modern Herbal: The Medicinal, Culinary, Cosmetic and Economic Properties, Cultivation and Folklore of Herbs, Grasses, Fungi, Shrubs and Trees with All Their Modern Scientific Uses* (New York: Dover Publications, 1971).

2. Aggarwal, Bharat B., and Debora Yost. *Healing Spices: How to Use 50 Everyday and Exotic Spices to Boost Health and Beat Disease* (New York: Sterling Pub., 2011).

3. Scholey, Andrew B., et al. "An Extract of Salvia (Sage) with Anticholinesterase Properties Improves Memory and Attention in Healthy Older Volunteers." *Psychopharmacology* 198, no. 1 (2008): 127–39. doi:10.1007/s00213-008-1101-3.

4. Akhondzadeh, S., et al. "Salvia Officinalis Extract in the Treatment of Patients with Mild to Moderate Alzheimer's Disease: A Double-blind, Randomized and Placebo-Controlled Trial." *Journal of Clinical Pharmacy and Therapeutics* 28, no. 1 (2003): 53–59. doi:10.1046/j.1365-2710.2003.00463.x.

5. Kennedy, David O., et al. "Effects of Cholinesterase Inhibiting Sage (Salvia officinalis) on Mood, Anxiety and Performance on a Psychological Stressor Battery." *Neuropsychopharmacology* 31, no. 4 (2005): 845–52. doi:10.1038/sj.npp.1300907.

6. Gerard, John. *The Herbal, or General History of Plants: The Complete 1633 Edition.* Revised by Thomas Johnson. (New York: Dover Publications, 1975), 766.

7. Kianbakht, S., and F. Hashem Dabaghian. "Improved Glycemic Control and Lipid Profile in Hyperlipidemic Type 2 Diabetic Patients Consuming Salvia Officinalis L. Leaf Extract: A Randomized, Placebo-controlled Clinical Trial." *Complementary Therapies in Medicine* 21, no. 5 (2013): 441–46. doi:10.1016/j.ctim.2013.07.004.

8. Sá, Carla M., et al. "Sage Tea Drinking Improves Lipid Profile and Antioxidant Defences in Humans." *International Journal of Molecular Sciences* 10, no. 9 (2009): 3937–50. doi:10.3390/ijms10093937.

9. Schapowal, A., et al. "Echinacea/Sage or Chlorhexidine/Lidocaine for Treating Acute Sore Throats: A Randomized Double-Blind Trial." *European Journal of Medical Research* 14, no. 9 (2009): 406–12.

10. Hubbert, M., et al. "Efficacy and Tolerability of a Spray with Salvia Officinalis in the Treatment of Acute Pharyngitis—A Randomised, Double-Blind, Placebo-Controlled Study with Adaptive Design and Interim Analysis." *European Journal of Medical Research* 11, no. 1 (2006): 20–26.

11. Bommer, S., P. Klein, and A. Suter. "First Time Proof of Sage's Tolerability and Efficacy in Menopausal Women with Hot Flushes." *Advances in Therapy* 28, no. 6 (2011): 490–500. doi:10.1007/s12325-011-0027-z.

12. Reuter, Juliane, et al. "Sage Extract Rich in Phenolic Diterpenes Inhibits Ultraviolet-Induced Erythema in Vivo." *Planta Medica* 73, no. 11 (2007): 1190–91. doi:10.1055/s-2007-981583.

13. Kuhn, Merrily A., and David Winston. *Winston & Kuhn's Herbal Therapy & Supplements: A Scientific & Traditional Approach.* 2nd ed. (Philadelphia: Lippincott Williams & Wilkins, 2008).

Chapter 19: Thyme

1. Romm, Aviva Jill. *Botanical Medicine for Women's Health* (St. Louis, MO: Churchill Livingstone/Elsevier, 2010).

2. Buhner, Stephen Harrod. *Herbal Antibiotics: Natural Alternatives for Treating Drug-resistant Bacteria* (North Adams, MA: Storey Pub., 2012).

3. Rajkowska, Katarzyna, et al. "The Effect of Thyme and Tea Tree Oils on Morphology and Metabolism of Candida Albicans." *Acta Biochimica Polonica* 61, no. 2 (2014): 305–10.

4. Thosar, Nilima, et al. "Antimicrobial Efficacy of Five Essential Oils against Oral Pathogens: An in Vitro Study." *European Journal of Dentistry* 7, no. suppl. 1 (2013): S71–77. doi:10.4103/1305-7456.119078.

5. Fadli, Mariam, et al. "Antibacterial Activity of Thymus Maroccanus and Thymus Broussonetii Essential Oils against Nosocomial Infection—Bacteria and Their Synergistic Potential with Antibiotics." *Phytomedicine* 19, no. 5 (2012): 464–71. doi:10.1016/j.phymed.2011.12.003.

6. Sienkiewicz, Monika, et al. "The Antimicrobial Activity of Thyme Essential Oil against Multidrug Resistant Clinical Bacterial Strains." *Microbial Drug Resistance* 18, no. 2 (2011): 137–48. doi:10.1089/mdr.2011.0080.

7. Kavanaugh, Nicole L., and Katharina Ribbeck. "Selected Antimicrobial Essential Oils Eradicate Pseudomonas spp. and Staphylococcus Aureus Biofilms." *Applied and Environmental Microbiology* 78, no. 11 (June 1, 2012): 4057–61. doi:10.1128/AEM.07499-11.

8. "Antibiotic Resistance Threats in the United States, 2013." Centers for Disease Control and Prevention. July 17, 2014. Accessed October 18, 2015.

9. Ross, Jeremy. *Combining Western Herbs and Chinese Medicine: A Clinical Materia Medica: 120 Herbs in Western Use* (Regensburg, Germany: Verlag Für Ganzheitliche Medizin, 2010).

10. Dioscorides. *De Materia Medica—Five Books in One Volume: A New English Translation.* Translated by T. A. Osbaldeston (Johannesburg: IBIDIS Press, 2000).

11. Kemmerich, B. "Evaluation of Efficacy and Tolerability of a Fixed Combination of Dry Extracts of Thyme Herb and Primrose Root in Adults Suffering from Acute Bronchitis with Productive Cough. A Prospective, Double-Blind, Placebo-Controlled Multicentre Clinical Trial." *Arzneimittel-Forschung* 57, no. 9 (2006): 607–15.

12. Kemmerich, B., R. Eberhardt, and H. Stammer. "Efficacy and Tolerability of a Fluid Extract Combination of Thyme Herb and Ivy Leaves and Matched Placebo in Adults Suffering from Acute Bronchitis with Productive Cough. A Prospective, Double-Blind, Placebo-Controlled Clinical Trial." *Arzneimittel-Forschung* 56, no. 9 (2005): 652–60.

13. Marzian, O. "[Treatment of Acute Bronchitis in Children and Adolescents. Non-Interventional Postmarketing Surveillance Study Confirms the Benefit and Safety of a Syrup Made of Extracts from Thyme and Ivy Leaves]." *MMW Fortschritte der Medizin* 149, no. 27-28 suppl. (2007): 69–74.

14. McIntyre, Anne. "Thymus vulgaris: Thyme." Anne McIntyre: Herbal Medicine, Ayurveda. Accessed April 20, 2015. http://annemcintyre.com/thymus-vulgaris-thyme.

15. Kuhn, Merrily A., and David Winston. *Winston & Kuhn's Herbal Therapy & Supplements: A Scientific & Traditional Approach.* 2nd ed. (Philadelphia: Lippincott Williams & Wilkins, 2008).

16. Ibid.

17. Ibid.

18. Gardner, Zoë, and Michael McGuffin, editors. *American Herbal Products Association's Botanical Safety Handbook.* 2nd ed. (Boca Raton, FL: CRC Press, 2013).

Chapter 20: Turmeric

1. Khansari, Nemat, Yadollah Shakiba, and Mahdi Mahmoudi. "Chronic Inflammation and Oxidative Stress as a Major Cause of Age-Related Diseases and Cancer." *Recent Patents on Inflammation & Allergy Drug Discovery* 3, no. 1 (2009): 73–80. doi:10.2174/187221309787158371.

2. Prasad, Sahdeo, and Bharat B. Aggarwal. "Turmeric, the Golden Spice: From Traditional Medicine to Modern Medicine." In *Herbal Medicine: Biomolecular and Clinical Aspects.* Edited by Iris F. F. Benzie and Sissi Wachtel-Galor (Boca Raton, FL: CRC Press/Taylor & Francis, 2011).

3. Patel, Deepak, and Adrian, Brian. "Do NSAIDs Impair Healing of Musculoskeletal Injuries?" Rheumatology Network. June 6, 2011. http://www.rheumatologynetwork.com/articles/do-nsaids-impair-healing-musculoskeletal-injuries.

4. Hauser, Ross. "When NSAIDs Make Pain Worse—A Significant Public Health Concern." Caring Medical Regenerative Medicine Clinics. Accessed September 26, 2015. http://www.caringmedical.com /prolotherapy-news/nsaids-chronic-pain-medications.

5. McNeil Consumer & Specialty Pharmaceuticals. "McNeil-FDA NSAID Briefing." September 20, 2002. http://www.fda.gov /ohrms/dockets/ac/02/briefing/3882b2_02_mcneil-nsaid.htm.

6. Biswas, Saibal K., et al. "Curcumin Induces Glutathione Biosynthesis and Inhibits NF-κB Activation and Interleukin-8 Release in Alveolar Epithelial Cells: Mechanism of Free Radical Scavenging Activity." Antioxidants & Redox Signaling 7, no. 1–2 (2004): 32–41. doi:10.1089/ars.2005.7.32.

7. Kim, Sang-Wook, et al. "The Effectiveness of Fermented Turmeric Powder in Subjects with Elevated Alanine Transaminase Levels: A Randomised Controlled Study." BMC Complementary and Alternative Medicine 13, no. 1 (2013): 58. doi:10.1186/1472-6882 -13-58.

8. Prucksunand, C., et al. "Phase II Clinical Trial on Effect of the Long Turmeric (Curcuma Longa Linn.) on Healing of Peptic Ulcer." Southeast Asian Journal of Tropical Medicine and Public Health 32, no. 1 (March 2001): 208–15. http://www.tm.mahidol.ac.th /seameo/2001_32_1/34-2714.pdf.

9. Hanai, Hiroyuki, et al. "Curcumin Maintenance Therapy for Ulcerative Colitis: Randomized, Multicenter, Double-Blind, Placebo-Controlled Trial." Clinical Gastroenterology and Hepatology 4, no. 12 (2006): 1502–6. doi:10.1016/j.cgh.2006.08.008.

10. Wickenberg, Jennie, Sandra Ingemansson, and Joanna Hlebowicz. "Effects of Curcuma Longa (Turmeric) on Postprandial Plasma Glucose and Insulin in Healthy Subjects." Nutrition Journal 9, no. 1 (2010): 43. doi:10.1186/1475-2891-9-43.

11. National Institute of Diabetes and Digestive and Kidney Diseases. "Kidney Disease of Diabetes." National Institutes of Health Publication No. 14-3925. April 2, 2014. http://www.niddk.nih.gov/ health-information/health-topics/kidney-disease/kidney-disease -of-diabetes/Pages/facts.aspx.

12. Khajehdehi, Parviz, et al. "Oral Supplementation of Turmeric Attenuates Proteinuria, Transforming Growth Factor-β and Interleukin-8 Levels in Patients with Overt Type 2 Diabetic Nephropathy: A Randomized, Double-Blind and Placebo-Controlled Study." Scandinavian Journal of Urology and Nephrology 45, no. 5 (2011): 365–70. doi:10.3109/00365599.2011.585622.

13. Wongcharoen, Wanwarang, et al. "Effects of Curcuminoids on Frequency of Acute Myocardial Infarction after Coronary Artery Bypass Grafting." American Journal of Cardiology 110, no. 1 (2012): 40–44. doi:10.1016/j.amjcard.2012.02.043.

14. DiSilvestro, et al. "Diverse Effects of a Low Dose Supplement of Lipidated Curcumin in Healthy Middle Aged People." Nutrition Journal 11, no. 1 (2012): 79.

15. Akazawa, Nobuhiko, et al. "Curcumin Ingestion and Exercise Training Improve Vascular Endothelial Function in Postmenopausal Women." Nutrition Research 32, no. 10 (2012): 795–99. doi:10.1016/j.nutres.2012.09.002.

16. Lee, Meei-Shyuan, et al. "Turmeric Improves Post-Prandial Working Memory in Pre-Diabetes Independent of Insulin." Asia Pacific Journal of Clinical Nutrition 23, no. 4 (2014): 581–91.

17. Li, William. "Can We Eat to Starve Cancer?" Ted Talk, presented February 2010. http://www.ted.com/talks/william_li?language=en.

18. Kuptniratsaikul, Vilai, et al. "Efficacy and Safety of Curcuma Domestica Extracts in Patients with Knee Osteoarthritis." Journal of Alternative and Complementary Medicine 15, no. 8 (2009): 891–97. doi:10.1089/acm.2008.0186.

19. Kuptniratsaikul, Vilai, et al. "Efficacy and Safety of Curcuma Domestica Extracts Compared with Ibuprofen in Patients with Knee Osteoarthritis: A Multicenter Study." Clinical Interventions in Aging 9 (March 20, 2014): 451–58. doi:10.2147/CIA.S58535.

20. Shoba, G., et al. "Influence of Piperine on the Pharmacokinetics of Curcumin in Animals and Human Volunteers." Planta Medica 64, no. 4 (1998): 353–56. doi:10.1055/s-2006-957450.

21. Kuhn, Merrily A., and David Winston. Winston & Kuhn's Herbal Therapy & Supplements: A Scientific & Traditional Approach. 2nd ed. (Philadelphia: Lippincott Williams & Wilkins, 2008), 449.

Chapter 21: Nettle

1. Weed, Susun. Healing Wise (Woodstock, NY: Ash Tree Publishing, 1989).

2. Pedersen, Mark. Nutritional Herbology: A Reference Guide to Herbs (Warsaw, IN: Wendell W. Whitman Company, 1998).

3. Ibid.

4. Helms, Steve, and A. Miller. "Natural Treatment of Chronic Rhinosinusitis." Alternative Medicine Review: A Journal of Clinical Therapeutics 11, no. 3 (2006): 196–207.

5. Roschek, Bill, et al. "Nettle Extract (Urtica Dioica) Affects Key Receptors and Enzymes Associated with Allergic Rhinitis." Phytotherapy Research 23, no. 7 (July 2009): 920–26. doi:10.1002/ptr.2763.

6. Bergner, Paul. "Urtica Dioica, Insulin Resistance and Systemic Inflammation." Medical Herbalism Journal 17, no. 1 (2014/2013): 1.

7. Namazi, N., A. Tarighat, and A. Bahrami. "The Effect of Hydro Alcoholic Nettle (Urtica Dioica) Extract on Oxidative Stress in Patients with Type 2 Diabetes: A Randomized Double-Blind Clinical Trial." Pakistan Journal of Biological Sciences 15, no. 2 (2012): 98–102.

8. Namazi, N., et al. "The Effect of Hydro Alcoholic Nettle (Urtica Dioica) Extracts on Insulin Sensitivity and Some Inflammatory Indicators in Patients with Type 2 Diabetes: A Randomized Double-Blind Control Trial." Pakistan Journal of Biological Sciences 14, no. 15 (2011): 775–79.

9. Kianbakht, Saeed, Farahnaz Khalighi-Sigaroodi, and Fataneh Hashem Dabaghian. "Improved Glycemic Control in Patients with Advanced Type 2 Diabetes Mellitus Taking Urtica Dioica Leaf Extract: A Randomized Double-blind, placebo-controlled Clinical Trial." Clinical Laboratory 59, no. 9–10 (2013): 1071–76.

10. Safarinejad, Mohammad Reza. "Urtica Dioica for Treatment of Benign Prostatic Hyperplasia: A Prospective, Randomized, Double-Blind, Placebo-Controlled, Crossover Study." Journal of Herbal Pharmacotherapy 5, no. 4 (2005): 1–11.

11. Rapp, Cathleen. "Special Saw Palmetto and Stinging Nettle Root Combination as Effective as Pharmaceutical Drug for Prostate Symptoms." American Botanical Council's Herbalgram 72 (2006): 20–21.

12. Culpeper, Nicholas. Culpeper's Complete Herbal: A Book of Natural Remedies for Ancient Ills (Ware, England: Wordsworth Editions, 1995).

13. Randall, C., et al. "Randomized Controlled Trial of Nettle Sting for Treatment of Base-of-Thumb Pain." Journal of the Royal Society of Medicine 93, no. 6 (2000): 305–9.

14. Weed, Susun S. Healing Wise (Woodstock, NY: Ash Tree Pub., 2003).

Chapter 22: Elder

1. Bertrand, Bernard, and Annie Bertrand. Sous la protection du sureau. 2nd ed. (Escalquens, France: Éditions de Terran, 2000).

2. Ho, Giang Thanh Thi et al. "Structure-Activity Relationship of Immunomodulating Pectins from Elderberries." Carbohydrate Polymers 125 (July 10, 2015): 314–22. doi:10.1016/j.carbpol .2015.02.057.

3. Balasingam, S., et al. "Neutralizing Activity of SAMBUCOL® against Avian NIBRG-14 (H5N1) Influenza Virus." In IV International Conference on Influenza, Preventing the Pandemic, Bird Flu Vaccines (London, June 2006), 23–24.

4. Zakay-Rones, Zichria, et al. "Inhibition of Several Strains of Influenza Virus in Vitro and Reduction of Symptoms by an Elderberry Extract (Sambucus Nigra L.) during an Outbreak of Influenza B Panama." *Journal of Alternative and Complementary Medicine* 1, no. 4 (1995): 361–69. doi:10.1089/acm.1995.1.361.

5. Zakay-Rones, Z., et al. "Randomized Study of the Efficacy and Safety of Oral Elderberry Extract in the Treatment of Influenza A and B Virus Infections." *Journal of International Medical Research* 32, no. 2 (2004): 132–40. doi:10.1177/147323000403200205.

6. Krawitz, Christian, et al. "Inhibitory Activity of a Standardized Elderberry Liquid Extract against Clinically-Relevant Human Respiratory Bacterial Pathogens and Influenza A and B Viruses." *BMC Complementary and Alternative Medicine* 11, no. 1 (2011): 16. doi:10.1186/1472-6882-11-16.

7. Roschek Jr., Bill, et al. "Elderberry Flavonoids Bind to and Prevent H1N1 Infection in Vitro." *Phytochemistry* 70, no. 10 (2009): 1255–61. doi:10.1016/j.phytochem.2009.06.003.

8. Jarzycka, Anna, Agnieszka Lewińska, Roman Gancarz, and Kazimiera A Wilk. "Assessment of Extracts of Helichrysum Arenarium, Crataegus Monogyna, Sambucus Nigra in Photoprotective UVA and UVB; Photostability in Cosmetic Emulsions." *Journal of photochemistry and photobiology. B, Biology* 128 (2013): doi:10.1016/j.jphotobiol.2013.07.029.

9. Harokopakis, Evlambia, et al. "Inhibition of Proinflammatory Activities of Major Periodontal Pathogens by Aqueous Extracts from Elderflower (Sambucus Nigra)." *Journal of Periodontology* 77, no. 2 (2006): 271–79. doi:10.1902/jop.2006.050232.

Chapter 23: Hawthorn

1. Hoffmann, David. *Medical Herbalism: The Science and Practice of Herbal Medicine* (Rochester, VT: Healing Arts Press, 2003).

2. Dalli, E., et al. "Crataegus Laevigata Decreases Neutrophil Elastase and Has Hypolipidemic Effect: A Randomized, Double-Blind, Placebo-Controlled Trial." *Phytomedicine* 18, no. 8–9 (2011): 769–75. doi:10.1016/j.phymed.2010.11.011.

3. Asgary, S., et al. "Antihypertensive Effect of Iranian Crataegus Curvisepala Lind.: A Randomized, Double-Blind Study." *Drugs under Experimental and Clinical Research* 30, no. 5–6 (2003): 221–25.

4. Walker, Ann F., et al. "Hypotensive Effects of Hawthorn for Patients with Diabetes Taking Prescription Drugs: A Randomised Controlled Trial." *British Journal of General Practice* 56, no. 527 (2006): 437–43.

5. Kane, Charles W. *Herbal Medicine: Trends and Traditions* (Tucson, AZ: Lincoln Town Press, 2009).

6. Tauchert, Michael, Amnon Gildor, and Jens Lipinski. "[High-Dose Crataegus Extract WS 1442 in the Treatment of NYHA Stage II Heart Failure]." *Herz* 24, no. 6 (1999): 465–74.

7. Habs, M. "Prospective, Comparative Cohort Studies and Their Contribution to the Benefit Assessments of Therapeutic Options: Heart Failure Treatment with and without Hawthorn Special Extract WS 1442." *Forschende komplementrmedizin und klassische Naturheilkunde [Research in Complementary and Classical Natural Medicine]* 11, no. suppl. 1 (2004): 36–39. doi:10.1159/000080574.

8. Kuhn, Merrily A., and David Winston. *Winston & Kuhn's Herbal Therapy & Supplements: A Scientific & Traditional Approach.* 2nd ed. (Philadelphia: Lippincott Williams & Wilkins, 2008).

Chapter 24: Lemon Balm

1. Akhondzadeh, S., et al. "Melissa Officinalis Extract in the Treatment of Patients with Mild to Moderate Alzheimer's Disease: A Double-blind, Randomised, Placebo-controlled Trial." *Journal of Neurology, Neurosurgery & Psychiatry* 74, no. 7 (2003): 863–66. doi:10.1136/jnnp.74.7.863.

2. Ballard, Clive G., et al. "Aromatherapy as a Safe and Effective Treatment for the Management of Agitation in Severe Dementia: The Results of a Double-Blind, Placebo-Controlled Trial with Melissa." *Journal of Clinical Psychiatry* 63, no. 7 (2002): 553–58.

3. Kennedy, D. O., et al. "Modulation of Mood and Cognitive Performance following Acute Administration of Melissa Officinalis (Lemon Balm)." *Pharmacology, Biochemistry, and Behavior* 72, no. 4 (2002): 953–64. doi:10.1016/S0091-3057(02)00777-3.

4. Kennedy, D. O., et al. "Modulation of Mood and Cognitive Performance following Acute Administration of Single Doses of Melissa Officinalis (Lemon Balm) with Human CNS Nicotinic and Muscarinic Receptor-Binding Properties." *Neuropsychopharmacology* 28, no. 10 (2003): 1871–81.

5. Taavoni, S., N. Nazem Ekbatani, and H. Haghani. "Valerian/Lemon Balm Use for Sleep Disorders during Menopause." *Complementary Therapies in Clinical Practice* 19, no. 4 (2013): 193–96. doi:10.1016/j.ctcp.2013.07.002.

6. Müller, S. F., and S. Klement. "A Combination of Valerian and Lemon Balm Is Effective in the Treatment of Restlessness and Dyssomnia in Children." *Phytomedicine* 13, no. 6 (2006): 383–87. doi:10.1016/j.phymed.2006.01.013.

7. Koytchev, R., R. G. Alken, and S. Dundarov. "Balm Mint Extract (Lo-701) for Topical Treatment of Recurring Herpes Labialis." *Phytomedicine* 6, no. 4 (1999): 225–30. doi:10.1016/S0944-7113(99)80013-0.

8. Khalsa, Kharta Purka Singh. Personal communication, September 10, 2015.

9. Zeraatpishe, Akbar, et al. "Effects of Melissa Officinalis L. on Oxidative Status and DNA Damage in Subjects Exposed to Long-Term Low-Dose Ionizing Radiation." *Toxicology and Industrial Health* 27, no. 3 (April 2011): 205–12. doi:10.1177/0748233710383889.

Chapter 25: Rose

1. Brenner, Douglas, and Stephen Scanniello. *A Rose by Any Name* (Chapel Hill, NC: Algonquin Books of Chapel Hill, 2009).

2. Allen, Kathy Grannis. "Cupid to Shower Americans with Jewelry, Candy This Valentine's Day." National Retail Federation. January 26, 2015. https://nrf.com/media/press-releases/cupid-shower-americans-jewelry-candy-this-valentines-day.

3. Andersson, U., et al. "Effects of Rose Hip Intake on Risk Markers of Type 2 Diabetes and Cardiovascular Disease: A Randomized, Double-Blind, Cross-Over Investigation in Obese Persons." *European Journal of Clinical Nutrition* 66, no. 5 (2012): 585–90. doi:10.1038/ejcn.2011.203.

4. T, Hongratanaworakit. "Relaxing Effect of Rose Oil on Humans." *Natural Product Communications* 4, no. 2 (2009): 291–96.

5. Winston, David. "Differential Treatment of Depression and Anxiety with Botanical and Nutritional Medicines." In *17th Annual AHG Symposium Proceedings Book.* Millennium Hotel, Boulder, Colorado, 2006.

6. Conrad, Pam, and Cindy Adams. "The Effects of Clinical Aromatherapy for Anxiety and Depression in the High Risk Postpartum Woman—A Pilot Study." *Complementary Therapies in Clinical Practice* 18, no. 3 (2012): 164–68. doi:10.1016/j.ctcp.2012.05.002.

7. Moerman, Daniel E. *Native American Ethnobotany* (Portland, OR: Timber Press, 1998).

8. Hoseinpour, H., et al. "Evaluation of Rosa Damascena Mouthwash in the Treatment of Recurrent Aphthous Stomatitis: A Randomized, Double-Blinded, Placebo-Controlled Clinical Trial." *Quintessence International* 42, no. 6 (2011): 483–91.

9. Kharazmi, Arsalan, and Kaj Winther. "Rose Hip Inhibits Chemotaxis and Chemiluminescence of Human Peripheral Blood Neutrophils in Vitro and Reduces Certain Inflammatory Parameters in Vivo." *Inflammopharmacology* 7, no. 4 (1999): 377–86. doi:10.1007/s10787-999-0031-y.

10. Rein, E., A. Kharazmi, and K. Winther. "A Herbal Remedy, Hyben Vital (Stand Powder of a Subspecies of Rosa Canina Fruits), Reduces Pain and Improves General Wellbeing in Patients with Osteoarthritis—A Double-Blind, Placebo-Controlled, Randomised Trial." *Phytomedicine* 11, no. 5 (2004): 383–91. doi:10.1016/j.phymed.2004.01.001.

11. Winther, K., K. Apel, and G. Thamsborg. "A Powder Made from Seeds and Shells of a Rose-hip Subspecies (Rosa Canina) Reduces Symptoms of Knee and Hip Osteoarthritis: A Randomized, Double-Blind, Placebo-Controlled Clinical Trial." *Scandinavian Journal of Rheumatology* 34, no. 4 (2005): 302–8. doi:10.1080/03009740510018624.

12. Willich, S. N., et al. "Rose Hip Herbal Remedy in Patients with Rheumatoid Arthritis—A Randomised Controlled Trial." *Phytomedicine* 17, no. 2 (2010): 87–93. doi:10.1016/j.phymed.2009.09.003.

13. Winther, K., E. Rein, and A. Kharazmi. "The Anti-Inflammatory Properties of Rose-Hip." *Inflammopharmacology* 7, no. 1 (1999): 63–68. doi:10.1007/s10787-999-0026-8.

14. Tseng, Ying-Fen, Chung-Hey Chen, and Yi-Hsin Yang. "Rose Tea for Relief of Primary Dysmenorrhea in Adolescents: A Randomized Controlled Trial in Taiwan, China." *Journal of Midwifery & Women's Health* 50, no. 5 (2005): e51–57. doi:10.1016/j.jmwh.2005.06.003.

Chapter 26: Tea

1. Xu, Renfan, Ke Yang, Jie Ding, and Guangzhi Chen. "Effect of Green Tea Supplementation on Blood Pressure: A Systematic Review and Meta-Analysis of Randomized Controlled Trials." *Medicine* 99, no. 6 (February 2020): e19047. doi:0.1097/MD.0000000000019047.

2. Mahdavi-Roshan, Marjan, Arsalan Salari, Zeinab Ghorbani, and Asieh Ashouri. "The Effects of Regular Consumption of Green or Black Tea Beverage on Blood Pressure in Those with Elevated Blood Pressure or Hypertension: A Systematic Review and Meta-Analysis." *Complementary Therapies in Medicine* 51 (June 2020): 102430. doi:10.1016/j.ctim.2020.102430.

3. Gomikawa, Syuzou, et al. "Effect of Ground Green Tea Drinking for 2 Weeks on the Susceptibility of Plasma and LDL to the Oxidation Ex Vivo in Healthy Volunteers." *Kobe Journal of Medical Sciences* 54, no. 1 (2008): E62–72.

4. Bahorun, Theeshan, et al. "Black Tea Reduces Uric Acid and C-Reactive Protein Levels in Humans Susceptible to Cardiovascular Diseases." *Toxicology* 278, no. 1 (2010): 68–74. doi:10.1016/j.tox.2009.11.024.

5. Narotzki, Baruch, et al. "Green Tea and Vitamin E Enhance Exercise-Induced Benefits in Body Composition, Glucose Homeostasis, and Antioxidant Status in Elderly Men and Women." *Journal of the American College of Nutrition* 32, no. 1 (2013): 31–40. doi:10.1080/07315724.2013.767661.

6. Basu, Arpita, et al. "Green Tea Supplementation Affects Body Weight, Lipids, and Lipid Peroxidation in Obese Subjects with Metabolic Syndrome." *Journal of the American College of Nutrition* 29, no. 1 (2010): 31–40.

7. Eshghpour, Majid, et al. "Effectiveness of Green Tea Mouthwash in Postoperative Pain Control following Surgical Removal of Impacted Third Molars: Double-blind Randomized Clinical Trial." *DARU Journal of Pharmaceutical Sciences* 21, no. 1 (2013): 59. doi:10.1186/2008-2231-21-59.

8. Awadalla, H. I., et al. "A Pilot Study of the Role of Green Tea Use on Oral Health." *International Journal of Dental Hygiene* 9, no. 2 (2011): 110–16. doi:10.1111/j.1601-5037.2009.00440.x.

9. Mohd, Razali Salleh. "Life Event, Stress and Illness." *Malaysian Journal of Medical Sciences* 15, no. 4 (2008): 9–18.

10. "Stress a Major Health Problem in the U.S., Warns APA." American Psychological Association press release. October 24, 2007. http://www.apa.org/news/press/releases/2007/10/stress.aspx.

Chapter 27: Artichoke

1. Holtmann, G., et al. "Efficacy of Artichoke Leaf Extract in the Treatment of Patients with Functional Dyspepsia: A Six-Week Placebo-Controlled, Double-Blind, and Multicentre Trial." *Alimentary Pharmacology & Therapeutics* 18, no. 11-12 (December 2003): 1099–1105.

2. Walker, A. F., R. W. Middleton, and O. Petrowicz. "Artichoke Leaf Extract Reduces Symptoms of Irritable Bowel Syndrome in a Post-Marketing Surveillance Study." *Phytotherapy Research* 15, no. 1 (February 2001): 58–61.

3. Bernard, Christophe. Personal communication, July 2, 2015.

4. Rondanelli, Mariangela, et al. "Beneficial Effects of Artichoke Leaf Extract Supplementation on Increasing HDL-Cholesterol in Subjects with Primary Mild Hypercholesterolaemia: A Double-Blind, Randomized, Placebo-Controlled Trial." *International Journal of Food Sciences and Nutrition* 64, no. 1 (February 2013): 7–15. doi:10.3109/09637486.2012.700920.

5. Lupatelli, G., et al. "Artichoke Juice Improves Endothelial Function in Hyperlipemia." *Life Sciences* 76, no. 7 (December 31, 2004): 775–82. doi:10.1016/j.lfs.2004.07.018.

6. Kuhn, Merrily A., and David Winston. *Winston & Kuhn's Herbal Therapy & Supplements: A Scientific & Traditional Approach.* 2nd ed. (Philadelphia: Lippincott Williams & Wilkins, 2008).

Chapter 28: Cacao

1. Szogyi, Alex. *Chocolate: Food of the Gods* (Westport, CT: Greenwood Press, 1997).

2. Shrime, Mark G., et al. "Flavonoid-Rich Cocoa Consumption Affects Multiple Cardiovascular Risk Factors in a Meta-Analysis of Short-Term Studies." *Journal of Nutrition* 141, no. 11 (2011): 1982–88. doi:10.3945/jn.111.145482.

3. Aggarwal, Bharat B., and Debora Yost. *Healing Spices: How to Use 50 Everyday and Exotic Spices to Boost Health and Beat Disease* (New York: Sterling Pub., 2011).

4. Desch, Steffen, et al. "Effect of Cocoa Products on Blood Pressure: Systematic Review and Meta-Analysis." *American Journal of Hypertension* 23, no. 1 (2010): 97–103. doi:10.1038/ajh.2009.213.

5. Sarriá, Beatriz, et al. "Regular Consumption of a Cocoa Product Improves the Cardiometabolic Profile in Healthy and Moderately Hypercholesterolaemic Adults." *British Journal of Nutrition* 111, no. 01 (2014): 122–34. doi:10.1017/S000711451300202X.

6. Grassi, Davide, et al. "Short-Term Administration of Dark Chocolate Is Followed by a Significant Increase in Insulin Sensitivity and a Decrease in Blood Pressure in Healthy Persons." *American Journal of Clinical Nutrition* 81, no. 3 (2005): 611–14.

7. Selmi, Carlo, et al. "The Anti-Inflammatory Properties of Cocoa Flavanols." *Journal of Cardiovascular Pharmacology* 47 (2006): S163–71.

8. Scholey, Andrew, and Lauren Owen. "Effects of Chocolate on Cognitive Function and Mood: A Systematic Review." *Nutrition Reviews* 71, no. 10 (2013): 665–81. doi:10.1111/nure.12065.

9. Desideri, Giovambattista, et al. "Benefits in Cognitive Function, Blood Pressure, and Insulin Resistance through Cocoa Flavanol Consumption in Elderly Subjects with Mild Cognitive Impairment: The Cocoa, Cognition, and Aging (CoCoA) Study." *Hypertension* 60, no. 3 (2012): 794–801.

10. Field, David T., Claire M. Williams, and Laurie T. Butler. "Consumption of Cocoa Flavanols Results in an Acute Improvement in Visual and Cognitive Functions." *Physiology & Behavior* 103, no. 3-4 (2011): 255–60. doi:10.1016/j.physbeh.2011.02.013.

11. Sathyapalan, Thozhukat, et al. "High Cocoa Polyphenol Rich Chocolate May Reduce the Burden of the Symptoms in Chronic Fatigue Syndrome." *Nutrition Journal* 9, no. 1 (2010): 55.

12. Miller, Kenneth B., et al. "Impact of Alkalization on the Antioxidant and Flavanol Content of Commercial Cocoa Powders." *Journal of Agricultural and Food Chemistry* 56, no. 18 (2008): 8527–33. doi:10.1021/jf801670p.

13. EFSA, NDA Panel. "Scientific Opinion on the Substantiation of a Health Claim Related to Cocoa Flavanols and Maintenance of Normal Endothelium-Dependent Vasodilation Pursuant to Article 13 (5) of Regulation (EC) No 1924/2006." *EFSA Journal* 10, no. 2809 (2012): b52.

Chapter 29: Chamomile

1. Gladstar, Rosemary. *Rosemary Gladstar's Medicinal Herbs: A Beginner's Guide* (North Adams, MA: Storey Pub., 2012).

2. Hardy, Karen, et al. "Neanderthal Medics? Evidence for Food, Cooking, and Medicinal Plants Entrapped in Dental Calculus." *Die Naturwissenschaften* 99, no. 8 (2012). doi:10.1007/s00114-012-0942-0.

3. Amsterdam, Jay D., et al. "Chamomile (Matricaria Recutita) May Have Antidepressant Activity in Anxious Depressed Humans—An Exploratory Study." *Alternative Therapies in Health and Medicine* 18, no. 5 (2012): 44–49.

4. Amsterdam, Jay D., et al. "A Randomized, Double-Blind, Placebo-Controlled Trial of Oral Matricaria Recutita (Chamomile) Extract Therapy for Generalized Anxiety Disorder." *Journal of Clinical Psychopharmacology* 29, no. 4 (2009): 378–82. doi:10.1097/JCP.0b013e3181ac935c.

5. Sharifi, Farangis, et al. "Comparison of the Effects of Matricaria Chamomila (Chamomile) Extract and Mefenamic Acid on the Intensity of Premenstrual Syndrome." *Complementary Therapies in Clinical Practice* 20, no. 1 (2014): 81–88. doi:10.1016/j.ctcp.2013.09.002.

6. Dos Reis, Paula Elaine Diniz, et al. "Clinical Application of Chamomilla Recutita in Phlebitis: Dose Response Curve Study." *Revista Latino-Americana de Enfermagem* 19, no. 1 (2011): 03–10. doi:10.1590/S0104-11692011000100002.

7. Charousaei, F., A. Dabirian, and F. Mojab. "Using Chamomile Solution or a 1% Topical Hydrocortisone Ointment in the Management of Peristomal Skin Lesions in Colostomy Patients: Results of a Controlled Clinical Study." *Ostomy/Wound Management* 57, no. 5 (2011): 28–36.

8. Batista, Ana Luzia Araújo, et al. "Clinical Efficacy Analysis of the Mouth Rinsing with Pomegranate and Chamomile Plant Extracts in the Gingival Bleeding Reduction." *Complementary Therapies in Clinical Practice* 20, no. 1 (2014): 93–98. doi:10.1016/j.ctcp.2013.09.002.

9. Becker, B., U. Kuhn, and B. Hardewig-Budny. "Double-Blind, Randomized Evaluation of Clinical Efficacy and Tolerability of an Apple Pectin-Chamomile Extract in Children with Unspecific Diarrhea." *Arzneimittel-Forschung* 56, no. 6 (2005): 387–93.

10. Kuhn, Merrily A., and David Winston. *Winston & Kuhn's Herbal Therapy & Supplements: A Scientific & Traditional Approach.* 2nd ed. (Philadelphia: Lippincott Williams & Wilkins, 2008).

Chapter 30: Coffee

1. Walsh, James K., et al. "Effect of Caffeine on Physiological Sleep Tendency and Ability to Sustain Wakefulness at Night." *Psychopharmacology* 101, no. 2 (1990): 271–73. doi:10.1007/BF02244139.

2. Muehlbach, Mark J., and James K. Walsh. "The Effects of Caffeine on Simulated Night-Shift Work and Subsequent Daytime Sleep." *Sleep: Journal of Sleep Research & Sleep Medicine* 18, no. 1 (1995): 22–29.

3. Pham, Ngoc Minh, et al. "Green Tea and Coffee Consumption Is Inversely Associated with Depressive Symptoms in a Japanese Working Population." *Public Health Nutrition* 17, no. 03 (2014): 625–33. doi:10.1017/S1368980013000360.

4. Smith, Andrew P. "Caffeine, Extraversion and Working Memory." *Journal of Psychopharmacology* 7, no. 21 (January 2013): 71–6. doi:10.1177/0269881112460111.

5. Wills, Anne-Marie A., et al. "Caffeine Consumption and Risk of Dyskinesia in CALM-PD." *Movement Disorders* 28, no. 3 (2013): 380–83. doi:10.1002/mds.25319.

6. Eskelinen, Marjo H., and Miia Kivipelto. "Caffeine as a Protective Factor in Dementia and Alzheimer's Disease." *Journal of Alzheimer's Disease* 20, no. suppl. 1 (2010): S167–S174.

7. Klatsky, Arthur L., et al. "Coffee, Cirrhosis, and Transaminase Enzymes." *Archives of Internal Medicine* 166, no. 11 (2006): 1190–95. doi:10.1001/archinte.166.11.1190.

8. Xiao, Qian, et al. "Inverse Associations of Total and Decaffeinated Coffee with Liver Enzyme Levels in National Health and Nutrition Examination Survey 1999–2010." *Hepatology* 60, no. 6 (2014): 2091–98. doi:10.1002/hep.27367.

9. Sasaki, Yachiyo, et al. "Effect of Caffeine-Containing Beverage Consumption on Serum Alanine Aminotransferase Levels in Patients with Chronic Hepatitis C Virus Infection: A Hospital-Based Cohort Study." *PLoS One* 8, no. 12 (2013): e83382. doi:10.1371/journal.pone.0083382.

10. Cardin, Romilda, et al. "Effects of Coffee Consumption in Chronic Hepatitis C: A Randomized Controlled Trial." *Digestive and Liver Disease* 45, no. 6 (2013): 499–504. doi:10.1016/j.dld.2012.10.021.

11. Killer, Sophie C., Andrew K. Blannin, and Asker E. Jeukendrup. "No Evidence of Dehydration with Moderate Daily Coffee Intake: A Counterbalanced Cross-Over Study in a Free-Living Population." *PLoS One* 9, no. 1 (2014): e84154. doi:10.1371/journal.pone.0084154.

12. Corrêa, Telma Angelina Faraldo, et al. "Medium Light and Medium Roast Paper-Filtered Coffee Increased Antioxidant Capacity in Healthy Volunteers: Results of a Randomized Trial." *Plant Foods for Human Nutrition* 67, no. 3 (2012): 277–82. doi:10.1007/s11130-012-0297-x.

13. Mišík, Miroslav, et al. "Impact of Paper Filtered Coffee on Oxidative DNA-Damage: Results of a Clinical Trial." *Mutation Research/Fundamental and Molecular Mechanisms of Mutagenesis* 692, no. 1–2 (2010): 42–48. doi:10.1016/j.mrfmmm.2010.08.003.

14. Van Dam, R. M., and F. B. Hu. "Coffee Consumption and Risk of Type 2 Diabetes: A Systematic Review." *JAMA* 294, no. 1 (2005): 97–104. doi:10.1001/jama.294.1.97.

15. Van Dam, Rob M., and Edith J. M. Feskens. "Coffee Consumption and Risk of Type 2 Diabetes Mellitus." *The Lancet* 360, no. 9344 (2002): 1477–78. doi:10.1016/S0140-6736(02)11436-X.

16. Bertoia, Monica L., et al. "Long-Term Alcohol and Caffeine Intake and Risk of Sudden Cardiac Death in Women." *American Journal of Clinical Nutrition* 97, no. 6 (June 2013): 1356–63. doi:10.3945/ajcn.112.044248.

17. Shechter, Michael, et al. "Impact of Acute Caffeine Ingestion on Endothelial Function in Subjects with and without Coronary Artery Disease." *American Journal of Cardiology* 107, no. 9 (May 1, 2011): 1255–61. doi:10.1016/j.amjcard.2010.12.035.

Chapter 31: Dandelion

1. Clare, Bevin A., Richard S. Conroy, and Kevin Spelman. "The Diuretic Effect in Human Subjects of an Extract of Taraxacum Officinale Folium over a Single Day." *Journal of Alternative and Complementary Medicine* 15, no. 8 (2009): 929–34. doi:10.1089/acm.2008.0152.

2. Piao, Taikui, et al. "Taraxasterol Inhibits IL-1β-Induced Inflammatory Response in Human Osteoarthritic Chondrocytes." *European Journal of Pharmacology* 756 (June 2015): 38–42. doi:10.1016/j.ejphar.2015.03.012.

3. Kuhn, Merrily A., and David Winston. *Winston & Kuhn's Herbal Therapy & Supplements: A Scientific & Traditional Approach.* 2nd ed. (Philadelphia: Lippincott Williams & Wilkins, 2008).

4. Ibid.

Chapter 32: Ashwagandha

1. Cooley, Kieran, et al. "Naturopathic Care for Anxiety: A Randomized Controlled Trial ISRCTN78958974." *PloS One* 4, no. 8 (2009): e6628. doi:10.1371/journal.pone.0006628.

2. Biswal, Biswa Mohan, et al. "Effect of Withania Somnifera (Ashwagandha) on the Development of Chemotherapy-Induced Fatigue and Quality of Life in Breast Cancer Patients." *Integrative Cancer Therapies* 12, no. 4 (July 2013): 312–22. doi:10.1177/1534735412464551.

3. Gannon, Jessica M., Paige E. Forrest, and K. N. Roy Chengappa. "Subtle Changes in Thyroid Indices during a Placebo-Controlled Study of an Extract of Withania Somnifera in Persons with Bipolar Disorder." *Journal of Ayurveda and Integrative Medicine* 5, no. 4 (December 2014): 241–45. doi:10.4103/0975-9476.146566.

4. Ahmad, Mohammad Kaleem, et al. "Withania Somnifera Improves Semen Quality by Regulating Reproductive Hormone Levels and Oxidative Stress in Seminal Plasma of Infertile Males." *Fertility and Sterility* 94, no. 3 (August 2010): 989–96. doi:10.1016/j.fertnstert.2009.04.046.

5. Gupta, Ashish, et al. "Efficacy of Withania Somnifera on Seminal Plasma Metabolites of Infertile Males: A Proton NMR Study at 800 MHz." *Journal of Ethnopharmacology* 149, no. 1 (August 26, 2013): 208–14. doi:10.1016/j.jep.2013.06.024.

6. Dongre, Swati, Deepak Langade, and Sauvik Bhattacharyya. "Efficacy and Safety of Ashwagandha (Withania Somnifera) Root Extract in Improving Sexual Function in Women: A Pilot Study." *BioMed Research International* 2015 (2015). doi:10.1155/2015/284154.

7. Pingali, Usharani, Raveendranadh Pilli, and Nishat Fatima. "Effect of Standardized Aqueous Extract of Withania Somnifera on Tests of Cognitive and Psychomotor Performance in Healthy Human Participants." *Pharmacognosy Research* 6, no. 1 (January 2014): 12–18. doi:10.4103/0974-8490.122912.

8. Chengappa, K. N. Roy, et al. "Randomized Placebo-Controlled Adjunctive Study of an Extract of Withania Somnifera for Cognitive Dysfunction in Bipolar Disorder." *Journal of Clinical Psychiatry* 74, no. 11 (November 2013): 1076–83. doi:10.4088/JCP.13m08413.

9. Mikolai, Jeremy, et al. "In Vivo Effects of Ashwagandha (Withania Somnifera) Extract on the Activation of Lymphocytes." *Journal of Alternative and Complementary Medicine* 15, no. 4 (April 2009): 423–30. doi:10.1089/acm.2008.0215.

10. Yance, Donald R. *Adaptogens in Medical Herbalism: Elite Herbs and Natural Compounds for Mastering Stress, Aging, and Chronic Disease* (Rochester, VT: Inner Traditions/Bear, 2013).

11. Khalsa, Karta Purkh Singh, and Michael Tierra. *The Way of Ayurvedic Herbs.*

12. Andallu, B., and B. Radhika. "Hypoglycemic, Diuretic and Hypocholesterolemic Effect of Winter Cherry (Withania Somnifera, Dunal) Root." *Indian Journal of Experimental Biology* 38, no. 6 (June 2000): 607–609.

13. Upton, Roy, and Petrone, Cathirose, eds. *Ashwagandha Root: Withania Somnifera—Analytical, Quality Control, and Therapeutic Monograph.* American Herbal Pharmacopoeia and Therapeutic Compendium (Scotts Valley, CA: American Herbal Pharmacopoeia, 2000).

14. Ibid.

15. Yance, Donald R. *Adaptogens in Medical Herbalism: Elite Herbs and Natural Compounds for Mastering Stress, Aging, and Chronic Disease* (Rochester, VT: Inner Traditions/Bear, 2013).

Chapter 33: Astragalus

1. Bergner, Paul. *Healing Power of Echinacea and Goldenseal and Other Immune System Herbs.* Healing Power Series (Roseville, CA: Prima Lifestyles, 1997).

2. Weng, X. S. "[Treatment of Leucopenia with Pure Astragalus Preparation—An Analysis of 115 Leucopenic Cases]." *Zhongguo Zhong Xi Yi Jie He Za Zhi* [*Chinese Journal of Integrated Traditional and Western Medicine*] 15, no. 8 (August 1995): 462–64.

3. Zwickey, Heather, et al. "The Effect of Echinacea Purpurea, Astragalus Membranaceus and Glycyrrhiza Glabra on CD25 Expression in Humans: A Pilot Study." *Phytotherapy Research* 21, no. 11 (November 2007): 1109–12. doi:10.1002/ptr.2207.

4. Poon, P. M. K., et al. "Immunomodulatory Effects of a Traditional Chinese Medicine with Potential Antiviral Activity: A Self-Control Study." *American Journal of Chinese Medicine* 34, no. 1 (2006): 13–21. doi:10.1142/S0192415X0600359X.

5. Lau, T. F., et al. "Using Herbal Medicine as a Means of Prevention Experience during the SARS Crisis." *American Journal of Chinese Medicine* 33, no. 3 (2005): 345–56. doi:10.1142/S0192415X05002965.

6. Duan, Ping, and Zai-mo Wang. "[Clinical Study on Effect of Astragalus in Efficacy Enhancing and Toxicity Reducing of Chemotherapy in Patients of Malignant Tumor]." *Zhongguo Zhong Xi Yi Jie He Za Zhi* [*Chinese Journal of Integrated Traditional and Western Medicine*] 22, no. 7 (July 2002): 515–17.

7. Chen, Kung-Tung, et al. "Reducing Fatigue of Athletes Following Oral Administration of Huangqi Jianzhong Tang." *Acta Pharmacologica Sinica* 23, no. 8 (August 2002): 757–61.

8. Zhou, Z. L., P. Yu, and D. Lin. "[Study on effect of Astragalus injection in treating congestive heart failure]." *Zhongguo Zhong Xi Yi Jie He Za Zhi* [*Chinese Journal of Integrated Traditional and Western Medicine*] 21, no. 10 (2001): 747–49.

9. Zhang, Jin-guo, et al. "[Effect of Astragalus Injection on Plasma Levels of Apoptosis-Related Factors in Aged Patients with Chronic Heart Failure]." *Chinese Journal of Integrative Medicine* 11, no. 3 (2005): 187–90.

10. Li, Shen, et al. "[Therapeutic Effect of Astragalus and Angelica Mixture on the Renal Function and TCM Syndrome Factors in Treating Stage 3 and 4 Chronic Kidney Disease Patients]." *Zhongguo Zhong Xi Yi Jie He Za Zhi* [*Chinese Journal of Integrated Traditional and Western Medicine*] 34, no. 7 (2014): 780–85.

INDEX

Page reference key: *Italics* indicate recipes; **bold** indicate summaries of herb facts (energetics, properties, uses, preparations, etc.); parentheses indicate non-contiguous references of topic.

Adrenal fatigue, 309

Allergic rhinitis, 100

Allergies, 6, 100, 191, 212, 289

Alzheimer's, 151–152, 160, 180, 280. *See also* Memory

Amenorrhea, 169, 191

Amounts of herbs to use, 29. *See also specific herbs*

Anemia, 307

Angiogenesis, 181

Antimicrobial support, 5. *See also* Bacteria, harmful/infections; Immune system support; Viral infections

Antioxidant properties, overview of herbs/spices providing, 4

Anxiety. *See* Stress and anxiety, relieving

Aphrodisiacs, 127, 251, 299

Appetite, improving, 135, 143, 171, 271

Arthritis, xix, 4, 39, 40, 42, 53, 56, 57, 59, 89, 100, 119, 151, 181, 189, 203, 232, 290, 301

Artichoke, 250, **251**–257
    about: historical perspective, 252; how to use (amounts, special considerations), 254; medicinal properties and energetics, 252–253

Artichoke and Orange Bitters, *256–257*

Bitter Artichoke Tea, *255*

Ashwagandha, 298, **299**–305
    about: historical perspective, 300; how to use (amounts, special considerations), 300–301; medicinal properties and energetics, 300–301

Ashwagandha Banana Smoothie, *305*

Ashwagandha Date Treats, *304*

Ashwagandha Ghee, *303*

Asthma, 77, 100, 168, 177, 192, 277, 299, 307

Astragalus, 306, **307**–313
    about: historical perspective, 308; how to use (amounts, special considerations), 310; medicinal properties and energetics, 309; types of, 308

Astragalus and Cardamom Rice, *312*

Astragalus Bone Broth, *313*

Astragalus Chai, *311*

Bacteria, beneficial, 5, 289

Bacteria, harmful, 5, 61, 79, 100, 107, 170, 203

Bad breath, 70, 135, 141

Banana, in Ashwagandha Banana Smoothie, 305

Bath salts, lavender, *113*

Bath salts, mustard and ginger, *123*

Bioavailability of other nutrients /herbs, 39, 41, 182

Bitter Fennel Digestive Pastilles, *74*

Bitter herbs, about, 21. *See also* Artichoke; Cacao; Chamomile; Coffee; Dandelion

Black pepper, 38, **39**-47
  about: historical perspective, 40; how to use (amounts, special considerations), 42; medicinal properties and energetics, 40-42; types of peppercorns, 40
    Chinese Five-Spice Blend, 46
    Peppery Borscht, 44-45
    Trikatu Pastilles, 43
Bladder infections, 229
Bleeding, 20, 49, 161, 170, 179
Bloating and gas, 41, 43, 45, 51, 71, 78, 89, 90, 100, 127, 135, 142, 152, 162, 171, 252, 271, 289
Blood movement, 59. See also Circulation
Blood pressure and hypertension, 49, 62, 80, 97, 99, 109, 127, 135, (211–213), 231, 240, 253, (259–261), 280, 288, 307
Blood, stagnant, 89-90. See also Circulation
Bone broth, astragalus, 313
Bone health, 191, 196
Book (this), using, 27–33, 315
Brain health, 99, 160–161, 261, 280, 301. See also Memory
Breastfeeding, herb precautions during, 128, 136, 144, 153, 163, 172, 182
Breast milk, 69, 144
Breath, bad, 70, 135, 141
Bronchial congestion, 77, 173
Bronchitis, 100, 119, 171
Bug bites, 111, 219
Burns, 110, 112, 169, 270. See also Sunburn
Butter, clarified, Ashwagandha Ghee, 303

Cacao, 258, **259**-265
  about: historical perspective, 260; how to use (amounts, special considerations), 262; medicinal properties and energetics, 260-261

    Cardamom Chocolate Mousse Cake, 263
    Chocolate Strawberry Pudding, 264
    Hot Chocolate, 265
Cancer, 20, 79, 100, 119, 132, 133, 135, 150, 181, 196, 240, 286, 290, 291, 300, 301, 308
Cardamom Chocolate Mousse Cake, 263
Cardamom, in Astragalus and Cardamom Rice, 312
Carrot cake, spiced, 130-131
Cayenne, 48, **49**-57
  about: historical perspective, 50; how to use (amounts, special considerations), 54; medicinal properties and energetics, 50-53; types of (chiles vs. peppers), 50
    Cayenne Salve, 57
    Cayenne Tea, 55
    Fire Cider, 56
Chai, astragalus, 311
Chamomile, 266, **267**-275
  about: historical perspective, 268; how to use (amounts, special considerations), 272; medicinal properties and energetics, 268-271; types of, 268
    Chamomile Eyewash, 273
    Chamomile Ice Pops, 275
    Chamomile Tea Blend with Roses and Vanilla, 274
Cheesecloth, 32
Chia Seed Pudding with Cinnamon-Maple Syrup, 66-67
Chicken
    Lemon Balm and Orange Chicken, 224-225
    Sage Chicken, 166-167
Chinese Five-Spice Blend, 46
Chocolate. See Cacao
Cholesterol levels, 62, 80, 91, 99, 119, 161, 180, 211, 213, 231, 241, 253, 259, 301
Choosing herbs. See Matching herbs to you

Cinnamon, 58, **59**–67
about: historical perspective, 60; how to use (amounts, special considerations), 63; medicinal properties and energetics, 61–62; types of, 60
Chia Seed Pudding with Cinnamon-Maple Syrup, 66–67
Cinnamon Tea for Soothing Throats, 65
Cinnamon Tooth Powder, 64
Circulation, 19, 41, 42, 49, 52, 61, 89, 95, 99, 119, 123, 151, 163, 171, 279
Citrus
Artichoke and Orange Bitters, 256–257
Ginger-Lemon Tea, 93
Lavender and Orange Custard, 115
Sage-Lemon Tea, 165
Coffee, 276, **277**–285
about: historical perspective, 278; how to use (amounts, special considerations), 281; medicinal properties and energetics, 279–280; types of, 278–279
Perfect Cup of French Press Coffee, 284–285
Spiced Cold-Brew Coffee, 282–283
Colds and flu, 40, 53, 55, 79–80, 81, 83, 90, 93, 100, 126, 143, 152, 171, 173, 177, (202–207), 229, 271, 272, (306–310).
See also Fevers
Colic, 69, 71, 75, 270
Colitis, 179
Compote, rose hip–cranberry, 236
Congestion, 40, 81, 93, 119, 144.
See also Colds and flu
Congestive heart failure, 309
Conjunctivitis, 70, 271, 273
Constipation, 71, 78, 90, 135, 191, 192, 252, 277
Constitution. See also Energetics of herbalism
assessing how herb/spice affects you, 23–25
discovering yours (quizzes for), 15–18

explanation of, 13–14
matching current energetics and plant energies with, 22–23
Coughs. See Colds and flu
Cough syrup, 175
Cranberries, in Rose Hip-Cranberry Compote, 236
Cystitis, 135

Dandelion, 286, **287**–295
about: historical perspective, 288; how to use (amounts, special considerations), 290–291; medicinal properties and energetics (leaves), 288; medicinal properties and energetics (root), 289–290
Artichoke and Orange Bitters, 256–257
Dandelion Pesto, 294–295
Dandelion Root Vinegar, 293
Roasted Dandelion and Reishi Tea, 292
Date treats, ashwagandha, 304
Degenerative diseases, 301
Depression, 49, 99, 110, 151, 231, 269, 279
Desserts. See Sweet treats
Detoxing, 192, 280
Diabetes, 53, 62, 63, 80, 91, 99, 101, 161, 180, 192, 203, 213, 241, 261, 280, 301. See also Neuropathy
Diarrhea, 49, 61, 71, 89, 127, 142, 171, 177, 232, 270, 275. See also Dysentery
Digestion. See also Appetite, improving; Bloating and gas; Constipation; Diarrhea; Heartburn; Nausea, treating; Ulcers
about: overview of herbs strengthening, 3–4
bitter herbs stimulating, 21
healthy gut flora, 289
poor, symptoms indicating, 4
sour herbs stimulating, 20

specific herbs helping, 51, 52, 61, (69–72), 74, 78, 89, 90, 93, 100, 110, 127, 128, 135, 140, 142, 144, 152, 162, 170, 171, 179, 212, 219, 252–253, (269–271), 279, (287–289). See also Black pepper

sweet spot of herbs for, 22–23

Diuretics, 19, 70, 135, 192, 212, 288. See also Astragalus; Coffee; Elder

DNA damage, preventing, 119, 150, 221, 260

Dry/damp and hot/cold, 12–13, 15–18

Dukkah, nettle leaf, 194–195

Dysbiosis, 87

Dysentery, 77. See also Diarrhea

Dyspepsia. See Digestion

Ear infections, 79, 91, 201. See also Dysbiosis

Earl Gray tea, making, 244

Eczema, xvi, xix, 177, 179, 192, 289

Edema, 70, 135, 213, 288

Eggnog, spiced, 129

Eggplant, in Nettle and Eggplant Sauté, 197

Elder, 200, **201**–209

about: historical perspective, 202; how to use (amounts, special considerations), 205; medicinal properties and energetics, 203–204

Elderberry Syrup, 206

Elderflower Facial Serum, 208–209

Elderflower Tea, 207

Emaciation, 299. See also Appetite, improving

Energetics of herbalism. See also Matching herbs to you; specific herbs and spices

constitutions of people and, 13–14

discovering your constitution, 15–18

hot/cold, dry/damp and, 12–13, 15–18

illness energetics and, 14

plant energetics and, 14

sweet spot of, 22–23

tastes of herbs and, 18–21

Energy, restoring/increasing, 20, 89, 143, 191, 239, 279, 300, 309

Experiences, tuning in to, 28–29

Eye health, 70, 203, 204

Eye infections. See Conjunctivitis

Eyewash, chamomile, 273

Facial products. See Skin

Fatigue, 51, 189, 213, 261, 279, 300. See also Energy, restoring/increasing; Sleep and relaxation

Feelings, tuning in to, 28–29

Fennel, 68, **69**–75

about: historical perspective, 70; how to use (amounts, special considerations), 72; medicinal properties and energetics, 70–71

Bitter Fennel Digestive Pastilles, 74

Fennel Tea, 75

Roasted Root Vegetables with Fennel, 73

Fevers, 23, 39, 49, 61, 119, 143, 152, 169, 204, 219, 271

Fibromyalgia, 301, 309

Fire Cider, 56

Fish, Xavier's Gingered Salmon, 94

Five-spice blend, Chinese, 46

Flu. See Colds and flu

Food as medicine

concept of, xv

One Solution Syndrome vs., xvi, xvii, xviii–xix, 11, 33

Food, preserving, 149

French press coffee, 284–285

Fried Sage Leaves, 164

Fungal infections, 49, 77, 79, 91, 100, 107, 149, 170

Funnels, 32

Garam Masala, 184

Garlic, 76, **77**–85
  about: historical perspective, 78; how to use
    (amounts, special considerations), 80–81;
    medicinal properties and energetics,
    78–80; types of, 78
  Garlic Honey, 84–85
  Garlic Oil, 83
  Smoky Garlic Hummus, *82*
Gas. *See* Bloating and gas
GERD (gastrointestinal reflux disease), 52, 144.
  See also Heartburn
Ghee, ashwagandha, 303
Ginger, 86, **87**–95
  about: historical perspective, 88; how to use
    (amounts, special considerations), 92;
    medicinal properties and energetics,
    88–91
  Ginger and Lavender Massage Oil, 95
  Ginger-Lemon Tea, 93
  Holy Basil-Ginger Julep, *102–103*
  Holy Basil-Ginger Syrup, *104*
  Mustard and Ginger Bath Salts, *123*
  Xavier's Gingered Salmon, *94*
Gingivitis. *See* Gums, bleeding/swollen
Glass jars, 32
Glossary, 319–324
Grief, 231
Grinder, for spices, 32
Gums, bleeding/swollen, 20, 161, 270

Hair health, 191, *196*
Hair loss, 152
Hair wash, 149
Hawthorn, 210, **211**–217
  about: historical perspective, 212; how to use
    (amounts, special considerations), 214;
    medicinal properties and energetics,
    212–213; types of, 212
  Hawthorn Cordial, *216*

Hawthorn Nourishing Infusion, *215*
  Hawthorn Vinegar, *217*
Hay fever, 100
Headaches, 49, 53, 90, 111, 143, *146*, 189, 193, 220,
  269, 277, 281, 289
Health benefits, of herbs/spices. *See* Herbs and
  spices, benefits of; *specific herbs and spices*
Heart, bitterness in/opening up, 127
Heartburn, 52, 81, 100, 144, 271, 281
Heart disease/heart health, 4, 52, 80, 99, 119,
  132, 135, 151, 159, 180, (211–214), 231, 239, 240,
  251, 253, 260–261, 262, 270, 280, 286, 309.
  See also Blood pressure and hypertension;
  Cholesterol levels; Diabetes
Heart/emotions, 231
Hemorrhoids, 39, 52
Hepatitis, 280, 307
Herbal teas, infusions, and other drinks. *See also*
  Coffee; Tea
  Artichoke and Orange Bitters, 256–257
  Astragalus Chai, *311*
  Bitter Artichoke Tea, 255
  Cayenne Tea, 55
  Chamomile Tea Blend with Roses and Va-
    nilla, *274*
  Cinnamon Tea for Soothing Throats, 65
  Elderflower Tea, *207*
  Fennel Tea, *75*
  Fire Cider, 56
  Ginger-Lemon Tea, *93*
  Hawthorn Cordial, *216*
  Hawthorn Nourishing Infusion, *215*
  Holy Basil-Ginger Julep, *102–103*
  Holy Basil Tea, *105*
  Hot Chocolate, 265
  Lemon Balm Nourishing Infusion, 223
  Lemon Balm Water, *226–227*
  Peppermint and Hibiscus Cooler, *147*
  Perfect Cup of Rosemary Tea, *154*

Roasted Dandelion and Reishi Tea, *292*

Rosebud Tea, *234-235*

Sage-Lemon Tea, *165*

Spiced Eggnog, *129*

Warm Golden Milk, *183*

Herbs and spices, 325-327. *See also* Energetics of herbalism; Medicine, plants as; *specific herbs and spices*

author's journey to yours, xviii–xix

balanced perspective on, 9

choosing. *See* Matching herbs to you

finding best ingredients, 30-31

harnessing the power of, xv

historical perspective, xvii, 7

measuring, 29-30

science today and, 8

tastes of, 18-21

this book and, xv, xvii, xx, 27-33, 315

tips for using, 325

Herbs and spices, benefits of. *See also* Antioxidant properties; Digestion; Immune system support; Nervous system support

about: overview of, xix, 3

flavoring and enhancing meals, xx

summary of health benefits, 3-6

Herpes virus (sores), 100, 203, 221, 222

Hiccups, 75, 142

History, of connection with plants as medicine, xvii

History of specific herbs, see *specific herbs*

HIV, 307. *See also* Immune system support

Holy basil, 96, **97**-105

about: historical perspective, 98; how to use (amounts, special considerations), 101; medicinal properties and energetics, 98-100; types of, 98

Holy Basil-Ginger Julep, *102-103*

Holy Basil-Ginger Syrup, *104*

Holy Basil Tea, *105*

Honey, bees and, 31

Honey, garlic, 84-85

Hormone levels, 289, 301

Hot Chocolate, *265*

Hot/cold and dry/damp, 12-13, 15-18

Hot flashes, 162, 182

Hypertension. *See* Blood pressure and hypertension

Hypothyroidism, 189, 299

IBS (irritable bowel syndrome), 142, 171, 253

Ice pops, chamomile, 275

Illness, energetics of, 14. *See also* Energetics of herbalism

Immune system support, 6, 20, 79, 100, 129, 170, 178, 203, 204, 212, 301, (306-309), 311, 313

Infections, 5-6, 59, 79, 91, 92, 159, 170, 179, 271. *See also* Colds and flu; Conjunctivitis; Fungal infections; Gums, bleeding/swollen; Urinary tract infections

Inflammation. *See also* Arthritis

anti-inflammatory drugs (NSAIDs) and, 178, 181

bitter herbs for, 21

heart health, cholesterol and, 151, 161, 213, 253, 261, 280

herbs/spices helping, 22, 49, 70, 79, 89, 91, 100, 110, 141, 143, *155*, (177-181), 192, 203, 204, 212, 232, 259, (267-272), 280, 289, 290, 299

skin, 141, 143, 162, 169

sour herbs for, 20

sweet herbs for, 20

Inflammatory bowel disease, xix, 78

Influenza. *See* Colds and flu

Infusions. *See* Herbal teas, infusions, and other drinks

Ingredients, finding best, 30-31

Insect (bug) bites, 111, 219

Insomnia. *See* Sleep and relaxation

Insulin resistance, 53, 62, 91, 161, 180, 192, 239, 253, 261, 280, 301. *See also* Diabetes

Irritability, 267

Jars, storage, 32

Kidney health, 180, 309

Kidney stones, 135

Lamb, rosemary, *156–157*

Lavender, 106, **107**–115

about: historical perspective, 108; how to use (amounts, special considerations), 112; medicinal properties and energetics, 109–111; types of, 108

Lavender and Clay Facial, *114*

Lavender and Orange Custard, *115*

Lavender Bath salts, *113*

Laxatives, 39, 277

Lemon balm, 218, **219**–227

about: historical perspective, 220; how to use (amounts, special considerations), 222; medicinal properties and energetics, 220–221

Lemon Balm and Orange Chicken, *224–225*

Lemon Balm Nourishing Infusion, *223*

Lemon Balm Water, *226–227*

Libido, 49, 299, 301

Liver health, 4, 21, 152, 171, 179, 192, (251–253), 280, 287, *292*, 309

Lung support, 100. *See also* Bronchial congestion; Bronchitis; Colds and flu

Matching herbs to you, 11–25. *See also* Energetics of herbalism

about: overview of, 11

assessing how herb/spice affects you, 23–25

choosing best herbs/spices, 28

constitutions of people and, 13–14

discovering your constitution, 15–18

finding best ingredients and, 30–31

measuring herbs and, 29–30

personalizing treatment, 12

putting pieces together, 22–25

Recommended Amounts sections and, 29

sweet spot for, 22–23

tastes of herbs and, 18–21

trusting your senses, 28

tuning in to feelings and experiences, 27–28

using this book and, 27–33, 315

Measuring herbs/spices, 29–30

Meat, best quality, 30. *See also specific meats*

Medicine, plants as

author's journey to yours, xviii–xix

historical perspective, xix, 7

One Solution Syndrome vs., xvi, xvii, xviii–xix, 11, 33

science today supporting, 8

summary of herb/spice benefits, 3–6. *See also specific benefits*

using this book and, 32, 315

Memory, 8, 99, 143, 151–152, 160–161, 180, 261, 280, 301

Menopause, 99, 162, 182, 189, 220

Menses, delayed, 133, 171

Menstrual cramps, 49, (69–71), 87, 89, 171, *174*, 191, 232, 269, 289. *See also* Premenstrual syndrome (PMS)

Mental stimulation, 143, 149. *See also* Brain health; Memory

Metabolic syndrome, 180, 241, 253. *See also* Diabetes

Metabolism, 52, 192, 301

Metric conversion chart, 316–317

Migraines, 90, 111

Milk, warm golden, *183*

Mint. *See Peppermint*

Mood, improving, 143, 160, 228, 261, 301

Mucus congestion, 39, 40, 43, 53, 55, 80, 90, 100, 119, *171*, *173*, 302

Muesli, rose hip and apple, *237*

Muscle spasms, 191, 192, 268

Muscles, sore, 57, 90, 95, *113*, 119, *123*, 144, 159

Muscle tension, 70, 89, 143, 268, 269

Mustard, 116, **117**-123

    about: historical perspective, 118; how to use (amounts, special considerations), 120; medicinal properties and energetics, 118-119; types of seeds, 118

    Homemade Mustard, *121*

    Mustard and Ginger Bath Salts, *123*

    Mustard Vinaigrette Salad Dressing with Parsley, *139*

    Squash Soup with Mustard Seeds, *122*

Nausea, treating, xix, 87, 91, 100, 141, 152, 289

Nervous system support, overview of herbs/spices providing, 4-5. *See also* Mood, improving; Sleep and relaxation; Stress and anxiety, relieving

Nettle, 188, **189**-197

    about: historical perspective, 190; how to use (amounts, special considerations), 193; medicinal properties and energetics, 191-192

    Nettle and Eggplant Sauté, *197*

    Nettle Leaf Dukkah, *194-195*

    Nourishing Nettle Infusion, *196*

Neuropathy, 53, 143

Nutmeg, 124, **125**-131

    about: historical perspective, 126; how to use (amounts, special considerations), 128; medicinal properties and energetics, 126-127

    Spiced Carrot Cake, *130-131*

    Spiced Eggnog, *129*

Nuts and seeds

    Muesli, rose hip and apple, *237*

    Nettle Leaf Dukkah, *194-195*

    Turmeric and Pumpkin Seed Paté, *184-185*

Oils

    about: olive oil, 31

    Garlic Oil, *83*

    Ginger and Lavender Massage Oil, *95*

Olive oil, 31

Olives, in Rosemary Tapenade, *155*

One Solution Syndrome, xvi, xvii, xviii-xix, 11, 33

Oolong tea, 245

Oral health. *See* Gums, bleeding/swollen; Tooth and gum health

Oxymel, thyme, *173*

Pain relief, 53, 57, 89-90, 95, 100, 110-111, *113*, 119, 143, 144, 151, *171*, 181, 192, 219, 221, 232, 269, 270. *See also* Arthritis; Digestion; Headaches; Menstrual cramps; Throat, sore

Parasites, 49, 77, 171

Parsley, 132, **133**-139

    about: historical perspective, 134; how to use (amounts, special considerations), 136; medicinal properties and energetics, 134-135; types of, 134

    Mustard Vinaigrette Salad Dressing with Parsley, *139*

    Parsley and Cilantro Pesto, *137*

    Parsley Potatoes, *138*

Pepper. *See* Black pepper; Cayenne

Peppermint, 140, **141**-147

    about: historical perspective, 142; how to use (amounts, special considerations), 144; medicinal properties and energetics, 142-143

Mint Raita, *145*

Peppermint and Hibiscus Cooler, *147*

Peppermint Fomentation for Headaches, *146*

Perfect Cup of French Press Coffee, *284-285*

Pesto, dandelion, *294-295*

Pesto, parsley and cilantro, *137*

Plague, 78, 79, 126

Potatoes, parsley, *138*

Premenstrual syndrome (PMS), 232, 269, 289

Prolapsed organs, 307

Pumpkin seeds, in Turmeric and Pumpkin Seed Paté, *184-185*

Pungent herbs, about, 19. *See also* Black pepper; Cayenne; Cinnamon; Fennel; Garlic; Ginger; Holy basil; Lavender; Mustard; Nutmeg; Parsley; Peppermint; Rosemary; Sage; Thyme; Turmeric

Quizzes, to discover constitution, 15-18

Raita, mint, *145*

Recipes
finding best ingredients, 30-31

metric conversion chart, 316-317

tools, supplies for, 32

using this book and, 32, 315

Reproductive health, 301. *See also* Hormone levels; Sex drive/libido

Restlessness, 204, 220, 271

Rice, astragalus and cardamom, *312*

Roasted Dandelion and Reishi Tea, *292*

Roasted Root Vegetables with Fennel, *73*

Rose, 228, **229**-237
about: historical perspective, 230; how to use (amounts, special considerations), 233; medicinal properties and energetics, 230-232; types of, 230

Chamomile Tea Blend with Roses and Vanilla, *274*

Green Tea and Rose Facial Cream, *246-247*

Rosebud Tea, *234-235*

Rose Hip and Apple Muesli, *237*

Rose Hip-Cranberry Compote, *236*

Rosemary, 148, **149**-157
about: historical perspective, 150; how to use (amounts, special considerations), 153; medicinal properties and energetics, 150-152

Perfect Cup of Rosemary Tea, *154*

Rosemary Lamb, *156-157*

Rosemary Tapenade, *155*

Sage, 158, **159**-167
about: historical perspective, 160; how to use (amounts, special considerations), 162-163; medicinal properties and energetics, 160-162

Fried Sage Leaves, *164*

Sage Chicken, *166-167*

Sage-Lemon Tea, *165*

Salmon, gingered, *94*

Salty herbs, about, 19. *See also* Nettle

Sauces and dressings
Dandelion Pesto, *294-295*

Mint Raita, *145*

Mustard Vinaigrette Salad Dressing with Parsley, *139*

Parsley and Cilantro Pesto, *137*

Scale, digital, 32

Senses, trusting when choosing herbs, 28

Sex drive/libido, 49, 299, 301. *See also* Aphrodisiacs

Shingles, 53, 143

Skin. *See also* Eczema; Wounds, healing
    about: eruptions, dandelion for, 287; pro-
      tecting, 151; protective shield just below,
      308; rashes, 289; softening and rejuve-
      nating, 204; soothing itching/inflamma-
      tion, 141, 162
        Elderflower Facial Serum, *208–209*
        Green Tea and Rose Facial Cream, *246–247*
        Lavender and Clay Facial, *114*
Sleep and relaxation, 20, 109–110, 127, 180, 220,
    269, 271, 281, 300
Small intestinal bacteria overgrowth, 77
Smoky Garlic Hummus, *82*
Smoothie, ashwagandha banana, 305
Soups
    Astragalus Bone Broth, *313*
    Peppery Borscht, *44–45*
    Squash Soup with Mustard Seeds, *122*
Sour herbs, about, 20. *See also* Elder; Hawthorn;
    Lemon balm; Rose; Tea
Spasms, 70, 71, 89, 141, 171, 192, 220, 268, 269,
    271
Spiced Carrot Cake, *130–131*
Spiced Cold-Brew Coffee, *282–283*
Spiced Eggnog, *129*
Spreads
    Rosemary Tapenade, *155*
    Turmeric and Pumpkin Seed Paté, *184–185*
Squash Soup with Mustard Seeds, *122*
Stagnant blood, 89–90. *See also* Circulation
Stimulants (herbal), about, 89
Storage jars, 32
Strainers, 32
Strawberries, in Chocolate Strawberry Pudding,
    264
Stress and anxiety, relieving, 4–5, 15, 20, 97,
    99, 110, *113*, 127, 220, 231, 241, 269. *See also*
    Mood, improving; Sleep and relaxation;

    Tension, releasing
Stress, oxidative, 4, 110, 119, 135, 151, 203, 212, 221,
    280, 301
Sugar, about, 31
Sunburn, 143, 151, 163, 232
Suribachi, 32
Sweating, excessive, 61, 162
Sweet herbs, about, 20. *See also* Ashwagandha;
    Astragalus
Sweet treats
    Ashwagandha Date Treats, *304*
    Cardamom Chocolate Mousse Cake, *263*
    Chamomile Ice Pops, *275*
    Chocolate Strawberry Pudding, *264*
    Lavender and Orange Custard, *115*
    Rose Hip-Cranberry Compote, *236*
    Spiced Carrot Cake, *130–131*
Synergists, 42, 89
Syrups
    Elderberry Syrup, *206*
    Holy Basil-Ginger Syrup, *104*
    Thyme and Cherry Bark Cough Syrup, *175*

Tapenade, rosemary, 155
Tea, 238, **239**–247. *See also* Herbal teas, infu-
    sions, and other drinks
    about: historical perspective, 240; how to
      use (amounts, special considerations),
      242–243; medicinal properties and ener-
      getics, 240–241; types of, 240
    Green Tea and Rose Facial Cream, *246–247*
    Make Your Own Earl Grey Tea, *244*
    Tea Break with Oolong, *245*
Tea, herbal. *See* Herbal teas, infusions, and other
    drinks
Teeth. *See* Gums, bleeding/swollen; Tooth and
    gum health

Teething, 220, 267

Tension, muscle, 70, 89, 268, 269

Tension, releasing, 107, 271. *See also* Mood, improving; Stress and anxiety, relieving

Throat, sore, 49, 65, *84*, 90, 91, 93, 100, 152, 161, 170, *173*

Throat, swollen, 20

Thyme, 168, **169**–175

about: historical perspective, 170; how to use (amounts, special considerations), 172; medicinal properties and energetics, 170–171

Thyme and Cherry Bark Cough Syrup, *175*

Thyme Oxymel, *173*

Tomatoes Provençal, *174*

Tomatoes Provençal, *174*

Tools and supplies, 32

Toothaches, 49, 59, 61, 159, 169

Tooth and gum health, 61, *64*, 191, *196*, 241. *See also* Gums, bleeding/swollen

Tooth powder, *64*

Trikatu Pastilles, *43*

Turmeric, 176, **177**–185

about: historical perspective, 178; how to use (amounts, special considerations), 182; medicinal properties and energetics, 178–181

Garam Masala, *184*

Turmeric and Pumpkin Seed Paté, *184-185*

Warm Golden Milk, *183*

Ulcerative colitis, 179

Ulcers, 52, 100, 110, 179, 232, 270

Ulcers, mouth, 161, 232

Upper respiratory infections, 52, 79, 90, 100, 168, 171, 204, 308, 309. *See also* Colds and flu

Urinary tract infections, 135, 170, 192

Using herbs. *See* Matching herbs to you

Vegetables, roasted root with fennel, *73*

Vinegar, dandelion root, *293*

Vinegar, hawthorn, *217*

Viral infections, 97, 100, 221, 309

Water retention, 287

Weight, gaining. *See* Appetite, improving

Weight loss, 52, 241

Whooping cough, 171

Wounds, healing, 20, 57, 79, 107, 110, 159, 169, 179, 181, 232, 270

Xavier's Gingered Salmon, *94*

Yeast infections, 170

ACKNOWLEDGMENTS

After writing my first book, I know now more than ever that while the author may get their name on the front cover, it takes a village of people to fully complete a book.

I feel incredibly lucky that I met John and Kimberly Gallagher so early on in my herbal path. From the very start they believed in me and gave me an outlet to continue learning and growing. Without their continued support over the years, you would not be holding this book in your hands. Likewise, the LearningHerbs and HerbMentor community has kept me inspired to keep coming up with new recipes and teachings. A major part of my own growth and learning has been alongside this grassroots community of herbalists. Thank you to Debbie, Althea, Jan, and Savannah for their behind-the-scenes help at LearningHerbs.

I was able to write this book because I have had the honor and privilege of studying with many wise herbal teachers, including, in order of appearance, Karen Sherwood, Michael and Lesley Tierra, Paul Bergner, Karta Purkh Singh Khalsa, jim mcdonald, and the P.H. Group.

It is an incredible honor to have the Foreword written by Rosemary Gladstar, as she has long inspired me with her many important contributions to the herbal world.

I've been lucky enough to travel to grassroots herbal conferences and learn from many talented herbalists, including 7Song, Rebecca Altman, Juliet Blankespoor, Robin Rose Bennett, Kristine Brown, Larken Bunce, Chanchal Cabrera, Todd Caldecott, Bevin Clare, Amanda McQuade Crawford, Sean Donahue, Cascade Anderson Geller, Kiva Rose Hardin, Christopher Hobbs, Phyllis Hogan, Phyllis D. Light, Guido Masé, Sajah Popham, Anna Rosa Robertsdottir, Robert Rogers, Christa Sinadinos, Cathy Skipper, John Slattery, Dr. Kevin Spelman, Susun Weed, David Winston, Matthew Wood, and Ben Zappin. Thank you, all.

It has been my good fortune to work alongside Hay House. Thank you to CEO Reid Tracy for believing in this book and taking a chance on a first-time author. Thank you to my editor, Nicolette Salamanca Young, who really whipped this book into shape with her organizational and editorial skills. I instantly fell in love with the cover for the book and offer my thanks to Tricia Briedenthal and the Hay House design team for coming up with the concept. Also thank you to Jan Bosman for his further help with the design.

Early on, I worked alongside Tracy Teel from Finesse Writing and Publishing, who helped me create the big-picture organization and contributed to the coherence of the book. Also in the beginning stages, Kurt Koenigs was instrumental in helping me frame key concepts in the book for added clarity.

Writing a book was not always easy. Thank you to my life coach, Lexi Koch, for her wise words and helping me to shift stagnation and dread into flow and gratitude.

A big part of this book was researching and citing many scientific studies. Thank you to Emer McKenna for compiling many of the scientific studies for me, and thank you to Stephany Hoffelt, who expertly whipped my Endnotes into shape.

Another facet of this book was the recipes. My deep gratitude goes out to Valorie Paul, who took on the big task of organizing and orchestrating the volunteer recipe testers (she helped me to find many of the quotes as well). My heart-felt thanks also goes out to the people who generously volunteered to test these recipes, as their feedback improved many of the recipes in this book immeasurably: Amber Tapley, Amy Marquardt, Amy Tompkins, Barbara Elder, Barbara Schmidt, Calla Harris, Cary & Anna Hayes, Cathy Izzi, Cathy Sciglibaglio, Charmaine Koehler-Lodge, Christeena Braucht, Christina Chencharik, Chris Durham, Christine Borosh, Cindy Aragon, Cora Anderson, Deb Soper, Deborah Kravig, Delinda Tonelotti, Dianne Brenner, Dianne Willett, Elaine Pollard, Emiko Luisi, Gabriela Rios, Gary Fisher, Gretchen Beaubier, Heather Davis, Ilka Mendoza, Jennifer Stanek, Jennifer Warnick, Jodi Howells, Kara Hughes, Karen Garcia, Karen Mezzano, Karen Vandergrift, Kate Briggs, Kathleen Payne, Keisha Forbes, Kelley Estes, Keri Mae Lamar, Kim Reid, Kimberly Padgett-Shaw, Kristina Cool, Krystal Beers, Laura Cole, Laurel Beck, Lauren Henderson, Laurie Murray, Leanne Holcomb, Lesa Wischmeyer, Lora Bonicelli, Lynne Lacroix, Mary Anne Leary, Mary Souder, Morgan Mays, Pamela Roberts, Rebecca Ingalls, Renée Otte, Shelly Langton,

Sofia Gonzales, Tamara White, Tanya Thampi Sen, Vanessa Nixon Klein, Victoria Sandz, Wendy Chu, and Wendy Joubert.

One of the hardest aspects of this book was doing a lot of the photography myself, but luckily I had behind-the-scenes help. Thank you to Matt Burke for giving me food photography lessons (while he was on vacation, no less) and for editing many of the photos himself—twice! Thank you to Matt Burke and Larken Bunce for allowing me to use their beautiful plant photos. And thank you to Sol Gutierrez for the photos of me and the fun, plant-centric photo shoots over the years.

Thank you to Rebecca Altman, Christophe Bernard, Dan Donohue, and Emily Han for contributing recipes. It's an honor to have each of you represented in this book. In addition, thank you to Emily Han, who gave me some great advice in regards to writing a book and recipe testers. And my deep gratitude to Rebecca Altman, who, during the writing of this book, often cheered me on with her friendship, laughter, and support. My heartfelt gratitude also goes to Stephanie Manteufel Beasley for our long conversations and for believing in me so much that she pre-ordered ten copies of this book before it was even finished!

Kari Bown, Ed Welch, Leslie Channing, Kosma Channing, Teague Channing, Anne LeFevre, and Ellen Brand either knowingly or unknowingly grew many of the plants in this book so that I was able to photograph them. I love having such heart-centered and hardworking farmers in my life.

There's a soft spot in my heart for the love and support (and great meals) I've gotten from the Myer Creek crew. A special thank you goes to Susie for sharing both her wisdom and honey from the bees. Writing is often easier with music, so thank you to Tori Amos and Ani DiFranco for being the sound track to this book (and to my life).

Thank you to my dad for his unwavering support of my unusual paths in life and for teaching me that the most delicious meals come from the best ingredients.

Some of the support I receive is no longer seen, but is still felt. In memory of my mother, my Papa Jack, Jay, Patrick, and Cole.

And lastly, my deepest gratitude goes to my husband and best friend, Xavier. He made this book possible in many logistical ways by being a sounding board, offering advice, and cooking many meals. But more than that, he inspires me to live my life in the best way I can; he shows up every day with his presence and love to make me feel like the luckiest woman on earth.

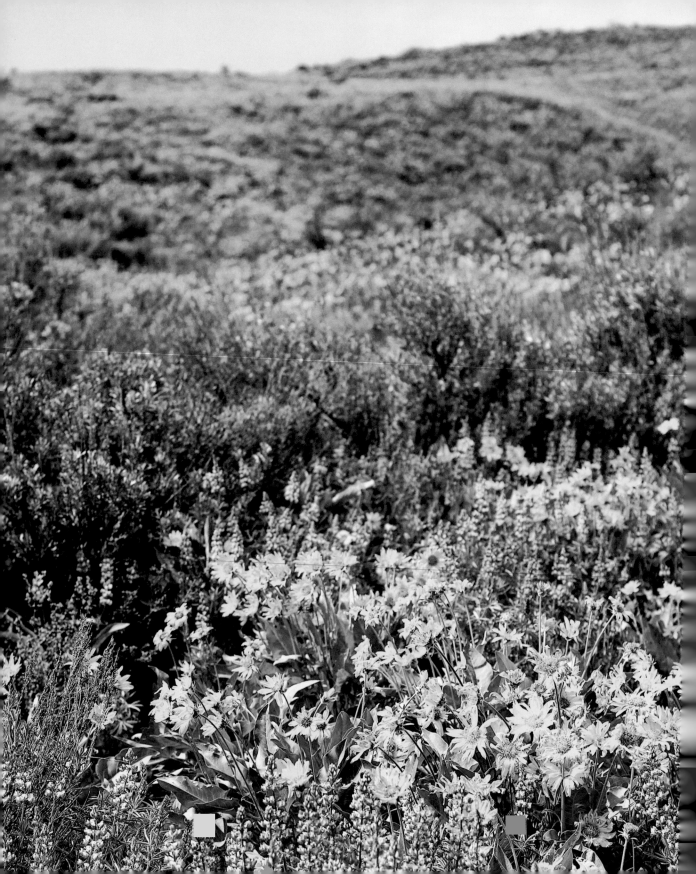

ABOUT THE AUTHOR

Rosalee de la Forêt, RH, is passionate about helping people discover the world of herbalism and natural health. She is a Registered Herbalist with the American Herbalist Guild and the Education Director at LearningHerbs. She is also the author of the online courses *The Taste of Herbs, Herbal Cold Care,* and *Apothecary: The Alchemy of Herbs Video Companion.* When she is not immersed in herbs, you can find her taking photos of nature, kayaking with her husband, or curled up in a hammock with a good book.

See more of Rosalee's articles and recipes at www.HerbsWithRosalee.com and www.LearningHerbs.com.

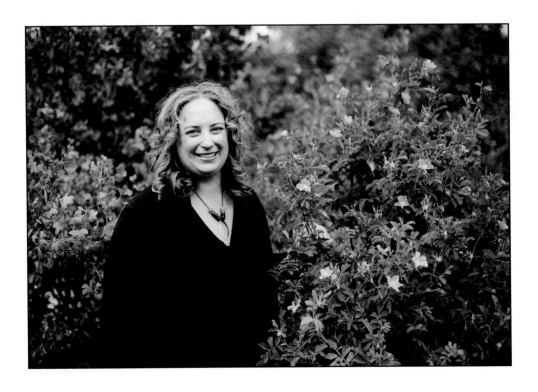

Hay House Titles of Related Interest

You Can Heal Your Life, the movie, starring Louise Hay & Friends
(available as an online streaming video)
www.hayhouse.com/louise-movie

The Shift, the movie, starring Dr. Wayne W. Dyer
(available as an online streaming video)
www.hayhouse.com/the-shift-movie

Clear Home, Clear Heart: Learn to Clear the Energy of People and Places, by Jean Haner

Cultured Food for Life: How to Make and Serve Delicious Probiotic Foods for Better Health and Wellness, by Donna Schwenk

The Earth Diet: Your Complete Guide to Living Using Earth's Natural Ingredients, by Liana Werner-Gray

The Mystic Cookbook: The Secret Alchemy of Food, by Denise Linn and Meadow Linn

All of the above are available at your local bookstore,
or may be ordered by contacting Hay House (see next page).

We hope you enjoyed this Hay House book. If you'd like to receive our online catalog featuring additional information on Hay House books and products, or if you'd like to find out more about the Hay Foundation, please contact:

Hay House, Inc., P.O. Box 5100, Carlsbad, CA 92018-5100
(760) 431-7695 or (800) 654-5126
(760) 431-6948 (fax) or (800) 650-5115 (fax)
www.hayhouse.com • www.hayfoundation.org

Published in Australia by: Hay House Australia Pty. Ltd.
18/36 Ralph St., Alexandria NSW 2015
Phone: 612-9669-4299 • ***Fax:*** 612-9669-4144 • www.hayhouse.com.au

Published in the United Kingdom by: Hay House UK, Ltd.
The Sixth Floor, Watson House, 54 Baker Street, London W1U 7BU
Phone: +44 (0)20 3927 7290 • ***Fax:*** +44 (0)20 3927 7291 • www.hayhouse.co.uk

Published in India by: Hay House Publishers India,
Muskaan Complex, Plot No. 3, B-2, Vasant Kunj, New Delhi 110 070
Phone: 91-11-4176-1620 • ***Fax:*** 91-11-4176-1630 • www.hayhouse.co.in

**Access New Knowledge.
Anytime. Anywhere.**

Learn and evolve at your own pace
with the world's leading experts.

www.hayhouseU.com

LearningHerbs® presents

Build your own
herbal medicine chest with...

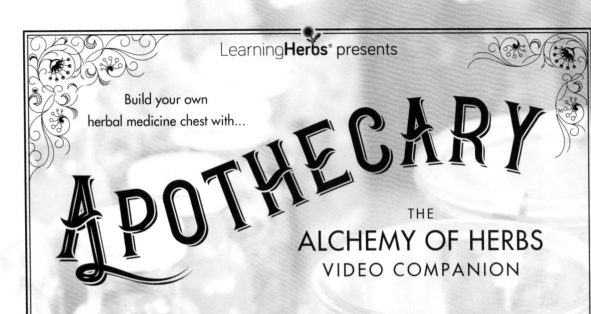

APOTHECARY™

THE
ALCHEMY OF HERBS
VIDEO COMPANION

ROSALEE DE LA FORÊT & JOHN GALLAGHER
BRING THIS BOOK TO LIFE
BY SHOWING YOU HOW TO CREATE
15 OF THE MOST ESSENTIAL HERBAL REMEDY PREPARATIONS,
FROM TEAS AND TINCTURES TO SYRUPS AND SALVES.

Be prepared for common everyday ailments by learning
exactly which remedies to create for your home apothecary.

EMPOWER YOURSELF TODAY AT
ALCHEMYOFHERBS.com/APOTHECARY

MEDITATE.
VISUALIZE.
LEARN.

Get the **Empower You**
Unlimited Audio *Mobile App*

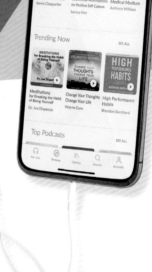

Get unlimited access to the entire Hay House audio library!

You'll get:

- 500+ inspiring and life-changing **audiobooks**

- 200+ ad-free **guided meditations** for sleep, healing, relaxation, spiritual connection, and more

- Hundreds of audios **under 20 minutes** to easily fit into your day

- ~~**Exclusive content** *only* for~~ subscribers

- No credits, **no limits**

New audios added every week!

 I ADORE this app. I use it almost every day. Such a blessing. – Aya Lucy Rose

Scan me with your phone camera!

HAY HOUSE

TRY FOR FREE!
Go to: hayhouse.com/listen-free

Free e-newsletters
from Hay House, the Ultimate
Resource for Inspiration

Be the first to know about Hay House's free downloads, special offers, giveaways, contests, and more!

 Get exclusive excerpts from our latest releases and videos from *Hay House Present Moments*.

 Our *Digital Products Newsletter* is the perfect way to stay up-to-date on our latest discounted eBooks, featured mobile apps, and Live Online and On Demand events.

 Learn with real benefits! *HayHouseU.com* is your source for the most innovative online courses from the world's leading personal growth experts. Be the first to know about new online courses and to receive exclusive discounts.

 Enjoy uplifting personal stories, how-to articles, and healing advice, along with videos and empowering quotes, within *Heal Your Life*.

Sign Up Now!

Get inspired, educate yourself, get a complimentary gift, and share the wisdom!

Visit www.hayhouse.com/newsletters to sign up today!

 HAY HOUSE

 HAY HOUSE online learning